RHEUMATIC DISEASES: REHABILITATION AND MANAGEMENT

Edited by

Gail Kershner Riggs, M.A.

Lecturer, Internal Medicine
Administrator, Southwest Arthritis Center
  and Division of Restorative Medicine
  University of Arizona College of Medicine, Tucson
Former President, Arthritis Health Professions Association,
  The Arthritis Foundation

and

Eric P. Gall, M.D.

Professor, Internal Medicine, Surgery (Orthopedics),
  and Family and Community Medicine
Chief, Section of Rheumatology, Allergy, and Immunology
  University of Arizona College of Medicine, Tucson
Former President, Arthritis Health Professions Association,
  The Arthritis Foundation

BUTTERWORTH PUBLISHERS
Boston • London
Sydney • Wellington • Durban • Toronto

*Every effort has been made to ensure that the drug dosage
schedules within this text are accurate and conform to standards accepted at time of publication. However, as treatment
recommendations vary in the light of continuing research and
clinical experience, the reader is advised to verify drug dosage
schedules herein with information found on product information sheets. This is especially true in cases of new or infrequently used drugs.*

Library of Congress Cataloging in Publication Data
Main entry under title:

Rheumatic diseases.

   Includes bibliographical references and index.
   1. Arthritics—Rehabilitation. 2. Arthritis—Treatment.
3. Rheumatism—Treatment. I. Riggs, Gail. II. Gall,
Eric P. [DNLM: 1. Arthritis—Therapy. 2. Arthritis—
Rehabilitation. 3. Rheumatism—Therapy.
4. Rheumatism—Rehabilitation. WE 344 R4713]
RC933.R37 1983   616.7'2206   83–15195
ISBN 0-409-95051-3

Butterworth Publishers
80 Montvale Avenue
Stoneham, MA 02180

10 9 8 7 6 5 4 3 2

Printed in the United States of America.

To my late father, Russell Kershner, who taught me the importance of always growing, loving, and searching for knowledge; to my mother, Evelyn, for instilling in me a spirit and motivation for life; to my brothers, Paul and Bob, for their continual support; and to Eric Gall, for believing in me.

Gail Kershner Riggs, M.A.

To Kathy, Gretchen, and Michael, who make my life and work meaningful and happy. To my late father, Edward A. Gall, who taught me the excitement of medicine and the importance of the written word and the human side of science.

Eric P. Gall, M.D.

CONTENTS

EDITORS

Gail Kershner Riggs, M.A., is Administrator of the Division of Restorative Medicine and Associate Director of the Southwest Arthritis Center at the University of Arizona Health Sciences Center. She received degrees in Biology Education and Guidance/Counseling from the University of Arizona in 1961 and Arizona State University in 1968. She is currently pursuing a doctorate in Rehabilitation and Health Care Administration. She is a past President of the Arthritis Health Professions Association, a former Vice-Chairman of the national Arthritis Foundation, a consultant to the National Institutes of Health, and Chairman of the Advisory Board of the National Arthritis Information Clearinghouse. Mrs. Riggs serves on numerous national, state, and local boards and committees. In 1983 she was awarded Arizona's Health Educator of the Year by the Arizona Public Health Association and Tucson's Woman of the Year by the Tucson Chamber of Commerce and Tucson Advertising Club.

Eric P. Gall, M.D., is Professor of Internal Medicine, Surgery (Orthopedics), and Family and Community Medicine at the University of Arizona College of Medicine. He is Associate Director of the Southwest Arthritis Center (a National Institutes of Health Multipurpose Arthritis Center). He is Chief of the Section of Rheumatology, Allergy, and Immunology at the University of Arizona College of Medicine. He received his A.B. and M.D. degrees from the University of Pennsylvania in 1962 and 1966, respectively. He served his medical internship and junior residency at the University of Cincinnati Medical Center, and his senior medicine residency and fellowship in rheumatology at the University of Pennsylvania. He is a past President of the Arthritis Health Professions Association and former Vice-Chairman of the national Arthritis Foundation. He is a member of the American Rheumatism Association, Chairman of Exhibits Subcommittee and a member of the Education Committee of the rehabilitation council of that organization.

CONTRIBUTORS

F. Paul Alepa, M.D., is Professor of Medicine at the University of Arizona College of Medicine and Chief of the Rheumatology Section at the Veterans Administration Hospital. He is former Chairman of the Rheumatology Section at Georgetown University, College of Medicine.

Frank C. Arnett, Jr., M.D., is Associate Professor of Medicine at the Johns Hopkins University School of Medicine. A Rheumatologist and Immunogeneticist, his major interests lie in the contribution of heritable factors to rheumatic diseases.

Barbara Figley Banwell, P.T., M.A., is the Program Leader in Physical Therapy at the University of Michigan Multipurpose Arthritis Center. She received her degrees in Physical Therapy and Guidance/Counseling from the University of Michigan in 1960 and 1978. Currently, she is pursuing a doctorate in Educational Psychology.

Michelle Boutaugh, M.P.H., is Vice-President for Patient Services at the National Arthritis Foundation in Atlanta. A nurse by training, she spent three years as Program Coordinator at the Diabetes Research and Training Center at the University of Michigan.

Marjorie C. Becker, P.T., Ph.D., earned her degree in physical therapy at the University of Michigan, her M.A. in counseling at Ohio State University, and her doctorate in education at the University of Michigan. She is now Assistant Dean and Director of Allied Health Professions and Assistant Professor in the Department of Physical Medicine and Rehabilitation at the University of Michigan Medical School and Hospital.

John T. Boyer, M.D., is a Professor of Internal Medicine and Family and Community Medicine at the University of Arizona's Health Sciences Center. He is Director of the Division of Restorative Medicine as well as Director of the National Institutes of Health Multipurpose Arthritis Center at the College of Medicine.

Mary P. Brassell, R.N., B.S., is Rehabilitation Arthritis Nurse Specialist in the Einstein-Moss Arthritis Center, Department of Nursing, at the Moss Rehabilitation Hospital in Philadelphia. Her interest in arthritis extends over many years, with a special interest in sexuality of the arthritis patient.

Clifford M. Clarke, C.A.E., is President of the Arthritis Foundation, which is headquartered in Atlanta, Georgia, and has seventy-one chapters and divisions across the country. Mr. Clarke, a certified association executive, is a member and past President of the American Society of Association Executives.

Solomon N. Forouzesh, M.D., F.A.C.P., is Chief of Rheumatology at Brotman Medical Center in Culver City in Los Angeles. He is also Assistant Clinical Professor of Medicine at UCLA School of Medicine.

William L. Fritz, R.Ph., M.S., is Director of Pharmacy and Supply, University Hospital; Assistant Dean, College of Pharmacy; and Instructor in the Department of Pharmacology, College of Medicine at the University of Arizona Health Sciences Center.

Lawrence M. Haas, M.D., is an Associate in Surgery at the University of Arizona Health Sciences Center and an Orthopedic and Hand Consultant for the Tucson Medical Center Rheumatology Clinic. He is a member of the American Society for Surgery of the Hand, American Academy of Orthopedic Surgeons, and American Board of Orthopedic Surgery.

Evelyn V. Hess, M.D., F.A.C.P., is McDonald Professor of Medicine and Director, Division of Immunology in the Department of Medicine, University of Cincinnati Medical Center. Dr. Hess is an Editorial Board member of several journals, including *Arthritis and Rheumatism*, and has served on numerous National Institutes of Health committees, the Food and Drug Administration Arthritis Advisory Committee, and Arthritis Foundation and American Rheumatism Association committees.

Joseph Lee Hollander, M.D., M.A.C.P., is Emeritus Professor of Medicine, Former Chief of the Arthritis Section, School of Medicine and Hospital of the University of Pennsylvania, and Master, American College of Physicians. He is a consultant in Rheumatology at the Veterans Administration Hospital, Children's Hospital, and Pennsylvania Hospital in Philadelphia.

Alan M. Jette, P.T., Ph.D., is Assistant Professor of Gerontology and Physical Medicine at the Massachusetts General Hospital Institute of Health Professions and is a Lecturer in Social Medicine and Health Policy at Harvard Medical School. He is the author of a number of articles on the subjects of long-term care of the elderly, functional status assessment, disability in the elderly, and health program evaluation.

Bob G. Johnson, Ed.D., is a Professor in the Department of Rehabilitation at the University of Arizona's College of Education. His interest in biofeedback and counseling are maintained through his teaching, articles, and private practice.

Kate Lorig, R.N., Dr.P.H., is Research Associate at the Stanford University School of Medicine and Director of the Arthritis Self-Management Patient Education Research Project, Stanford Arthritis Center. She is a former Fellow of the Arthritis Health Professions Association of the Arthritis Foundation.

Jeanne Lynn Melvin, O.T.R., M.S.Ed., F.A.O.T.A., is Director of the Arthritis and Health Resource Center, Wellesley, Massachusetts. She is author of *Rheumatic Disease: Occupational Therapy and Rehabilitation* and a former Fellow of the Arthritis Health Professions Association of the Arthritis Foundation.

Carolee Moncur, P.T., Ph.D., is Clinical Assistant Professor in the Division of Physical Therapy, University of Utah, and Research Consultant at the LDS Hospital, Department of Physical Therapy. Currently, she is President of the Utah Chapter of the Arthritis Health Professions Association.

Karen Moutevelis, O.T.R., is Staff Occupational Therapist at Brigham and Women's Hospital in Boston and was formerly Staff Occupational Therapist in the Arthritis-Immunology Center at the Veterans Administration Medical Center in Philadelphia. She holds a degree in Occupational Therapy from Tufts University.

Anneli H. Navarro, R.P.T., M.Ed., is Assistant in Medicine at the Johns Hopkins University School of Medicine and Instructor in the Department of Physical Therapy at the University of Maryland School of Medicine. A former Arthritis Health Professions Association Fellow of the Arthritis Foundation, she has lectured and written extensively on rheumatology topics. Her clinical interests are quantitation of muscle strength in rheumatic disease and public education in arthritis.

Catherine A. Novak, R.N., M.S.N., holds degrees from The Johns Hopkins Hospital School of Nursing and the University of Maryland School of Nursing. A former Rheumatology Nurse Specialist, she is now conducting clinical trials research at the EMMES Corporation in Potomac, Maryland.

Marilyn Gross Potts, M.S.W., is Community Component Director of the Indiana University Multipurpose Arthritis Center and doctoral student in medical sociology. She is a former clinical social worker with the Rheumatology Division of Indiana University School of Medicine and has just completed a two-year Arthritis Health Professions Association Fellowship with which she evaluated education support groups for rheumatic disease patients.

Amos P. Sales, Ed.D., is Department Head and Professor in the Department of Rehabilitation, College of Education, at the University of Arizona. His professional expertise, publications, and presentations concern rehabilitation psychology, administration, and education. He is a recipient of the National Rehabilitation Association's W.F. Faulkes Award for Excellence in Professional Service to the Handicapped.

H. Ralph Schumacher, M.D., is Professor of Medicine at the University of Pennsylvania School of Medicine and Director of the Arthritis-Immunology Center at the Veterans Administration Medical Center in Philadelphia. He is a clinician, teacher, and basic researcher.

Helen Schweidler, O.T.R., is currently affiliated with Hand Surgery Associates in Phoenix, Arizona. Her professional experience spans fifteen years with arthritis patients in home health, hospital, and long-term care facilities.

Melinda Wayne Seeger, B.S., O.T.R., is Associate Chief of Rehabilitation Services at the University of California Medical Center. Treatment, research, and teaching in rheumatic diseases is the major focus of her career. The author of numerous publications, she currently serves on the Arthritis Foundation Professional Education and National Arthritis Health Professions Association Executive Committees.

Dena M. Shapiro-Slonaker, O.T.R., M.S.Ed., is a therapist for the outpatient rheumatology population at the University of California, Los Angeles, Rehabilitation Center and has a private practice as a consultant in rheumatology rehabilitation. A frequent lecturer, she coordinates the UCLA short-term Arthritis Health Professions Fellowship in Rheumatology.

Marlin N. Shields, R.P.T., is Director of Physical Therapy, LDS Hospital and Clinical Assistant Professor in the Division of Physical Therapy at the University of Utah. A past President of the Arthritis Health Professions Association and member of the National Arthritis Advisory Board, Mr. Shields is a 1983 recipient of the Kendall Award for Outstanding Achievement in Clinical Practice from the American Physical Therapy Association.

Martin Snyder, D.P.M., is Chief of Podiatric Services at the Tucson Veterans Administration Medical Center and Associate in the Departments of Internal Medicine and Surgery at the University of Arizona Health Sciences Center. Dr. Snyder is a member of the American College of Foot Surgeons and a Diplomate in the American Board of Podiatric Orthopedics. He is currently serving as Chairman of the Medical and Scientific Committee of the Southern Arizona Chapter of the Arthritis Foundation.

Timothy M. Spiegel, M.D., is Assistant Professor of Medicine and Director of the Rheumatology Rehabilitation Unit, Division of Rheumatology at the University of California, Los Angeles, College of Medicine. He is the Medical Director of Physical and Occupational Therapy and Co-Director of the Arthritis Clinic at U.C.L.A.

Terence W. Starz, M.D., is a Clinical Instructor in Medicine at the University of Pittsburgh College of Medicine and in private practice and research in rheumatology in Pittsburgh, Pennsylvania.

Mary Betty Stevens, M.D., is the Director of the Rheumatology Division at Johns Hopkins University where she received her medical training. Her research has focused on the systemic rheumatic diseases.

Joan D. Sutton, R.N., M.S.N., is an Instructor in Medicine at the Johns Hopkins University School of Medicine. She is past President of the Arthritis Health Professions Association of the Arthritis Foundation.

Robert L. Swezey, M.D., F.A.C.P., is Clinical Professor of Medicine at the University of California, Los Angeles, School of Medicine and Medical Director of the Arthritis and Back Pain Center, Inc. He is the author of numerous publications, including *Arthritis: Rational Therapy and Rehabilitation.*

Betty A. Wickersham, B.S., R.P.T., is affiliated with the Southern Arizona Chapter of the Arthritis Foundation and the Southwest Arthritis Center, University of Arizona, Tucson. She has specialized in physical therapy treatment and education of rheumatology patients for the past 18 years.

Nina Wolchasty, L.P.T., B.S., was formerly Staff Physical Therapist in the Arthritis-Immunology Center at the Veterans Administration Medical Center in Philadelphia. She is now a medical student at Philadelphia College of Osteopathic Medicine.

William L. Woods, Jr., B.S.M.E., is a Clinical Engineer at the University of Arizona Health Sciences Center in Tucson. A mechanical engineer by training, he has specialized in biomedical engineering, with particular interest in specifying, designing, and building technological aids for arthritis patients. He has been principle investigator on three research projects funded by the National Institutes of Health and the National Bureau of Standards studying the architectural requirements of the handicapped.

Elizabeth J. Yerxa, Ed.D., O.T.R., F.A.O.T.A., received a degree in Occupational Therapy from the University of Southern California and her master's and doctoral degrees in Educational Psychology from Boston University. She is currently Professor and Chairwoman of the Department of Occupational Therapy at the University of Southern California.

Beth Ziebell, Ph.D., is a psychologist in private practice and consultant to the Arthritis Foundation, Southern Chapter, and the Multipurpose Arthritis Center at the University of Arizona Health Sciences Center. Her book, *Wellness: An Arthritis Reality,* reflects an interest in stress and pain management.

ACKNOWLEDGMENTS

We sincerely acknowledge the efforts of the multipurpose arthritis center at the University of Arizona's College of Medicine. The Southwest Arthritis Center staff as well as the staff of the Section of Rheumatology, Allergy, and Immunology at the College of Medicine have been most supportive in this work. We especially would like to express our thanks to Jane Palmer, Ida Miller, Laurie Smith, and Cindy Olney for their hard work and many hours that they gave to the production of this book. We would also like to acknowledge the staff of the National Arthritis Foundation and its professional organizations, the Arthritis Health Professions Association and the American Rheumatism Association. Special acknowledgments go to John T. Boyer, M.D., Director of the Southwest Arthritis Center, Professor of Internal Medicine and Director of the Division of Restorative Medicine at the University of Arizona College of Medicine; and to Rubin Bressler, M.D., Professor and Head of Internal Medicine for allowing us the time to pursue this endeavor. Acknowledgments also go to the Butterworth people for their guidance.

ACKNOWLEDGMENTS

Philosophy of Rehabilitation

Gail Riggs, M.A., and Eric P. Gall, M.D.

Disability is a problem of coordination (of resources) rather than limitation.
Debbie Gately-McKeen
Counseling Student at
Southwest Arthritis Center

In this age of expanding knowledge, increasing specialization, and complexity of health care regimens, no one profession can be expected to provide all the services required for comprehensive care. This is especially true of the care needed by the person who has arthritis. Interdisciplinary cooperation is what is needed.

Cooperation demands an understanding of the responsibilities, capabilities, and role of each health professional in the care of both acutely and chronically ill patients. Yet the health care system, particularly in its training programs for professionals, deemphasizes chronic care and colleagial cooperation.

The medical system has made remarkable progress in scientifically based and crisis-oriented medicine. Physician-training programs provide experience mostly on inpatient acute problems; attention is paid to ambulatory and chronic debilitating disease only secondarily. The family practice specialty has made inroads into this problem, but such specialists comment that they are unsure how best to utilize other members of the health care team.

This book addresses in a professional way how individual physicians, nurses, and allied health professionals can best approach patients with rheumatic diseases. The area of arthritis and rheumatic disease care is particularly suited to a study of rehabilitation principles and a team approach to treatment. The mildly involved patient is concerned about a future of disability. This patient needs great attention to good diagnosis, treatment, and psychosocial concerns. The patient with more disabling disease requires a comprehensive approach in order to be restored to a physically and functionally optimal role in society.

Many members of the health care system—nurses, physical therapists, occupational therapists, counselors, rehabilitation engineers, speech and hearing professionals, and a myriad of others—receive their education, for the most part, in a setting separate from medical students. They usually have access to patients through entirely different routes than the physician. All too often the allied health professional has a different concept of health and disease than does the physician, and communication between members of different health specialties is not common.

With the aging of the population, the crowding of this country, the recent recognition of the rights to a full life on the part of the handicapped, it is most important to shift the focus of the American health care system from crisis care to chronic care. It would be helpful to students of particular health care disciplines to be exposed to other, related disciplines at various times in their training. The ultimate goal should be to include in medical students' curricula the development of expertise in the complicated management of chronic care and rehabilitation, including the use of and cooperation with allied health personnel.

The primary care physician (family practitioner, general practitioner, internist, or pediatrician) as well as most medical specialists and subspecialists have little exposure to the health care team during training. The exception to this rule is occasional interaction with office, ward, or clinic nurse and social worker in nursing home placement. Even with these people, however, the doctor has little knowledge of their training and capabilities. A recent survey conducted in preparing for this book indicated a widespread misunderstanding of what members of the health care team do and how they are best utilized.

In this survey 61 replies were received from 225 individuals listed as primary care physicians in Tucson. There were 42 internists and 19 family and general practitioners in the responding group. Table 1 shows which allied health personnel were utilized by these physicians. Several of the specialists were not used by many of these physicians. Comments made most often indicated that the physicians did not know what allied health specialists did and that physicians believed that the services offered by them cost too much and were not covered by insurance, that they were not readily accessible, that they did not communicate well with physicians and that they either threatened the MD's authority or were not assertive enough. Table 2 delineates how four groups of allied health profes-

Table 1. Allied Health Professionals Utilized by 61 Primary Care Physicians in Tucson

	Have	Make Use	Refer To	Never Use
Nurse	46	31	8	13
Physical therapist	21	44	46	2
Occupational therapist	8	4	39	15
Social worker	20	16	36	25
Vocational rehabilitation counselor	0	3	33	46
Psychology counselor	15	20	28	28
Pharmacist	26	34	26	12

Table 2. How Allied Health Disciplines Are Used by the Primary Care Physicians (61 Doctors)

Nurses		Physical Therapists		Occupational Therapists		Social Workers	
Office (vitals, chief complaint)	26	Referral for musculo-skeletal problems	32	Never use	12	Never use	20
Home care	10	Exercise prescription or training	17	Seldom use	17	Seldom use	17
Patient education	13	Heat	9	Hospital only	7	Hospital setting only (discharge planning)	6
Injections	7	Massage	4	Refer patients to them	11	Referral	5
History taking	4	Traction	4	ADL training	6	Locate community resources	9
Physical exam	3	Hydrotherapy	7	Hand function and therapy	5	Nursing home placement	7
Gold and penicillamine follow-up	3	ADL training	2	Splints	2	Financial problems	9
Triage	2	Gait training	3	Vocational rehabilitation	2	Living arrangements	4
Counseling	2	Splinting	3	Same as PT	1	Counseling	3
PT	1	Patient education	5	For patient boredom	1	Emotional support	2
Medication review	1	Physician training	1	Home evaluation	1	Meals	1
Drug studies	1					Transportation	1
Make flow charts	1						

sionals were used by local physicians. In the doctors' individual comments there was obvious lack of knowledge of the proper roles of these individuals in the health care of the arthritis patient. These role definitions are addressed in part I of this book.

On the other hand allied health professionals in some cases learn many skills but are not prepared to apply these skills to arthritis care. Even the physical therapist and the occupational therapist have limited exposure to rheumatic disease in their curricula.[1] Yet they have the potential *skills* to treat such patients.

It is not practical to have all patients tended to by physician subspecialists in rheumatic disease. Likewise it is impractical to have a multitude of allied health personnel specialize in rheumatic disease. It is the purpose of this book to outline the skills available to various members of the health care team and to suggest ways to apply these skills practically in the primary care setting.

REHABILITATION DEFINED

The health professional needs to keep in mind the World Health Organization's definition of rehabilitation: "the combined and coordinated use of medical, social, educational, and vocational measures for training and retraining the individual to the highest possible level of functional ability."[2] Rehabilitation, then, is the restoration to function, the return to normality, the helping to achieve work, self-reliance, self-respect. Rehabilitation is synonymous with comprehensive medical care. Rehabilitation in many settings must be practiced by the primary care practitioner, the health care team, and the patient and family—not by an arthritis specialist. This book describes how the person who has arthritis can be helped to achieve a useful life through education and therapy.

Acton defines rehabilitation as the coordinated application of medical, educational, vocational, and social measures to enable a disabled individual to achieve maximum independence and to participate as fully as possible in the society of which he or she is a part. Moreover, "As members of the rehabilitation community, as well as members of the communities and societies in which we live, we have the additional challenge to enlighten those people with distorted and retarded attitudes so that the successes of the rehabilitation professions will not be drowned in the swamps of prejudice, discrimination, and apathy."[3]

The concept of rehabilitation has broad scope. The patient's environment often is created by conditions that are irreversible even with excellent medical care. The arthritis may result in significant long-term loss of function. "To adapt to such a loss the patient needs to make a physiological adaptation, and also to make psychological, social, educational, and, if of working age, vocational adjustment. Therapy obviously also includes any medical care that may reduce the irreversible portion of the condition. This is frequently called functional restoration, in contrast to comprehensive rehabilitation. It may also include maintenance care."[4]

The primary care physician and allied health professional share the responsibility for setting up the best, most comprehensive treatment program available. They should remember, though, that "TLC (tender, loving care), which is so frequently considered an inherent part of medical care, can undermine rehabilitation efforts, however, if it allows the patient to remain in the sick role for too long."[5] The patient has the responsibility for carrying out prescribed activities. The treatment, then, is an equal partnership involving collaboration, communication, and cooperation.

THE GOALS OF REHABILITATION

The goal of rehabilitation is to enable patients to obtain maximum usefulness in terms of themselves, their family, and their community. This goal includes relief of symptoms, restoration of mobility and strength, and increase in the sense of self-worth.

Most medicine, but especially rehabilitative medicine, depends for its ultimate utility on patients who expect the best of themselves. Rehabilitative medicine is a paradigm of what medicine should become. It is collaborative work—with which few doctors have much experience—and the collaboration often involves not only other health professionals but the patient's family and the community. The patient must be motivated to participate in the most efficacious manner. In the past "we have perceived disability as being primarily a problem of the individual who is impaired, and the solution as being primarily to eliminate, reduce, or compensate for the impairment. Only slowly have we begun to understand the crucial flow of the environment and society as causes of handicapped lives."[3]

Many types of arthritis are prolonged illnesses, with a relatively short time spent in the hospital or with the physician. This means that physicians have limited exposure to the effects of the disease. The bulk of patients' difficulties occur at home or in the vocational and social milieu and their ability to function depends on the right kinds of aids, home modifications, and support systems (friends, family, work). People with arthritis need a variety of resources in order to remain as independent as possible and functioning in the least restrictive lifestyle. This involves a delicate balance between the need for a complex of services adaptable to the patient's needs and the tendency to oversupport and produce dependency, as in acute care settings.

THE SIGNIFICANCE OF THE USE OF THE TEAM

A theme repeated in many of the chapters of this book is the importance of interpersonal communication and listening skills of health professionals who are treating chronically ill patients. It is common for members of different health professions to be brought together to provide coordinated services to persons with chronic illnesses.[6,7] In this age of expanding knowledge, increasing specialization, and complexity of care regimens, no one profession can be expected to provide all of the services needed for comprehensive care.[8-10]

Teamwork depends on mutual respect, clarity of individual roles, shared goals, and skill in communication and decision making.[8,11,12] "Team rehabilitation" is more difficult to define because of the broadness of the phrase, which could refer to almost any group of health professionals working in any type of arrangement. The composition may be justified on the basis of meeting the needs of the patient or determined by practice specialty and presenting symptoms.[13] The community and its resources and the type of practice setting in which care is being provided must be considered. In some instances certain allied health specialists are not present or are not readily available. Other professionals may have to learn some of their skills with occasional guidance from distant consultants. Physicians in a rural setting, for instance, or their office nurses, may need to know and prescribe basic physical therapy and occupational therapy modalities.

THE ROLE OF THE PATIENT ON THE TEAM

Throughout this book the phrase *arthritis patients* is used rather than *arthritics* or *arthritic patients*. The word *arthritic* is avoided because it tends to be a label, a somatotype. The preferred terminology is *people who have arthritis* or *arthritis patients*. The concept of this book is that people who have arthritis should focus on the positive aspects of their lives and themselves and not focus disproportionately on the disease. Although the disease must be fully understood and coped with, it should not become the first priority. When a person is labeled arthritic, then that person becomes synonymous with "disease." The bearer of the label then becomes a "diseased person" with a sickness-oriented viewpoint rather than a healthy one.

Many patients do not have a model for coping with physical illness and few will have one for coping with rheumatoid arthritis. After the severity of the disorder has been assessed and interventions proposed, the patient must become an active member of the rehabilitative team. Membership of the team varies, depending on potential availability[1] and interest in the case, but the professional personnel can include a physician, physical therapist, occupational therapist, pharmacist, nurse, public health nurse, social worker, and others. The team (as well as the patient) must believe that the patient is able to learn to cope and to manage adaptive tasks.

The team approach requires that the patient take an active and central role as a team member and coleader and be an equal partner on the team. Primary care providers and specialists in various aspects of health care delivery must interact not only with one another but with the patient. No matter how much effort is expended on the patient's behalf, without the patient's own active participation, the care plan will not work. In the management of a disease that is not curable and that lasts a long time, education of the patient for independence must be emphasized. This goal cannot be achieved without full cooperation of the patient who must come to realize that "The key to coping with one's disability is to receive enough satisfaction and rewards to make life worthwhile. All the hard work of living with a disability must pay off to the individual."[14] Of course, no one can guarantee that the hard work of living (with or without a disability) will pay off, but the authors of this book show many ways to help the arthritis patient experience those much needed satisfactions and rewards.

REFERENCES

1. Jette AM, Becker MC. Nursing occupational therapy, and physical therapy preparation in rheumatology in the United States and Canada. J Allied Health 1980;9: 268–275.

2. World Health Organization (WHO) 1980. The international classification of impairment, disabilities and handicaps: a manual of classification relating to the consequences of disease. Geneva: WHO.

3. Acton N. The world's response to disability: evolution of a philosophy. Arch Phys Med Rehab 1982;63:145–149.

4. Lehmann JF. Rehabilitation medicine: past, present and future. Arch Phys Med Rehab 1982;63:291–297.

5. Grzesiak RC, ed. Chronic pain: a psychobehavioral perspective. Baltimore: Williams and Wilkins, 1980.

6. Halstead L. Team care in chronic illness: a critical review of the literature of the past 25 years. Arch Phys Med Rehab 1976;61:507–511.

7. Nason F. Team tension as a vital sign. Gen Hosp Psychiatry 1981;3:32–36.

8. Brill N. Teamwork: working together in the human services. Philadelphia: JB Lippincott, 1976.

9. Nagi S. Teamwork in health care in the United States: a sociological perspective. Milbank Memorial Fund Quart 1975;53:75–89.

10. Wise H, Beckhard R, Rubin I. Making health teams work. Cambridge, Mass.: Ballinger, 1974.

11. Given B, Simmons S. The interdisciplinary health care team: fact or fiction? Nursing Forum 1977;16:165–184.

12. Lynch B. Team building: will it work in health care? J Allied Health 1981;10: 240–247.

13. Rothberg J. The rehabilitation team: future directions. Arch Phys Med Rehab 1981; 62:407–410.

14. Trieschmann KB. Coping with disability: a sliding scale of goals. Arch Phys Med Rehab 1974;55:556–560.

The Interdisciplinary Team Approach

Gail Riggs, M.A.

The multidisciplinary team or interdisciplinary team concept is given much lip service. Why and how each works receives little attention, however. What we are talking about when we refer to the multidisciplinary team is a coordinated pattern of interaction. Scribner describes this process as subdividing a problem such that its parts can be treated separately by persons from different disciplines.[1] The interdisciplinary process, on the other hand, is characterized by focusing on a commonly acceptable definition of a problem such that its resolution does not distinguish the individual contributions of separate disciplines. The interdisciplinary team is the ideal mechanism for organizing health professionals to provide services to people with arthritis. Realistically, it is not possible to organize such teams in every setting and in some settings they would not be cost effective.

 The roles of health professionals involved in the rehabilitation of the arthritis patient and the interaction among members of the health care team are the subjects of part I of this book. Role descriptions and interdisciplinary team interactions can be presented only as a model. Implementation must be left to the creativity and resources of the many health professionals in their varied settings who care for the chronically ill arthritis patient.

WHY IS A TEAM NECESSARY IN ARTHRITIS REHABILITATION?

Management of arthritis must follow a logical progression incorporating multiple therapies. The *pyramid approach* to the management of rheumatic disease requires the input of many health professionals.[2,3] Management is designed to help the patient lead a comfortable, productive life while relieving much of the physician's burden by utilizing services of other trained health professionals.[4] The basic arthritis treatment includes patient and family education, salicylates in most cases, and exercise, rest, and adequate follow-up. Those patients unresponsive to the basic program may respond to other more toxic or expensive drugs or a number of adjunctive therapies (figure I.1). To put the pyramid approach into practice, the primary care physician must work with many members of the team who are experts in various aspects of care and who can suggest and carry out various portions of the plan.

Looking at team involvement another way, health professionals need to know their craft well to contribute something to the team and participate actively in it. Nurses or physical therapists learn all they can in order to excel at their chosen career. It is going to be their profession for 20, 30, or even 40 years. Similarly, persons with arthritis must also learn all they can, not only to become active in their own health care and rehabilitation but because they are going to be living with this unchosen, complex disease for the rest of their lives. Education of the person with arthritis and management of a chronic illness over a period of decades requires creative integration of the individual functions of the team as well as a supreme effort to facilitate communication among team members. It is the cornerstone of the pyramid.

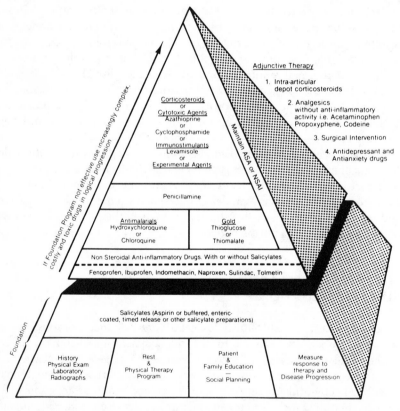

Source: Gall EP, Gall EA, Boyer JT, Rheumatoid Arthritis: Concepts in Evolution. Ariz Med 1979;36:55–59.

Figure I.1. Pyramid for the therapy of rheumatoid arthritis.

WHAT IS A TEAM?

Webster's dictionary defines teamwork as work done by a number of associates each doing a part but all subordinating personal prominence to the efficiency of the whole. Halstead defines *team care* not as a single treatment variable, but rather as a broadly defined concept, encompassing such elements as assessment, common objectives, continuity of care, coordination, regular communication, and comprehensiveness.[5] We would define a team as a group of individuals including the patient, the primary care physician, the patient's family, and other health professionals (as needed and available) who contribute their expertise in devising a comprehensive care program for and with the patient. Ideally the team would function in a conference format or collaborative way; however, this is unrealistic in many, if not most settings. In the less than ideal format good communication then is essential among the many practitioners who may be involved in the care of the arthritis patient.

Rubin shows health team members, in a self-instructional workbook, how to identify coordinating problems that claim their time and energy and offers proven techniques for solving them so that a team's total effort can be centered on actual patient care.[6] Many share McCann's belief that the success of a coordinated team approach is dependent upon respect and communication among all members, all directed toward the individual patient's goal.[7]

The patient and primary care doctor are the team leaders and coordinate and sift input, suggestions, and activities of the various members. The team may only consist of doctor and patient or may consist of many specialists and providers depending on the geographic location, extent of the disease, and financial and health resources available.

The team can consist of the rheumatologist, internist, family practitioner, the nurse, physical therapist, occupational therapist, orthopedic surgeon, podiatrist, counselor, social worker, nutritionist, even the biomedical engineer, and, of course, the most important person on the team: the patient. Joining this team means striving for mutual goals. The team is like a family building its own home, which soon realizes that the plumbers, carpenters, electricians, and architect are *all* important and that without the unique contribution and input of each, the house may not be built the way the family wants it.

COST OF TEAM CARE VERSUS INDIVIDUAL CARE

Having analyzed the literature on the subject, Halstead has pointed out that coordinated team care appears to be more effective than the usual fragmented care that is generally received by persons with long-term illnesses.[5] But team care is usually associated with increased utilization of health care services, which increases overall health costs. The question then might be asked, does team care in the long run save money? Yelin et al. show that the indirect cost of illness due to lost wages exceeds the cost of medical services by a large margin.[8] Meenan et al.

show that people with rheumatoid arthritis were earning only 50 percent of the income predicted for them had they not had arthritis.[9] Sixty-three percent experienced a major change in psychosocial status as a result of the disease. Work disability appears to be the most important sociologic impact of rheumatoid arthritis since it is associated with significantly greater income and psychosocial losses. This evidence raises questions of emphasis and approach for physicians involved in the clinical care of chronic rheumatic disease patients. Thus it is suggested while the actual medical cost of team care of the individual may be higher, actual cost to the community overall may be less if such care is effective in returning the patient to the work force. Further studies are needed in this area.

TEAM COMMUNICATION

Communication is the key to success in the team approach to arthritis care. Each team member must share information freely with other members, including the patient. "If we don't have genuine health teams, the reasons begin with problems in communication. Problems of communication revolve around perceptions of various roles," as Epstein has observed.[10] He points out that different perceptions of various health professional qualifications also may interfere with communication among these professionals, and the more we find fault with others, the less we are reminded of our own deficiencies.

It is important to remember that communication has two purposes. First, it is the means whereby a plan can be implemented and action coordinated toward a common end. And second, it is the means whereby the members of a team can be motivated to execute the plans willingly and enthusiastically.

How a person uses communication—whether physician, nurse, physical therapist, or counselor—largely determines how effective he or she is. A simple model, the Johari Window, named after its originators Joseph Luft and Harrington Ingram, represents a way to look at the self and to help individual members of the team improve communication by

- Exposing one's views and feelings to others more openly, thus reducing facades.
- Actively soliciting feedback of feelings and opinions of others (especially the patient's), thus reducing blind spots.

Concepts of communication are treated further in chapter 28.

TEAM LEADERSHIP AND THE ROLE OF THE PRIMARY CARE PHYSICIAN

In the management of rheumatoid arthritis, the primary care physician ideally works with a multidisciplinary team.[11] The real leader of a health team need not be the doctor. As Epstein points out, the leader can be any person sensitive to the individual needs of the members. Moreover, team members should bear in mind that "Real leadership should not be vested in only one person. Different members should take on the leadership role when their own particular skills are especially needed to solve a particular problem. Thus, leadership becomes a shared function."[10]

Today there are many different types of health professionals, and it is apparent that these same health professionals do not always understand the roles of others in the health industry. Some disparage other professions for one reason or another. These negative attitudes do not encourage open communication among members of different health care professions or allow them to profit from one another's special knowledge and skills.

For the smooth running of a health care team, as Epstein advocates, every therapeutic technique that comes into dispute must be evaluated from the point of view of its efficacy rather than its identification with a person on the staff. Every member of the team should be encouraged to give information relevant to the technique being studied. Every meeting should have time scheduled for pointing out the strengths of individual team members (as well as the patient) and the things they have done right since the last session.

Years ago Lillywhite enumerated some factors that help develop the team into a smooth working unit:

1. Coordination of the team takes time.
2. Procedures and patterns of operation result largely from group decision rather than from forces above or outside. There is a need for flexibility to allow for changes that are necessary with a widely diversified group.
3. Mutual respect for each individual member on the team is emphasized. It is important to recognize the contributions of each in the past and to look ahead to increase this effectiveness.
4. The central purpose of the team should be better care for the patient and help in all that is done.
5. Careful handling of staffing and clinic sessions is of course necessary and should be planned and carried out with some precision and with an understood purpose.
6. It is necessary to make careful reports and good follow-up and to see that all specialists involved with any one patient know what all of the others are doing.
7. As much as possible face-to-face situations, the telephone, and group work should be used to keep in contact with one another and to keep one another informed. In doing this, written reports, memos, notes, formal requests, and written instructions can be played down. This helps to increase understanding among the specialists once they have talked with each other face to face.
8. Attention should be paid to pleasantness and convenience in the examining rooms, the group meeting rooms, and to providing a friendly, informal relaxed atmosphere.[12]

Another view on what makes such teams work was provided by Bole, who said, "Health care practice revolves around the critical relationships between persons providing and receiving care. Unified efforts of health professionals to build relationships (as on a team) could improve patient education, satisfaction, and compliance."[13]

A recent study identified problems in the provision of team care, such as unclear goals and role expectations, competition for team leadership, limited time, team conferences that are lectures rather than group problem-solving sessions; values that support individual rather than team practice.[14] Several recommendations resulted from the study: Patients should write down their questions before visits and develop goals for each visit with the physician or team. Each patient should receive a copy of the written evaluation. Written physical therapy prescriptions, in addition to descriptions of exercise procedures, should include both rationale for exercise and expectations for outcome. Psychosocial support in the form of referrals to a counselor is an important part of treatment for chronically ill patients. And patients need to learn how to define their treatment expectations at regular intervals.

WHAT DEGREE OF TEAM CARE IS REALISTIC?

All members of the team are not always available, especially in rural settings. One allied health professional may have to do dual duty, even triple duty. An office nurse might be able to offer some psychological or emotional support to an anxious patient as well as teach range-of-motion exercises. The primary care physician in a solo practice might depend on the patient's family as an important support unit in the care of the arthritis patient. Not only do family members share the problems of the arthritis patient, but they can offer social and emotional support, administer medication, assist with home therapy, and make home improvements to allow more independent functioning of the person with arthritis. An integral portion of the team, the family generally must supplement other attempts to improve the care of their own loved one.[15] In areas where resources are limited, an occasional well-planned trip by the patient to consult specialists in different disciplines may be of great value to patient and doctor. If this is not possible, telephone consultation may also prove worthwhile.

SUMMARY

Most health professionals can define what a team should be and why it is necessary especially in the care of the chronically ill arthritis patient who may require multiple rehabilitative techniques. However, effective team functioning in the present health care system seems to evade practical application. Necessary ingredients for successful team operation are inclusion of the patient on the team as an equal partner, sharing of knowledge, development of good communication skills, and dedication of the health care team to a common goal.

REFERENCES

1. Scribner R. Interdisciplinary research management. AAAS Report 77-R-6, American Association for the Advancement of Science, Washington, DC, October 1977.
2. Gall EP, Gall EA, Boyer JT. Rheumatoid arthritis: concepts in evolution. Ariz Med 1979;36:55–59.
3. Gall EP, Johnson SA. Arthritis: altered levels of mobility. Chronic health problems. St. Louis: CV Mosby, 1981;146–176.
4. Duff IF, Newkom JE. Patient with rheumatoid arthritis. Slide presentation from media library, University of Michigan, Ann Arbor, 1975.
5. Halstead LS. Team care in chronic illness: a critical review of the literature of the past 25 years. Arch Phys Med Rehab 1976;57(11):507–511.
6. Rubin I, Plovnick MS, Fry RE. Improving the coordination of care, a program for health team development. Cambridge, Mass.: Ballinger, 1975:279.
7. McCann V, Philips CA, Quigley R. Preoperative and postoperative management: the role of allied health professionals. Orthopedic Clin North Am 1975;6(3):881–906.
8. Yelin E, Nevitt M, Epstein W. Toward an epidemiology of work disability. Milbank Memorial Fund Quart 1980;58(3):386–415.
9. Meenan RF, Yelin EH, Nevitt M, Epstein WV. The impact of chronic disease: a sociomedical profile of rheumatoid arthritis. Arthritis Rheum 1981;24(3):544–549.
10. Epstein D. Breaking the barriers to communication on the health team. Nursing 1974;4(9):65–68.
11. Bartholomew LE, Rynes RI, Hedberg SA, Commach CJ. Management of rheumatoid arthritis. Am Fam Physician 1976;13(2):116–125.
12. Lillywhite H. Communication problems in a medical rehabilitation team. J Commun 1956;167–173.
13. Boles BK. Interpersonal skills development in health professions education. J Allied Health 1976(Fall):23–29.
14. Ziebell B, Wickersham EA, Boyer JT. Team arthritis consultation. Phys Ther 1981;61(4):519–522.
15. Pigg, J, Gall E. The family tree. Permanent Exhibit of the American Rheumatism Association. Atlanta, 1980.

ADDITIONAL READING

Beckhard R. Organizational issues in the team delivery of comprehensive health care. Milbank Memorial Fund Quart 1972;50:287–316.
Rubin I, Beckland R. Factors influencing the effectiveness of health teams. Milbank Memorial Fund Quart 1972;50:317–335.
Wise H, Beckhard R, Rubin I, Dyte A. Making health teams work. Cambridge, Mass.: Ballinger, 1974.

1

The Role of the Rheumatology Nurse

Joan D. Sutton, R.N., M.S.N.

Rheumatology, a subspecialty of medical-surgical nursing, has emerged since the mid-1970s as an increasingly popular specialty for nurses. Its popularity may be explained in part by passage of the Arthritis Act of 1974, which provided the necessary resources for the development of Multipurpose Arthritis Centers (MAC). Underlying the MAC concept is a focus on an interdisciplinary approach to the problems of rheumatic disease. Subsequently, opportunities became available for nurses and other health professionals to specialize in rheumatology. The Arthritis Act also paralleled a trend in nursing for increasing numbers of nurses electing to specialize rather than to generalize. As rheumatology continues to gain increased recognition as a subspecialty of medicine, and as rheumatologists continue to increase in numbers, so also are increasing numbers of nurses selecting rheumatology as their specialty of choice.

A national survey in 1979 revealed that rheumatology is given a low level of priority in most schools of nursing.[1] Nurses generally are not prepared to function in a rheumatology setting and therefore require an internship, preceptorship, or a similar educational program prior to assuming major nursing responsibilities. In 1976 a report to the Congress of the United States by the National Commission on Arthritis and Related Musculoskeletal Diseases stated "specialized training programs are virtually nonexistent for nurses, physical therapists and the other health professionals who are essential to the comprehensive care of arthritis patients."[2] In this same report it was recommended that top priority be given to training nurses and other allied health professionals who are committed to academic careers in teaching and the study of arthritis.[3] Although the implementation of this priority has not been fully realized, there has been an increase in the numbers of nurses selecting rheumatology as a specialty area of practice.

Nurses with expertise in rheumatology are functioning in a variety of settings.[4] In physicians' offices and in outpatient settings, nurses play an important role in coordinating services that the patient may need, in assuming responsibilities for patient care, and in providing patient and family education. In addition it has been demonstrated that in those settings where waiting lists for new patients must be established, an office nurse with expertise in rheumatology is able to assess accurately the urgency of a patient's need for an appointment.[5] With the use of an abbreviated telephone screening protocol, completed by a secretary, this process requires little secretarial time and even less for the nurse's interpretation of the completed protocol.

In a rheumatology office or ambulatory care setting patients whose disease activity and therapeutic regimens are relatively stable often are referred to nurse practitioners (nurses with additional formal education in physical assessment skills) for ongoing care. In addition to assessing, planning, and implementing a care program for the patient, nurse practitioners are also proficient in monitoring disease activity. Likewise clinical nurse specialists (nurses with a master's degree in a specialty area) are well qualified to follow physician-referred patients in an outpatient or office setting. In addition to patient care, clinical nurse specialists are often expected to assume major responsibilities for education at all levels and for research.

For the nurse employed in a family practitioner's or internist's office, exposure to patients with a rheumatic disease is understandably more limited. These nurses may find the local chapter of the Arthritis Foundation an invaluable resource with regard to patient education materials, professional education opportunities, professional resources, and so on. In addition, information and assistance may be sought from professional colleagues working at Multipurpose Arthritis Centers, located nationwide.

Inpatient rheumatic disease units require the expertise of nurses with a solid medical-surgical nursing background, a base upon which rheumatology content can be built. As the health care provider who spends the most time with the patient, the rheumatology staff nurse is concerned not only with the physical needs of patients, but also with the educational needs of both the patient and his family. The staff nurse may recognize the need for referral of patients to other health care providers and after referral assume the role of reinforcing prescribed therapeutic regimens.

Nurses with expertise in rheumatology are also extremely valuable in the public health setting (home, school, industry, and so on). Modifications in the home and work setting, working with schoolteachers to develop an appropriate activity program for a child with arthritis, and educating leaders in industry regarding the problem of arthritis are but a few examples of the activities of rheumatology nurses in public health. Nurses with extensive experience in rheumatology are assuming roles as nursing consultants working as administrators, planners, coordinators, and advisors.

The role of the nurse varies considerably depending upon setting, educational preparation, and experience of the individual. Perceptions of physicians regarding roles and responsibilities of a nurse are likewise quite variable. Selected results of a recent survey of primary care physicians regarding their perceptions of nurses revealed that physicians employ nurses for the following reasons: patient education and instruction, psychological support and reassurance of patients, physical evaluation and assessment, appraisal of the home situation, and administration of medication.[6]

In addition to nursing roles and responsibilities aforementioned, office and ambulatory care nurses may assume major responsibility for patients entered into nurse management programs. Patients with rheumatoid arthritis[7] treated with gold, penicillamine, or methotrexate, patients with degenerative joint disease,[8] and those with gout[9] can be effectively managed by a rheumatology nurse.

Patients receiving gold, penicillamine, or methotrexate are initially evaluated every 1 to 2 weeks. At the time of these visits the nurse assesses the following: (1) physical condition of the musculoskeletal system in order to monitor disease activity; (2) side effects or untoward reactions to prescribed medication (bone marrow depression, nephrotoxicity, abnormal liver function, skin rash, mouth ulcers, or hypogeusia); (3) the need for referral to other health care professionals, such as a physical therapist, occupational therapist, or social worker; (4) the educational needs of both patient and family; and (5) the patient's level of acceptance of the disease. Based upon a complete assessment and with involvement of both the patient, other health professionals, and the nurse, a comprehensive plan of care is developed and implemented. The opportunities for continuous reevaluation are numerous due to the frequency of required patient visits. Reevaluations by a physician are scheduled at regular intervals or as the patient's situation dictates.

The condition of patients with degenerative joint disease may also be successfully managed by a nurse. Because of the nonsystematic nature of this disorder and secondary to the slow progression of the disease process, the interval between patient visits may be long. In addition to completing a nursing assessment (as outlined), the nurse is frequently in a position to monitor other health problems, such as hypertension, diabetes, and vascular insufficiency. The principles of adequate nutrition and of weight reduction, in addition to the need for joint protection and ambulatory/assistive devices are often included in a plan of care. The needs of the older individual may be complex, and meeting those needs may require additional nursing time and involvement.

In the majority of instances, gout, once diagnosed, should be totally controlled by medication. Due to the episodic nature of gouty attacks and the feeling of total well-being between attacks, some patients discontinue their medications, which results in emergency room visits for subsequent acute attacks or progression of destructive arthritis. It has been shown that patients with gout in telephone contact with a nurse every six weeks can do extremely well: compliance with medication increases; emergency room visits decrease; and emerging problems, medical and other, can be dealt with effectively.[10]

Although the aforementioned relates primarily to the role of the nurse, it must be emphasized that optimal care and outcome for the patient with a rheumatic disease is dependent upon coordination and communication by multiple health professionals involved with that patient's care.

SUMMARY

Rheumatology is a specialty that is appealing to increasing numbers of nurses with a variety of interests and talents. Rheumatic Disease Nursing Standards[10] have recently been accepted by both the American Nurses' Association and the Arthritis Health Professions Association of the Arthritis Foundation. It is hoped that certification for rheumatology nurses by the American Nurses' Association will soon become a reality. In the meantime the primary care nurse, when adequately educated in rheumatic disease care, is also a valuable asset to patient management.

REFERENCES

1. Jette A, Becker M. Nursing, occupational therapy and physical therapy preparation in rheumatology in the United States and Canada. J Allied Health 1980;9(4): 268–275.
2. Arthritis: out of the maze, the arthritis plan. Report to the Congress of the United States, vol. 1. U.S. Department of Health, Education and Welfare 1976:53.
3. Ibid., p. 55.
4. White J, Pigg J, Heiss M, Raish M, Sutton J. Rheumatology nursing: a specialty you can tailor to your talents. Nursing '79 1979;9(9):108–112.
5. Sutton J, Schaffhauser D, Stevens MB. Program-entry priorities—an AHP judgement. Abstract and presentation, 16th Annual Meeting of the Arthritis Health Professions Association, Boston, 1981.
6. Gall E, Riggs G. Survey of primary care physicians in Tucson, Arizona, 1981.
7. Brown-Skeer V. How the nurse practitioner manages the rheumatoid arthritis patient. Nursing '79 1979;9(6):26–35.
8. Sutton J, Novak C, Zizic T, Stevens MB. Nursing intervention in degenerative joint disease. Abstract and presentation, 13th Annual Meeting of the Allied Health Professions Section, New York, 1978.
9. The Johns Hopkins Hospital. Arthritis clinic. Baltimore, 1976 (unpublished).
10. Heiss M, Pigg J. Co-chairs, Task force on development of rheumatic disease nursing standards, in press.

2

The Role of the Physical Therapist

Anneli H. Navarro, R.P.T., M.Ed.

The physical therapist shares with other members of the health care team the responsibility of helping each patient with rheumatic disease lead as close to normal, satisfying, and productive a life as possible. The unique contribution of physical therapy toward this ultimate goal centers around specific aspects of assessment, treatment, and education: yet the general goals guiding physical therapy intervention are shared by most health disciplines striving for comprehensive management of the case of the patient with rheumatic disease.

GOALS AND PHYSICAL THERAPY RESPONSIBILITIES

Suppression of Inflammation

Suppression of inflammation in rheumatic disease is mainly achieved through appropriate anti-inflammatory drug therapy, as prescribed and monitored by the physician. The physical therapist can aid this process by providing and teaching rest as an added treatment modality.[1] An acutely inflamed joint may be rested by temporary reduction of exercise and activity, as well as by splinting.[2] Increased fatigue often associated with exacerbation of disease can be counteracted by increasing the number of hours of rest each night and by adding brief rest periods during the day. Each patient also needs to know how to maintain a proper balance between rest and activity as changes in disease status occur.

There is evidence that not only physical, but also emotional stress may trigger a flare-up of rheumatic disease.[3] Helping the patient to recognize and cope with potential sources of stress in daily life may reduce the frequency and severity of flare-ups.

13

Relief of Pain

Pain and stiffness are major features of arthritis, causing much discomfort and disability. For temporary relief of pain, reduction of muscle spasm, and in preparation for exercise, the physical therapist will select among many thermal modalities.[4] Not only the degree of disease activity, site, and number of joints involved, specific contraindications, and general practical considerations, but also patient preference and tolerance should determine the type of heat or cold selected. Special attention is given to teaching safe, simple, and effective use of inexpensive heat at home. Dealing with morning stiffness through timing of medication combined with the use of moist heat and active range-of-motion exercise is also emphasized in patient education. The potential role of stretch gloves, sleeping bag, electric blanket, warm clothing, as well as of weather and climate upon arthritis is discussed with the patient.

Other techniques used by physical therapists to obtain temporary relief of pain in rheumatic disease may include relaxation, biofeedback, and transcutaneous nerve stimulation. The recent discovery of endorphins, opiatelike substances released in the brain, may clarify the mechanism behind some traditional methods and perhaps open new avenues for pain control.[5]

Prevention of Deformity

Ongoing synovitis leads to a gradual erosion of joint surfaces as well as a weakening of periarticular structures rendering the joint vulnerable to internal and external forces acting upon it.[6] It is the responsibility of the physical therapist to teach the patient methods to minimize abnormal forces particularly on the metacarpophalangeal and proximal interphalangeal joints, wrists, knees, ankles, and feet during transfer and locomotion activities. Such joint protection measures need to be incorporated into a patient's life-style long before the onset of instability and malalignment of a joint. Deformity, when established, cannot be reversed by any such measures.

Recent advances in joint replacement surgery combined with appropriate pre- and postoperative physical therapy aimed to restore optimum comfort and function have provided gratifying results,[7] also in the setting of advanced disease especially of the hip and the knee.[8]

Maintenance of Function

Chronic disease such as rheumatoid arthritis may lead to impairment of physical as well as psychological functioning.[9] Sensitivity by the physical therapist to psychosocial factors and referral for appropriate help will minimize the interruption of the rehabilitation process.

The physical therapist possesses expertise in the assessment of articular and muscular status affecting the patient's ability to function, that is, to perform needed activities of daily life. Functional activities of particular concern to the physical therapist comprise all aspects of mobility, including the ability to move in bed, get safely in and out of bed and bathtub, get on and off the commode and chairs, and stand, walk, and negotiate steps—all in a safe manner. The actual and perceived functional problems experienced by patients in their own particular environments determine their true functional needs. Several well-tested assessment tools are now available to the physical therapist to quantify and serially follow function in rheumatic disease.[10-13]

The need for special devices such as canes, crutches, and raised toilet seats to enhance safety, independence, and joint protection in transfers and locomotion, as well as the need for functional footwear are evaluated by the physical therapist. The physical therapist is also trained to assess the status and needs of the rheumatology patient with regard to self-care, including bathing, personal hygiene, grooming, dressing, and eating.

On the basis of carefully established needs through the initial evaluation, specific treatment goals and a treatment plan can be developed and implemented by the physical therapist. A physical therapy program may range from instruction in a simple, preventive home exercise program and patient education to intensive long-term rehabilitation combining thermal modalities, hydrotherapy, exercise strategies, functional skills training, and training in the correct use of needed equipment and devices.[14]

OUTCOME FACTORS IN PHYSICAL THERAPY

In spite of the largely unpredictable clinical course for the individual patient, there are several means available within the control of the referring physician and the physical therapist to maximize the effectiveness of physical therapy intervention in the comprehensive long-term management of the patient with rheumatic disease.

Early Intervention. It is estimated that only 15 percent of persons with rheumatoid arthritis have a rapid, relentless course of the disease, responding poorly to therapy.[15] In the great majority disability can be prevented through early institution of appropriate therapy. Patient education, close monitoring of parameters relative to function, and institution of a preventive home exercise regimen designed to maintain optimum joint range of motion, muscle strength, physical condition, and function should be implemented at the time of diagnosis of chronic rheumatic disease.[16]

Team Approach. In a complex chronic disease such as rheumatoid arthritis, often affecting multiple systems, the expertise of various members of the health care team will need to be called upon. An important part of the integral core is made up of the physical therapist teamed with the patient and physician.

One of the most frequently identified obstacles to true team care is poor communication between the physical therapist and the physician.[17] The physical therapist is expected to provide written documentation of initial evalution, treatment goals, and a treatment plan followed by progress notes. Written and verbal communication is needed to keep all parties well informed of patient progress (or its lack) as well as to promote recognition among the various disciplines of one anothers' contributions to the comprehensive management in rheumatic disease.

Individualized Care. The great spectrum of disease manifestations as well as variability within the same individual over time demands sensitivity and flexibility on the part of the physical therapist. What is appropriate treatment may soon become inappropriate as the disease status and patient needs change. Also, what is appropriate for one patient may not be appropriate for another with the same disease. Thus knowledge, understanding, and good judgment in applying established principles of management must be exercised in each situation.

Patient and Family Education. The responsibility of patient and family education and ongoing reinforcement is equally shared by all members of the health care team. With sometimes major misconceptions and poor understanding about the disease and its management, as has been found also in persons with long-standing disease, the basic rationale for compliance with a therapeutic program may be totally lacking.[18]

In addition to helping the patient understand the basics of the disease process and basic medical management, the physical therapist needs to help the patient understand the proper use of heat and cold, prescribed exercise, rest and physical activity, and specific joint protection and energy conservation measures. Patients need to know what are the things within their own control that they can do in daily life to maintain optimum long-term function and independence.[19,20]

Continuity of Care. In diseases characterized by exacerbations and remissions it is particularly tempting for the patient to discontinue prescribed therapy during periods of remission, in the hopes that a cure has been achieved. Ongoing monitoring with periodic adjustment of the physical therapy program as needs change, and reinforcement of the need for continuity of care during remission are essential features of management of chronic disease.

An examination of the foregoing may suggest a positive outlook for the patient with rheumatic disease, and realistically so; yet many individuals with arthritis are not able to obtain the needed physical therapy services. Limited professional preparation in rheumatology and inadequate health insurance coverage, particularly for outpatient physical therapy services, constitute major obstacles.

Most physical therapists in practice have a bachelor's degree with a certificate of proficiency in physical therapy. The professional curriculum focuses on anatomy, physiology, pathology, physical therapy theory and practice, basic rehabilitation, and clinical sciences and education.

A recent survey of undergraduate preparation in rheumatology indicated that although virtually all students of physical therapy trained in the United States do receive some exposure to rheumatology during the course of their professional training, few of the programs actually offer formal courses that focus on the rheumatic diseases.[21]

There is a need for greater emphasis on rheumatology in professional preparation, which is only partially offset by available rheumatology continuing education. The local, regional, and national components of the Arthritis Health Professions Association, a professional section of the Arthritis Foundation, and the Multipurpose Arthritis Centers are attempting to meet this need through a variety of continuing education activities and programs. The Arthritis Foundation AHP fellowship program offers a rare opportunity for advanced preparation in rheumatology for nonphysician health professionals, including physical therapists.

Limitations in third-party reimbursement for physical therapy may also prevent the patient from obtaining needed services. While most health insurance policies provide coverage for physical therapy and certain prescribed assistive devices for the hospitalized patient, few programs include outpatient physical therapy services. Medicare has established an annual ceiling for outpatient physical therapy, currently set at $500 per person. Persons confined to the home may be eligible for visits by a physical therapist when arranged by the doctor and a Medicare-authorized home health agency is used to provide the service.

SUMMARY

The foremost roles of the physical therapist in the comprehensive long-term management of the patient with rheumatic disease is as health care provider and educator. As a health care provider the physical therapist performs clinical assessments of the patient's disease activity, articular, muscular and functional status, on the basis of which specific treatment goals and plans are developed and then implemented. Patient and family education and reinforcement are integral components of physical therapy intervention in rheumatic disease. Professional education on the role of physical therapy and open lines of communication with other members of the health care team serve to improve patient care. As solid scientific evidence on the efficacy of various forms of therapeutic intervention in arthritis is still scarce, the physical therapist must ultimately also be a contributing member of the interdisciplinary health services research team in rheumatology.

REFERENCES

1.   Smith RD, Polley HF. Rest therapy for rheumatoid arthritis. Mayo Clin Proc 1978; 53:141–145.

2.   Feinberg J, Brandt KD. Use of resting splints by patients with rheumatoid arthritis. Am J Occup Ther 1981;35(3):173–178.

3.   Moskowitz RW. Psychosocial aspects of rheumatoid arthritis. J Albert Einstein Medical Center 1971;19(Spring):36–39.

4.   Lehmann JF, Warren CG, Scham SM. Therapeutic heat and cold. Clin Orthopedics Related Res 1974;99(March–April):207–245.

5.   Stewart D. Turning on the endorphins. Am Pharmacy 1980;NS 20(10):50–54.

6.   Swezey RL. Dynamic factors in deformity of the rheumatoid arthritic hand. Bull Rheum Dis 1971–72;22(1,2):649–656.

7.   McCann VH, Philips CA, Quigley TR. Preoperative and postoperative management: the role of allied health professionals. Orthopedic Clin North Am 1975;6(3): 881–906.

8.   Box JH, Turner R, Box P, et al. Total knee and total hip replacement in arthritis therapy. North Carolina Med J 1978;39(6):364–374.

9.   Vignos PJ. Psycho-social problems in the management of chronic arthritis. In: Ehrlich GE. Total management of the arthritic patient. Philadelphia: Lippincott, 1973: ch. 5.

10. Convery FR, Minteer MA, Amiel D, et al. Polyarticular disability, a functional assessment. Arch Phys Med Rehab 1977;58(11):494–499.

11. Fries JF, Spitz P, Kraines RG. Measurement of patient outcome in arthritis. Arthritis Rheum 1980;23(2):137–145.

12. Meenan RF, Gertman PM, Mason JH. Measuring health status in arthritis, the arthritis impact measurement scales. Arthritis Rheum 1980;23(2):146–152.

13. Jette AM. Functional status index: reliability of a chronic disease evaluation instrument. Arch Phys Med Rehab 1980;61(9):395–401.

14. Swezey RL. Arthritis, rational therapy and rehabilitation. Philadelphia: W.B. Saunders, 1978.

15. Duthie JJR, et al. Course and prognosis in rheumatoid arthritis. Ann Rheum Dis 1964;23:193–204.

16. Scott FE. Arthritis: a patient's view. Phys Ther 1969;49:373–376.

17. Gall E, Riggs G. Survey of primary care physicians in Tucson, Ariz., 1981.

18. Ferguson K, Bole GG. Family support, health beliefs, and therapeutic compliance in patients with rheumatoid arthritis. Patient Counseling Health Ed 1979 (Winter/ Spring):101–105.

19. Kaye RL, Hammond AH. Understanding rheumatoid arthritis, evaluation of patient education program. JAMA 1978(June);239(23):2466–2467.

20. Rand PH. Evaluation of patient education programs. Phys Ther 1978;58(7):851–856.

21. Jette AM, Becker MC. Nursing, occupational therapy and physical therapy preparation in rheumatology in the United States and Canada. J Allied Health 1980(November);9(4):268–275.

3

The Role of the Occupational Therapist

Elizabeth J. Yerxa, Ed.D., O.T.R., F.A.O.T.A.

The term *occupational therapy* was first coined in 1914 to describe a new health profession that employed "occupations" in the treatment of those who were physically or mentally ill.[1] In this sense "occupations" does not mean employment but rather encompasses the gamut of activities human beings perform in their daily lives. Occupational therapy uses a wide range of "occupations," defined as purposeful activities, in order to reduce the incapacity of persons who are chronically disabled by illness or injury. Occupational therapists, OTRs, are registered by the American Occupational Therapy Association when they have met the qualifications for practice. Their major goal is to increase function in everyday activities. In some settings occupational therapists may be augmented by certified occupational therapy assistants (COTAs) who share the same goals but receive primarily technical training. This chapter is limited to discussion of the role of the registered occupational therapist.

Occupational therapy is the use of self-initiated, purposeful, and meaningful activity to reduce the incapacity caused by pathology.[2,3] Occupational therapists work to help the patient increase his or her adaptive skills in meeting the demands of the environment in a satisfying way. Through occupational therapy patients learn the skills required to perform their expected roles in society whether as preschooler, student, homemaker, worker, or retiree, in spite of often severe and chronic impairments. Occupational therapists are employed in hospitals, rehabilitation centers, extended care facilities, outpatient clinics, private practice clinics, and in home health service agencies such as the Visiting Nurses' Association.

EDUCATIONAL PREPARATION

Occupational therapists complete a bachelor's or master's degree, a six months' supervised internship, and a written national certification examination in order to

19

practice. In some states occupational therapists are also required to be licensed. The occupational therapy curriculum is accredited jointly by the American Occupational Therapy Association and the Council on Allied Health Education Accreditation of the American Medical Association.[4]

Building upon a strong liberal arts foundation, course content reflects a bio-psychosocial view of the person, who is seen as in a stage of continual development across the life span. The major organizing curriculum concept is therefore human development viewed as a continuum from conception through death. Biological sciences include biology, anatomy, physiology, kinesiology, neurology, and medical pathology. The psychosocial foundational subjects include psychiatry, anthropology, and sociology. Occupational therapy theories address the development of adaptive skills in persons of all ages and with all types of disabilities.[5] Finally course work teaching occupational therapy interventions includes such approaches as the use of arts and crafts to improve function, task analysis, use of work simplification techniques, teaching activities of daily living, designing, fabricating, and applying splints and other orthotic devices, providing adapted equipment and adapting the patient's home or work environment for improved function.

OCCUPATIONAL THERAPY FOR ARTHRITIS

With the patient who has arthritis as with any other disease, occupational therapy focuses on the reduction of incapacity and development of maximum independence in real life (see table 3.1). Specific approaches are influenced by the pathology and sequelae of arthritis along with the unique life-style of the patient.[6] After evaluating the patient to determine expected levels of function, occupational therapists enlist techniques of energy conservation, such as grouping tasks in one room, and work simplification, such as using devices that improve efficiency, to enable the person with arthritis to continue to perform the expected

Table 3.1.   Role of the Occupational Therapist with the Patient Who Has Arthritis

Reduce incapacity, increase function in daily living
Conserve energy, simplify patient's work
Train in independent living skills (self-care, homemaking, community adaptation)
Adapt environment to improve function
Evaluate patient for, design, and fit hand splints and assistive devices
Develop motivation for independence
Develop interests and skills in leisure pursuits
Restore time management, balance between rest and activity
Educate patient for self-management toward independence
Help prevent institutionalization due to dependency
Provide information of help in deciding whether to elect surgery

skills of independent living that are still feasible (see chapters 22 and 23). These might include personal self-care, home-making, community living, and problem-solving, social-recreational skills, and school or vocational skills.[7] Occupational therapists employ purposeful activity, patient instruction, or splints to protect weakened joints and to help prevent deformities.[7] In general occupational therapists teach the patient to adapt to environmental demands by doing common activities in new ways including through the use of assistive devices (such as dressing aids) when necessary (see chapter 23). In addition, occupational therapists instruct the patient in how to adapt the home or work environments to save energy and increase function.[8] For patients who are despondent because of the effects of their disease, occupational therapy may provide some relief through restoring a balance between activity and rest and helping the patient organize time and energy. This is done so that the patient can continue to perform those activities that bring satisfaction and a sense of accomplishment. Occupational therapists may be asked to perform an occupational therapy evaluation, which may include an assessment of strength, range of motion, endurance, and function in daily life, and to recommend whether occupational therapy services are required for specific patients who have arthritis. Occupational therapists can also contribute their knowledge of function to the team decision-making process regarding the predicted outcomes of reconstructive surgery.

CRITERIA FOR REFERRAL TO OCCUPATIONAL THERAPY

The following are indications that a patient might benefit by referral to occupational therapy:

1.   Difficulty in or inability to perform daily living tasks or meet occupational role expectations (such as an employee or homemaker)
2.   Fatigue or pain preventing function at home or in the community
3.   Danger of developing or exacerbating deformities, particularly to the hands or upper extremities
4.   Lack of apparent motivation to retain independence
5.   Need to improve function in a variety of environments such as work, school, home, community, or new and unfamiliar settings
6.   Being in danger of institutionalization because of inability to care for self
7.   Need to develop new skills, interests, or organization in the use of time
8.   Problems of loss of function complicated by the aging process
9.   Potential for reduced ability to function

WHO PAYS FOR IT AND WHERE TO FIND IT

Reimbursement for occupational therapy services is provided under Medicare, Medicaid, the Department of Rehabilitation Services, and many private insurance carriers under specified conditions, which usually include provision of a physician's referral. In rural areas or smaller cities it may be difficult to locate an occupational therapist. Information regarding the availability of services in such communities might be obtained by contacting the local chapter of the Arthritis Foundation, which has a list of OTRs concerned with arthritis care, the state occupational therapy association, or the nearest occupational therapy university program. Additional information regarding occupational therapy may be obtained by writing to the American Occupational Therapy Association Inc., 1383 Piccard Drive, Rockville, Md. 20850.

SUMMARY

Occupational therapy can help improve the patient's ability to perform expected daily living activities with satisfaction, conservation of energy, prevention of unnecessary losses of function, and maintenance of a positive patient outlook regarding potential abilities. Occupational therapists reduce incapacity in patients who have arthritis by teaching them to meet environmental demands in new and more effective ways. Patients should be referred to an occupational therapist if they exhibit problems in the ability to perform daily living tasks, the potential to lose function, or reduced motivation to remain independent.

REFERENCES

1. Mock HE, Abbey ML. Occupational therapy. JAMA 1928;91:797–801.
2. Reilly M. The educational process. Am J Occup Ther 1969;23:299–307.
3. Yerxa E. Authentic occupational therapy. Am J Occup 1967;21:1–9.
4. American Occupational Therapy Association. Essentials of an accredited program for the occupational therapist. Adopted June 1973. (Unpublished.)
5. Llorens L. Facilitating growth and development: the promise of occupational therapy. Am J Occup Ther 1970;24:93–101.
6. Hopkins HJ, Smith A. Willard and Spackman's occupational therapy. 5th ed. Philadelphia: JB Lippincott, 1978.
7. Melvin J. Rheumatic disease: occupational therapy and rehabilitation. Philadelphia: FA Davis, 1977.
8. Cordery J. Joint protection. Am J Occup Ther 1965;19:285–294.

4

The Role of the Counselor

Beth Ziebell, Ph.D.

There is an emotional component to the life of every person. Even in the healthiest of humankind, this emotional component occasionally requires some extra attention and focus—in order to cope with depression, smooth out marriage or other family relationships, or face difficult career decisions.

The person who has a chronic disease like arthritis has an even greater range of possible emotional concerns. In addition to the universal conflicts everyone might experience, the person with arthritis must often deal with chronic pain, changing body image, and a loss of self-esteem from becoming a less contributing member of the household or of society.

A counselor or psychologist who is trained to work with chronic disease patients can help put these concerns back into perspective and assist with discovering solutions and alternatives. Dictionaries define *counselor* as an advisor. In this setting the advisor can be a person with a degree in counseling and guidance or psychology or social work or rehabilitation. Probably more important than the specific degree is the individual's ability to be a good listener and to relate well with many different kinds of people.

Allen[1] and Syme[2] have discussed the role of a counselor in a health care setting. Recognition of the value of counseling in medicine has come about largely because of the recent emphasis on the role of stress in physical illness. The sources of stress are primarily in the areas of life generally considered to be the counselor's domain—that is, home, school, job, and personal relationships.

Counseling for a patient with chronic disease can take many forms and be for many purposes. Some typical reasons for referral are depression, anxiety, pain management, difficulties in marriage or other personal relationships, sleep disturbance, problems with communication in general and with health care providers in particular, and employment concerns.

If a counselor is functioning as a member of a health care team, he or she might see individual patients upon referral from the other team members but preferably would routinely see each patient in order to evaluate their psychological status or adjustment. In a study conducted in 1979, my colleagues and I dis-

that every patient we interviewed had some degree of emotional discomfort that would probably have been ameliorated by counseling.[3]

Counselors who are trained to work in medical settings may not always be available in local communities. However, if there are qualified mental health professionals available who are interested in the problems of chronic disease, encouraging them to learn about your patients with arthritis and to become involved with their management would be worthwhile.

Physicians can also be excellent counselors, but their schedule restrictions generally prevent them from spending enough time with each patient to deal adequately with very involved personal concerns. Therefore, making referrals to qualified mental health professionals is often appropriate.

Physicians with no referral resources, of course, must do the best job possible in the time available. In any case, every physician needs good listening skills in order to pick up the sometimes subtle messages about the emotional distress a patient may be experiencing.

The counselor can perform many and varied functions that contribute to the care of the rheumatic disease patient. Another dictionary definition for *counselor* is advocate, and indeed the counselor working in a medical setting often functions as an advocate for the patient. The counselor as advocate may be explaining, orienting, or facilitating the patient's sometimes difficult journey through the health care system.

The counselor is an educator, teaching about parenting, providing reading materials, instructing in the art of good communication and assertiveness and explaining to people how they can gain more control over their own lives. If there is planned arthritis patient education in the community, the counselor can contribute information about the emotional aspects of life.

Counselors sometimes find themselves in the position of needing to intervene in a school or community agency on the part of a patient with arthritis. School personnel often do not have enough information about children with arthritis and do not always deal effectively with the problems that come up, such as taking medication during school hours or negotiating an appropriate adaptive physical education class. Expectations are often either too high or too low for kids with arthritis; school personnel need to understand both the ups and downs of rheumatic disease and the very human reaction of using illness to avoid difficult tasks. In this type of intervention the counselor is also an educator.

Through a lack of understanding or communication, a patient may not be receiving available community services such as transportation, visiting nurses, or home-delivery of meals. Sometimes a brief intervention by the mental health professional who is familiar with the case can clear up the misunderstanding.

Acting as a liaison between patients (or the parents of child patients) and their physician is an important part of advocacy. Patients and physicians usually both benefit from improved communication. Patients do not always ask the right questions, and physicians do not always provide enough information. Patients can be encouraged to tell doctors of their concerns by developing written lists of specific questions. Physicians can be encouraged to develop the listening skills that will help patients to feel understood. Restating what the doctor tells the patient can help clarify and also reinforce the treatment program.

Counseling in a formal sense can be for individuals, couples, families, or groups, depending on the needs of the patients. The patient whose physician talks about counseling in a calm, matter-of-fact way is more likely to accept the suggestion that counseling be sought without feeling as though he or she is being sent to a "shrink" because he or she is "crazy." Counseling is usually acceptable when it is treated as a customary part of the disease management.

Support groups for people with rheumatic disease have become a popular phenomenon across the country. These groups are often sponsored by local chapters of the Arthritis Foundation as well as by clinics and hospitals serving a population of people with arthritis. There are groups for adult patients, for teenagers with arthritis, and for parents of children with arthritis. Support groups are sometimes led by professional counselors but may also have lay leadership. People without professional training should limit their activity to group leadership and should not attempt personal counseling. People attending these groups offer support and encouragement to each other. They may discuss common experiences and propose solutions to mutual problems.

Teenagers with arthritis who have participated in support groups have reported deeply appreciating feeling understood in a "less emotional" environment than within their family group.[4] These young people also stated that they felt less alone when they could talk to other youths with arthritis.

Counselors in a medical setting may work with both adults and children. The primary difference in working with children is that their parents are also involved in their disease management. The home environment has a strong emotional impact on a child and must be taken into consideration when planning the treatment program. For example, telling the parents that a child should lead as normal a life as possible is useless advice if "normal" to that family means pampering and specialness for an ill child.[5] And instructing the parent in an involved home physical therapy program may not be successful in a one-parent family where all the energies are being devoted to survival. If the counselor has some understanding of the child's family and home environment, the treatment program can be planned realistically.

With the new emphasis on patient education and understanding, the counselor has a role to play in helping patients develop better participation in their own health care. Because of the chronic nature of arthritis, people can easily feel like helpless victims and passively wait for a cure that has yet to be invented.[6] But the entire burden for wellness does not fall on the health care practitioner. The patients themselves have the responsibility for the creation of an individual life-style conducive to optimum health and personal fulfillment.

When counselors have the opportunity to help arthritis patients learn the skills to deal with depression, improve their communication, understand how too much stress can affect their health, learn stress reduction and pain management techniques, these patients are much better equipped to stay on an even emotional keel. If these skills are combined with a plan for improved physical health by developing an awareness of the importance of diet and exercise and understanding the effects of drinking and smoking, and so on, this combined effort will surely produce a healthier human being. And all of these considerations are efforts patients must make for themselves. Traditional medicine is obviously very important too, but patients themselves must be key members of the health care team in order to achieve the best possible results.

The physical and the emotional parts of people are constantly interacting.[7] What affects the mind, affects the body, and what affects the body, affects the mind. Treating only the physical symptoms of rheumatic disease is like treating half a person. The physician and the mental health professonal can work together to treat the whole human being.

SUMMARY

The counselor or psychologist provides patient education; facilitation; liaison between patient and doctor; and advice to individuals, couples, families, and groups. Reasons for counseling include depression, anxiety, pain management, stress management, parenting, personal relationships, career decisions, communication problems, and life-style analysis.

REFERENCES

1. Allen T. Physical health: an expanding horizon for counselors. Personnel Guidance J 1977;56(1):40–43.
2. Syme S. Behavioral factors associated with the etiology of physical disease: a social epidemiological approach. Am J Public Health 1974;64:1043–1045.
3. Ziebell B, Wickersham E, Boyer J. Team arthritis consultation. Phys Ther 1981;61(4):519–522.
4. Ziebell B. Psychosocial needs of adolescents with arthritis. Allied Health Professions Section of the Arthritis Foundation Newsletter 1978;11(4):5–10.
5. Ziebell B. As normal as possible. Tucson, Ariz.: Arthritis Foundation, 1976.
6. Ziebell B. Wellness: an arthritis reality. Dubuque, Iowa: Kendall/Hunt, 1981.
7. Pelletier K. Holistic medicine, vol. 2. New York: Delacorte Press, 1979:32,35.

5

The Role of the Social Worker

Marilyn Gross Potts, M.S.W.

The skills of the social worker may be utilized in the comprehensive management of cases of patients with chronic rheumatic disease in two ways. Social workers can provide counseling regarding social and emotional concerns of people with chronic illness in patients not requiring the attention of mental health professionals. They can also locate available community resources to meet environmental needs. Social workers are available in hospitals, community mental health clinics, family service associations, and church-related counseling agencies such as Catholic Social Services and Lutheran Social Services. Some public health departments, visiting nurses' associations, and extended care facilities have social workers on their staff. Finally, many social workers engage in private practice.

Social workers may have a baccalaureate or master's degree, and several states require licensing. Use of the affiliation ACSW (Academy of Certified Social Workers) after the person's name indicates that a social worker has passed a written examination and obtained at least two years' experience in practice.

Social workers are trained in interviewing and counseling techniques suitable for work with individuals or families. Many have received instruction in group work techniques. Schools of social work may provide a generic training program or various tracks directed toward practice in particular organizations or with particular populations (community planning agencies, corrections, psychiatric settings, child welfare agencies). Courses about abnormal and normal human development and about social problems such as crime, poverty, and racism are typically offered.

Although many schools of social work offer curricula relevant to practice in medical settings, most social workers in practice today have received little instruction specifically about arthritis. Therefore it may be incumbent upon the physician to provide information to the social worker regarding the physical aspects of arthritis and its prognosis, treatment, and so on, in addition to specific information about an individual patient. For example, the social worker intervening with a patient who expresses frustration over lack of an immediate response to penacillamine should know that this is a slow-acting drug. The social worker discussing employment concerns with a patient with rheumatoid arthritis should be aware of how employability may be affected by morning stiffness, pain, fatigue, limited strength and mobility, and by the possible variability of the disease from day to day or week to week.

COMMUNITY RESOURCES

Finances for Daily Living Expenses

Successful alleviation of the financial concerns of arthritis patients can reduce a major stress. A social worker who is intervening with a patient who needs financial assistance may first gather information from the patient, the physician, and other health professionals regarding the patient's employability—his motivation and goals, functional ability and mobility, the prognosis of the disease, and more. If the patient is unable to continue in his present job but may engage in some other type of employment, the social worker may suggest that he contact the state department of vocational rehabilitation (DVR). Although the resources allotted by various states to vocational rehabilitation services vary greatly, arthritis patients may be able to receive job counseling, aid in seeking further education or training, or aid in locating employment through the DVR.

If the patient is unable to work in any capacity, the social worker may encourage him to contact the Social Security Administration. Arthritis patients may be eligible for Social Security Disability or Supplemental Security Income (SSI) benefits if their disabling condition is expected to continue for at least 12 months, or to end in death, *and* if they are unable to engage in *any* substantial gainful employment (work usually done for pay and requiring significant physical or mental ability). The patient may be denied benefits if he is considered employable or retrainable in a capacity other than his former occupation. Laboratory and x-ray findings, functional ability, age, and educational and vocational background are among the factors considered in determining the patient's eligibility.[1]

In general a disabled person with arthritis who has worked for 5 of the past 10 years may receive a monthly Social Security Disability benefit, the amount of which is based on the individual's prior earnings. In contrast, disabled people may receive SSI if they have never worked or do not have a sufficient recent work history. In addition, disabled people with small Social Security or other income may receive a monthly SSI benefit to supplement their other income. States are allowed to provide SSI recipients additional benefits above a federal maximum (as of July 1983, the federal maximum was $304.30 per month for an individual with no other income). Finally, some low-income patients may receive food stamps, which may be redeemed for groceries, or Aid to Families with Dependent Children (AFDC), which provides a minimal monthly income. Eligibility for these programs is established by county welfare or public assistance departments.

Finances for Medical Care

Patients may refuse aspects of their care because they think they cannot afford them. A recent survey has shown that in Indianapolis 56 percent of elderly sufferers of arthritis with Medicare or Medicaid were unaware that those programs would pay *any portion* of the cost of care for their joint problems.[2] Thus the social worker or hospital financial officer may need to explain to the patient the extent of his insurance coverage or to clarify methods for obtaining reimbursement.

Patients who are age 65 or over or who have received Social Security Disability benefits for 2 years may receive Medicare benefits.[3] With the exception of a deductible amount and certain copayments, Medicare hospital insurance (Part A) pays the "allowable" charges (an amount based on the average cost of a service in a locale) for inpatient hospital care, including physical and occupational therapy, laboratory tests and x-rays, skilled nursing care and posthospitalization skilled home health care. Medicare medical insurance (Part B) pays the allowable charges for physical services and outpatient treatment, including diagnostic tests and procedures, x-rays, drugs that cannot be self-administered (such as gold injections), durable medical equipment, physical and occupational therapy, and skilled home health care. Medicare, however, does *not* pay for drugs that can be self-administered (aspirin and other nonsteroidal anti-inflammatory medications, for example), patient education, routine physical examinations, or orthopedic shoes that are not part of leg braces. Many patients purchase private health insurance supplements that pay a portion of the deductible and copayments required by Medicare.

Certain arthritis patients who are "medically indigent," which means they have a low income relative to their medical expenses, may qualify for Medicaid (MediCal in California), which is administered by county welfare or public assistance departments. Although the types of services paid for by Medicaid vary among the states, in general this program pays for *most* of a wide variety of medical costs, including hospital and outpatient care, medication, physical and occupational therapy, home care, and nursing home care.

Other Needs

Supplemental Home Care.   The social worker may work with other health providers to coordinate a home care plan involving a community agency referral. Many areas have public health departments or Visiting Nurses' Associations that can provide home care by a nurse or a home health aide. Some agencies also provide physical or occupational therapy services. In addition, the social worker may be able to locate handyman, homemaker, or companion services for the arthritis patient who needs additional assistance at home but does not require care by a health care professional.

Alternate Housing.   The social worker can often help arthritis patients locate a public or private facility designed for disabled or elderly people. Such facilities commonly provide meal services, "panic buttons," and group recreational activities. If extended care in a rehabilitation facility or nursing home is required, the social worker can work with the patient and family to arrange a suitable placement.

Other Environmental Needs.   Numerous miscellaneous problems may require referral of the arthritis patient to community resources. Social workers should be aware of transportation services such as special buses for the handicapped and taxi discounts for elderly people. They may refer patients to meals-on-wheels programs, which in many localities provide home delivery of two meals per day for a minimal fee. In addition, social workers are aware of free food programs and sources through which patients may obtain low-cost or free clothing and household items. Finally, social workers should have contact with community service organizations, such as the Arthritis Foundation, churches, Rotary Clubs, and sororities, which can provide various services to patients.

PSYCHOSOCIAL ASSESSMENT AND COUNSELING

Social workers are trained in counseling techniques for individuals and families. In many medical settings the social worker has the primary responsibility for addressing the psychosocial needs of patients. This responsibility may be assigned by the physician or determined by mutual decision on the part of all professionals working with an arthritis patient. Of course, physicians, psychologists, nurses, chaplains, and others frequently play a major role in counseling patients regarding emotional and interpersonal issues as well.

One study attempted to define roles of the clinical nurse specialist and the social worker by surveying 45 members of each profession.[4] All of the social workers were employed in hospitals of over 400 beds; 93 percent of the nurses practiced in a hospital with 300 beds or more. All respondents had had actual work experience with a member of the other profession. Seventy-one percent of the respondents agreed that the clinical nurse specialist should be solely responsible for physical care of the patient, and the majority agreed that the social worker's role was to help patients locate improved housing and financial assistance (80 percent and 85 percent, respectively). However, 60 percent viewed the task of helping the patient and family accept emotional and physical aspects of disability as a collaborative responsibility, falling upon both nurses and social workers.

Although collaboration among health care professionals can have a beneficial effect on patient care (individuals may reinforce each others' instructions and provide feedback to each other regarding patient misunderstandings of information), role conflict should be avoided. If several people intervene with an arthritis patient regarding psychosocial issues, roles should be clarified and individual treatment plans coordinated.

THE PSYCHOSOCIAL ASSESSMENT

The basis for the social worker's intervention with a patient is the psychosocial assessment: the psychosocial diagnosis and treatment plan. This assessment addresses four issues: the patient's roles, reactions, relationships, and resources.[5] In addition to outlining the social worker's intervention, information from the psychosocial assessment may be relevant to planning and implementation of treatment by all individuals working with the patient.

Roles

By analyzing the roles of the patient (mother, father, spouse, homemaker, bread-winner, student, manual worker, professional) and the patient's view of these roles, the social worker gathers information that may highlight potential problems in coping with the illness. If the patient is the mother of small children, the arthritis may affect her ability to provide child care. Such patients may need the social worker's help in locating a day care center or a resource for homemaker services, or the occupational therapist's advice regarding ways of accomplishing child care tasks. The patient may feel guilty for being unable to meet her own expectations in her role as a mother and require reassurance that she still is valued by her family despite her reduced physical ability. In such instances the social worker may convene a family conference. If the patient is a manual laborer, the arthritis may affect his ability to continue employment. Referral to vocational counseling may be warranted. If the patient is a student it may be necessary to instruct his teachers about arthritis and the patient's treatment plan. Often the social worker is the liaison between the school and the medical professionals working with a child with juvenile arthritis.

Is the patient's role as a sexual partner affected by the illness? Sexual counseling may need to be provided by the social worker, the physician, or another health care professional with expertise regarding the specific sexual problem. Team interaction is important here.

Reactions

One must assess how the patient views arthritis and its consequences. Patients who view the disease as inevitably crippling may need considerable reassurance from all individuals involved in their care regarding the benefits of treatment before agreeing to comply with the health care plan. The patient's emotional reactions (denial, anger, depression) should be documented. Although the social worker or counselor may be primarily responsible for helping the patient deal with these reactions, other health professionals should also take them into account. For example, individuals working with a patient who is denying the illness may need to clarify their instructions more than once; those working with an angry patient may need to allow him to vent frustrations openly.

Has the arthritis reactivated prior personal conflicts? For example, an adolescent who is struggling to gain independence from his family may rebel strongly against the need for increased dependence imposed by the arthritis. This patient may need to be provided as much control as possible over such aspects of his care as timing of treatments and sequence of exercises. The patient who is able to secure his spouse's attention only when he is ill may use the illness for secondary gain, be unmotivated to follow the treatment plan, and thus require counseling from the social worker regarding expression of his needs in a more direct manner.

Relationships

How does the arthritis affect the patient's interactions with others, and how do these interactions affect the patient's ability to cope with the arthritis? The social worker will analyze the patient's significant relationships. Are family members supportive, or are they resentful of the need to undertake some of the patient's tasks? If family members are unsupportive because of lack of knowledge about arthritis and its treatment, family education by the physician or other health care professionals may be especially important. If deep-seated communication problems exist between the patient and the family, extensive family counseling may be warranted. This may be provided by the medical social worker, or the social worker may recommend that the patient be referred to a counseling agency.

How are the patient's social relationships affected by the illness? If an unemployable patient's work was a main social outlet, the social worker may need to suggest alternate opportunities for interaction with others, like senior citizens' centers, community centers, or patient support groups. As another example, many patients' relationships with friends and acquaintances are strained because the patient perceives that these individuals do not understand his arthritis. The social worker may encourage such patients to explain to their friends that arthritis is often not visibly apparent but may be unpredictable and variable from time to time and from person to person.

RESOURCES

The social worker should assess the patient's strengths and weaknesses regarding environmental and social resources—the adequacy of finances, housing, home care, and so on. The patient's psychological strengths and weaknesses should be analyzed as well and prior mechanisms for coping with stress determined. For example, the patient who tends to avoid problems may be unwilling to comply with care plans. The social worker or other health care professional may need to confront the patient regarding this maladaptive coping mechanism.

Adaptive coping mechanisms may be encouraged, but some modification may be warranted. If the patient tends to sublimate anxieties by engaging in physical activity, arthritis may preclude utilization of this coping mechanism. Such patients may need aid in redirecting their energies and finding new hobbies that do not impose stress on affected joints. Or a patient may be skillful in analyzing problems and determining a fixed course of action. However, due to the uncertainty and unpredictability of some forms of arthritis, such patients may need help in learning to devise flexible goals. An individual may overdo exercises on days when the arthritis is flaring because of an overzealous determination to comply fully with the exercise program. This patient needs instruction from the physician or therapist regarding the effects of excessive exercise. The social worker may support this patient's high level of motivation but encourage him to modify any maladaptive behavior.

SUMMARY

Social workers are available in most medium-sized hospitals and in various community agencies to help patients locate resources to meet their environmental needs. In addition social workers provide counseling regarding the social and emotional concerns of patients. Problems that may require a referral by the social worker to a community resource include need for finances for daily living or medical expenses, inadequate home care or housing, and lack of transportation.

The psychosocial assessment—an analysis of the patient's roles, relationships, reactions, and resources—is the basis for the social worker's intervention regarding psychosocial concerns. The information provided by the social worker in the psychosocial assessment may guide other health care professionals in their interactions with the patient. Because psychosocial counseling is often viewed as a collaborative effort among professionals of different disciplines, roles should be clearly defined to preclude role conflict.

REFERENCES

1. Disability examination under social security: a handbook for physicians. SSA Publication 79-10089. Social Security Administration, U.S. Department of Health and Human Services.
2. Potts M, Nichols D, Brandt KD, Weinberger M. Educational needs of ambulatory arthritics attending senior citizens centers. Submitted for publication.
3. Your Medicare Handbook. SSA Publication 05-10050, Social Security Administration, Health Care Financing Administration, U.S. Department of Health and Human Services.

4.   Mullaney JW, Fox RA, Liston MF. Clinical nurse specialist: clarifying the roles. Nurs Outlook 1974;22:712–718.
5.   Doremus BL. The four Rs: social diagnosis in health care. Health Soc Work 1976;1: 121–139.

6

The Role of the Vocational Counselor

Amos P. Sales, Ed.D.

The vocational counselor's raison d'être is to assist the patient to reach optimal work or career adjustment. This is often done in conjunction with an occupational therapist who addresses the specific functions that help the patient carry out his or her work or pursue a career. The vocational counselor works in this capacity while being fully aware that one cannot isolate vocational adjustment from personal and social adjustment. Counseling emphasizes involvement of the patient, or client, as an active participant in effecting the changes necessary to move toward a more successful personal and vocational adjustment. Individual needs determine to a great extent the type of counselor-client interaction.

There are three fundamental courses of action available when a disability like arthritis imposes limitations that handicap the individual: the causes of the person's handicap can be remedied by restoring ability; the handicap can be compensated for by enhancing other characteristics of the person; or the environmental circumstances can be changed so that the impact of the disability is avoided, lessened, or negated. The best foundation for vocational counseling incorporates all of these approaches, utilizing and developing all needed resources of the community and embracing all professions that can contribute to the process.[1]

Vocational counseling as a professional field is usually considered to have begun just after the turn of the century with the work of Frank Parsons, who identified the goal of vocational guidance as the selection of a vocation, sufficient preparation for it, and the achievement of vocational effectiveness.[2] Parsons considered three factors necessary for a systematic occupational choice: (1) a sound knowledge of the individual's personality, abilities, and limitations; (2) understanding of the demands and rewards of various types of work; and (3) a clearer conception of how these two sets of data are related. This concept of vocational decision making has prevailed and has significantly affected federally funded training efforts through the Rehabilitation Act of 1965 to develop professional rehabilitation counselors to work as vocational counselors specifically with the disabled. Two-year master's degree programs in rehabilitation counseling exist in every one of the United States. These professional education programs provide for competency and skill development in the areas of psychosocial and medical aspects of disability, vocational diagnosis, development of a plan for reaching vocational goals, principles of rehabilitation, and a sequence of practicum and internship. The unique competencies of the rehabilitation counselor are an invaluable resource in the total treatment plan of the arthritis patient.

Quality vocational counseling requires a theoretical knowledge that can assist in providing structure through which the vocational counselor can synthesize and analyze the vast amount of data about the individual and the world of work and assist the client to make the best choice. The variety of theoretical approaches include trait-factor theory, need-strive theories, psychoanalytic theory, social learning theories, self-concept theory, and eclectic points of view. No matter what the theoretical model, the vocational counselor is concerned with five basic constructs: (1) the individual's background (physical and psychosocial); (2) work personality (the psychological characteristics such as vocational self-image and motivation that mediate adaption to work); (3) work competencies (behaviors, skills, interpersonal relationships in the work setting); (4) work choice (appropriateness and completeness of career plans); and (5) work adjustment (satisfaction and effectiveness on the job). Arthritis can directly affect the work competency and the mental or emotional status of the patient who has trouble adjusting to it. The extent of vocational adjustment to arthritis depends upon the prior nature of these five constructs and their interrelationships, how far into the individual's career development the onset of arthritis occurred, and its specific impact on each of the elements. Thus for the vocational counselor the emphasis is on determining how disability has disrupted work adjustment.[1] Utilizing diagnostic data in promoting self-understanding and commitment on the part of the client in relation to occupational choice is the most challenging task in the vocational counseling process.

THE VOCATIONAL COUNSELING PROCESS

Several principles need to be firmly in mind for the vocational counselor if the counseling is to be effective. The foremost concerns the counselor-client relationship. Regardless of setting, the vocational counselor must develop a helping relationship with clients characterized by rapport, confidence, understanding, and permissiveness. This relationship begins with the initial interview and should continue throughout the counselor-client contact. The second principle relates to communication. Valid communication occurs when the counselor respects the client and is both an active listener and an accurate sender of information. True communication facilitates mutual understanding. The third principle is individualization of the process. Recognition of the client as an unique individual worthy of respect and possessing special qualities is essential if the counseling process is truly to be individualized. A fourth principle relates to participation, or involvement of the client in the process, which is considered essential for success. Self-direction and self-determination on the part of the patient lead ultimately to independent functioning and hence are the keys to success in vocational counseling. The vocational counseling process can be outlined as follows:

Intake (initial interview)

Assessment (interview, vocational evaluation, medical information, psychological information, etc.)
Individual strengths
Individual problems

Planning
Participation
Service identification
Individualization

Implementation
Monitor progress
Deliver a range of service
Encourage independence

Placement (rehabilitation and other programs)

Follow-up

Termination

The counselor must be skillful in obtaining a diagnostic knowledge of the client and the impact of that client's specific disability and be able to influence the client positively to bring about the changes necessary to move the client toward employment.

SPECIAL CONSIDERATIONS WITH THE ARTHRITIS PATIENT

Client need will determine to a great extent the type and emphasis of counselor-client interaction in working with arthritis patients. No unique counseling technique or theory has to be developed for the rehabilitation counselor to provide services to individuals with arthritis. There are special areas of knowledge that the counselor must have in order to be truly effective within the full range of contacts with such clients, the most basic being the medical implications of the disability. Other considerations assist the counselor in anticipating the full range of vocational restrictions posed by the particular disorder. The referring physician should make clear exactly what the local articular problem and systemic psychosocial issues are.

As is noted within other chapters of this text, classification of arthritis diseases results in broad categories. An attempt to provide special vocational counseling considerations in relation to each is outside the scope of this chapter. However, discussion of psychosocial, rehabilitation, educational, physical demand, and environmental considerations by Nicholas[3] is utilized in identifying special considerations regarding vocational counseling with individuals with rheumatoid arthritis.

Psychosocial Considerations

Psychologists frequently characterize clients with rheumatoid arthritis as hostile, repressed, angry, and frustrated. While the cause-and-effect relationship of such clients' psychology is not known, it is believed that these characteristics are related to constant pain with movement rather than the propensity for hostile or repressed persons to develop rheumatoid arthritis.[4] Some patients adapt to their disease and disability and function well with limited abilities, whereas others seem incapacitated by fairly minimal involvement. Adapting to rheumatoid arthritis requires the client to modify greatly a former self-image and life-style, without giving up the efforts required to achieve and sustain maximum independence. Maintenance of effort requires a tolerance for pain.

Many people who are in almost constant pain may never entirely give up the hope that one morning the pain will vanish. This type of denial may lead to unrealistic expectations and resistance to altering behavior patterns. The patients may presume that once the pain goes away and their strength returns, their vocational problems will disappear. The vocational counselor should be alert to another possible reaction. Faced with the prospect of progressive deformities and pain on movement, the client may decide to avoid pain and give up trying to remain active by increasingly depending on others for care. Frustration and depression occur also when limitations of the disability are not accepted. Frustration occurs because, despite the effort, it becomes increasingly difficult or impossible to maintain previous activities, due to the accumulation of deformities. Patients become particularly frustrated when they discover that certain physical outlets are no longer feasible. Their inability to accept diminished activity and continued pain often leads to depression.

The rheumatoid arthritis patient needs understanding during adjustment to disability as well as help and support during the transition to a more limited range of activities. It is not sufficient for the vocational counselor simply to tell him to get out and do things differently. The counselor needs to be understanding and listen to the exact nature of the particular problems the patient may have. The counselor must also attempt to help achieve a resolution of the problems and an alteration in the type and degree of physical activity to conform to the patient's limitations. The patient should also be encouraged to avoid those activities believed to increase deformities and disabilities and helped to find vocational and other activities that will make up as active a life as the arthritis will allow.

REHABILITATION POTENTIAL

The longevity of rheumatoid arthritis patients is somewhat less than that of the normal population because of an apparent increased susceptibility to infection and other complications. Life expectancy is sufficient, however, so that the counselor can plan in terms of tenure of years rather than months for possible education or retraining.

After appropriate consultation and evaluation have been obtained from physicians and allied health personnel, several factors must be considered. The problem is not how long that the patient will live, but how he will function. The prognosis for work is of course much better for patients who possess highly trained skills that do not depend on manual dexterity or strength. Those who possess more intellectual skills before the onset of the disease will more likely maintain these skills afterward.

Unlike the person with an amputation, paraplegia, or a stroke, the individual with rheumatoid arthritis has a condition that varies from day to day. The counselor therefore must observe and understand the client's changing condition and provide vocational goals and support appropriate to the more difficult periods so that employment can be sustained.

Most rheumatoid arthritis patients do not progress to severe disability. The client with limited involvement or remission is more easily provided with vocational goals and supports. This discussion of specific vocational goals and supports assumes, however, that the client has a persistent generalized involvement with a slow, steady, but progressive course. Patients with other types of arthritis may have either a limited or a more global type of disease and must be treated in this context.

EDUCATION

There is nothing inherent in the disability to indicate that educational goals should not be a strong consideration both for clients with recent-onset rheumatoid arthritis and those with long-standing disease. Vocational training or college courses should be considered. If the patient is in the third or fourth decade of life, a common age of onset of rheumatoid arthritis, educational goals should be guided by past intellectual skills and experience, rather than limited by the fear of death or total disability.

Rheumatoid arthritis does not affect the client's intellect, learning ability, verbal skills, numerical skills, color discrimination, or form and space perception. It can adversely affect motor coordination, finger and hand dexterity, and eye-hand-foot coordination. Loss of motion and pain on motion certainly slow the client's movements and diminish coordination.

PHYSICAL DEMANDS

The counselor must remember that the rheumatoid arthritis patient is likely to be in his 30s or 40s. By the fifth or sixth decade, the client may have progressed from the inflammatory phase to the stage of persistent deformity where movement is limited by mechanical failure of the joints to support weight and allow motion. The counselor thus will have to guide the interests of younger clients into areas where frequent use of joints will not aggravate the disease.

Most patients with rheumatoid arthritis will be better employed in vocations with sedentary, or, at most, light work. While most of the individuals who respond to treatment will be able to perform medium or heavy work, the counselor must keep in mind that possible progression of the disease may cause further crippling and disability. Thus a client who initially may do medium work (lift 25 to 50 pounds) or even heavy work (lift 100 pounds) may not be able to do so throughout his or her working career. Many patients may be able to continue sedentary or light work until retirement and probably should not be encouraged to continue medium or heavy work, which will perhaps further inflame their joints and result in total disability before the usual age of retirement.

Ligament, tendon, and muscle weakness can affect coordination late in the course of the disease. Deformities subsequent to destruction decrease mechanical ability (for example, weakening of the grip when the wrist is subluxed in a palmar direction and when the fingers are distorted or stiff). Patients can lose the ability to raise their arms and hands above shoulder level due to contractures of the shoulder joint. The loss of stability of the thumb decreases the force of pinch. Vocational goals dependent upon fine, dexterous, or coordinated movement of the hand are therefore not good choices for people with rheumatoid arthritis. The operation of machines requiring percussive, rapid, repeated movements probably also is a bad choice. Nevertheless, if the force required is quite low, dexterous tasks, including the use of an electric typewriter, may be accomplished. Patients with diseases such as degenerative joint disease may have only one or two joints involved, which makes the choice of work much easier. Then only the function of particular joints affected need be considered.

Jobs with continuous stresses, both to the joints and to the person, are not recommended. They may exacerbate both the disease and the patient's frustration. The management of rheumatoid arthritis usually requires rest periods, and a combination of rest and exercise often must be available on the job as well as at home. Some clients may even require a nap at noon or in the afternoon. In addition, they also benefit from frequent changes of position.

Climbing skills, balancing skills, stooping, and kneeling are all hampered by pain on weight bearing or with motion. All these activities may be accomplished by some patients with rheumatoid arthritis, but activities that repeatedly overuse joints without periods of rest and recovery should be avoided. Reaching, handling, and fingering will be clumsy, painful, weak, and awkward in clients whose hand joints are inflamed.

A further consideration concerns which joints are the most seriously involved. Unfortunately, at onset this is somewhat difficult to predict or determine. However, if the arthritis seems to attack particular joints and spare others, the counselor may consider recommending vocations that utilize the less affected joints. Thus if the fingers are spared but the hips and knees are seriously involved, a sedentary clerical job might be appropriate.

ENVIRONMENT

It is usual for patients with rheumatoid arthritis to detect changes in humidity, temperature, or barometric pressure. An indoor climate where the environment is relatively controlled is therefore well advised. Extremes of weather or temperature with abrupt variation probably should be avoided when possible (but a patient should not disrupt his or her life and support system in order to move to a more climatically suitable location). Whether the climate is wet, humid, dry, warm, or cold is apparently less important to a client's comfort than the frequency of abrupt changes. The occurrence of excessive noise, vibration, fumes, gases, dust, and poor ventilation has no specific effects on clients with rheumatoid arthritis.

Some patients with rheumatoid arthritis may not be industrially competitive but are able to work in a sheltered workshop. This experience may enable them to work in an environment consistent with their level of productivity and may also support them until they acquire the skills that enable them to gain access to the competitive commercial world.

Above all, the counselor must realize that the client with rheumatoid arthritis does not have a static disability with clearly defined limits, but rather a changing disability with frequent pain, varying from day to day. Such individuals require a combination of adequate evaluation, effective treatment, and creative vocational placement.

SUMMARY

The vocational counselor plays an important role in a comprehensive program for the care and treatment of the arthritis patient. Towen has indicated that, "Job placement of disabled arthritics remains the most difficult objective to attain."[4] Whereas the medical, social, and psychological assessments of the treatment team identify what the individual patient may be capable of doing, it is the vocational counselor who must pull these facts together into a workable vocational plan that the client can accept and that the family and future employer will permit to come to fruition. The vocational counselor who successfully meets this challenge is amply rewarded.

REFERENCES

1. Wright GN. Total rehabilitation. Boston: Little, Brown, 1980.
2. Parsons F. Choosing a vocation. New York: Houghton Mifflin, 1909.
3. Nicholas JJ. Rheumative disease. In: Stokov WC, Clowery MR, eds. Handbook of severe disability. US Department of Education, RSA, 1981.
4. Seidenfeld MA. Arthritis and rheumatism. In: Garrett JF, Levine ES, eds. Psychological practices with the physically disabled. New York: Columbia University Press, 1962.
5. Lowen EW, ed. Arthritis, general principles, physical medicine, rehabilitation. Boston: Little, Brown, 1959.

7

The Physician Team

Mary Betty Stevens, M.D.

In recent years it has become clear that problem solving for patients with rheumatic disorders is a multidisciplinary issue. The reasons for this evolution in the approach to diagnosis and management are multiple and diverse. With the emergence of rheumatology as a recognized subspecialty in medicine, there has been increased interest in the spectrum of rheumatic disease by clinicians and investigators alike. The explosion in knowledge of disease mechanisms in recent decades has led not only to more sensitive diagnostic methods but also to a continuing expansion of interventions to suppress the inflammatory processes affecting the articular skeleton and supporting structures. New medical and psychosocial problems have surfaced with the modulation of these disease processes and with reparative surgical procedures, which have extended potentially productive years of life for the arthritis patient. Thus especially in those new chronic articular and connective tissue disorders, the one-doctor approach is no longer viable; and the team concept becomes not a choice but a necessity if optimal management is to be realized. The doctor-only approach is as invalid as the one-doctor concept when it comes to the surveillance and management of patients with rheumatic disorders.

RHEUMATIC DISORDERS

The Processes

The spectrum of rheumatic disease can encompass virtually all of medicine (see table 7.1). Articular problems alone are both acute (septic arthritis, trauma) and more often chronic (degenerative joint disease) or recurrent (microcrystalline synovitis). Very different management problems arise in those with arthritis primarily associated with extraarticular lesions (psoriasis, Crohn's disease, solid tumors). In these patients, treatment is necessarily directed as much toward the associated lesion as the arthritis itself. Furthermore, certain primary articular

Table 7.1.   Rheumatic Disorders

Articular
  Arthropathy alone
  Arthritis with extraarticular lesions
  Systemic disease
Periarticular
Nonorganic syndromes

---

problems become associated with such complications as the iritis and aortic insufficiency of ankylosing spondylitis, to which the physician must remain alert in the longitudinal follow-up of such individuals. Finally, among the arthropathies are the systemic disorders, namely, those like rheumatoid arthritis, in which joint involvement dominates the clinical problems and those systemic connective tissue disorders in which synovium is but one end-organ involved in the inflammatory process.

Although periarticular problems (bursitis, tendonitis) are most often acute, even self-limited, some patients have established contractures and other soft tissue changes requiring prolonged rehabilitative measures. No less imperative is the need of those with functional illness clinically expressed in rheumatic pain-syndrome terms, which, without appropriate intervention, can be as invaliding as any tissue-destructive process.

Thus if one considers the vastness of rheumatic disease, the difficulty lies not with the recognition of need for a physician team but rather with the definition of its limits; and, in truth, there is no single formula encompassing the needs of all patients or even an individual with chronic disease over time.

The Problems

Throughout the course of any rheumatic disorder, patients present problems in diagnosis and management (table 7.2). In the earliest stages the issue of sorting out one disease from the others and establishing as specific a diagnosis as possible is of key importance. With time, as new clinical problems arise, the concern is whether such reflect the underlying disease, complications of its therapeutic program, or an intercurrent, unrelated process. It must be remembered that those with chronic disorders of the musculoskeletal system and connective tissue require general health maintenance as well as therapies directed toward rheumatic problems.

Management goals similarly vary with time and stage of disease. Suppression of the disease process when possible or at least the removal of aggravating factors in the attempt to halt progression is key to prevention of loss of tissue integrity and skeletal function. Furthermore, such is the major route to relief of pain. In some circumstances prompt control of systemic features outweighs con-

Table 7.2.   Problems in Rheumatic Disease

Diagnostic
  Specific rheumatic disorder
  Basis of clinical problem
    Underlying disease
    Complication of therapy
    Intercurrent illness
  Psychosocial factors
Management
  Suppression or retardation of disease process
  Prevention of structural damage and/or loss of function
  Improvement in musculoskeletal function
  Repair of structural damage and deformities
  Psychosocial factors

cern for musculoskeletal problems. Systemic lupus erythematosus or the arthritides are good examples. Irrespective of specific diagnostic label, however, the early intent is to prevent if possible, or to improve if not, total patient functional capacity. Finally, in those with tissue loss and deformity, as well as those with intractable pain, reconstruction of the part surgically may become a major focus of the rehabilitative process.

From both diagnostic and management points of view, the recognition of psychosocial factors and their role in the presentation and course of disease must be given high priority in the planning and evaluation process. Failure to give appropriate weight to the human dimension of rheumatic disease not only makes unlikely the patient's compliance with prescribed regimens but also dooms to failure educational programs at every level.

Thus it becomes apparent from the spectrum of disorders and, even more, the clinical problems they determine, that the medical expertise and input must be broad and diverse and changeable in focus from time to time.

THE PHYSICIANS

The roster of physicians entering into the care programs for patients with acute and chronic forms of arthritis and connective tissue disease is a lengthy one. In table 7.3 are shown which physician-specialists are seen in consultation for a rheumatic disease-related problem by 100 consecutive patients admitted to a rheumatic disease unit. All the patients entered the rheumatologist's service on referral by their physicians, who were usually in family practice or internal medicine. In most instances the patient-specialist encounter was a limited consultation for diagnostic opinion regarding a specific disease manifestation or therapeutic complication. Approximately 25 percent of the patients were seen by three or more clinical consultants; an equal number required none other than their attending rheumatologist supported by radiology/pathology services and

Table 7.3.   Percentage of 100 Patients Consulting Physicians in Various Specialities

---

Group I (100%)[a]
  Family practitioner and/or internist, rheumatologist
Group II (>50%)
  Orthopedist,[a] radiologist, pathologist
Group III (>25%)
  Physiatrist,[a] ophthalmologist, gastroenterologist, dermatologist
Group IV (<10%)
  Hematologist, neurologist, cardiologist, general and vascular surgeons,[a] nuclear
  medicine specialist, pulmonary specialist, psychiatrist,[a] infectious disease specialist.

---

[a]Extended continuing care as opposed to a single diagnostic consultation.

arthritis health professionals' involvement. Between these extremes are the coordinated physician groups (or "physician teams") which, except for family physician and rheumatologist, phase in and out of care programs during the course of disease.

Several factors govern the design of the physician team for the individual patient (table 7.4) in practical terms. Perhaps the disease process is most determinant, with the more systemic disorders having increased consultative need over those like degenerative joint disease or microcrystalline synovitis, which focus on articular problems alone. Within any single disorder, however, the spectrum of clinical problems is so great that, realistically, the physician team varies broadly as illustrated by the schematic course of two patients with rheumatoid arthritis (figure 7.1.) who have followed in our program since onset of their disease 20 years ago. One (A), after discrete flares of synovitis in the first decade, has been maintained in near remission ever since. The other (B) has had a progressive, per-

Table 7.4.   Factors Influencing Design of the Physician Team

---

Disease process

Professional resources
  Sensitivity of primary physician
  Availability of specialists
  Philosophy of rheumatologist
Patient factors
  Awareness
  Understanding
  Acceptance
  Compliance
Societal issues
  Facilities for care
  Socioeconomic status of patient and community

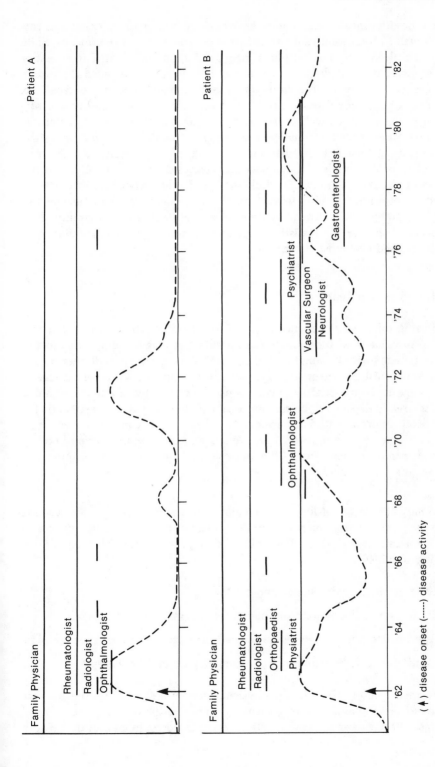

Figure 7.1.   Course of rheumatoid arthritis

sistent synovitis since onset, requiring orthopedic intervention for tendon ruptures as well as total joint replacements, management for rheumatoid vasculitis with its leg ulcerations and peripheral neuropathy, and psychiatric intervention when stress of disease, therapy, and social complications exceeded the professional capacity of private practitioner and rheumatologist. The disease label does not define a professional team membership formula. The availability and attitudes of professionals as well as patient and societal factors similarly enter into the program design at the practical level despite the ideal of universal patient multispecialty assessment. Furthermore, divorce of the physician team from other health professionals (nursing specialists, physical and occupational therapists, social workers, clinical psychologists, and others) is unrealistic and ill-advised. Professional roles overlap on the one hand and are flexible and changeable on the other, depending on professional needs and availability. Thus only a core team can be realistically defined in terms of need, specific roles, availability, and even cost effectiveness.

The Physician Team

In analyzing our own experience and that reported by others, there is a core group of physicians who dominate the essentials of diagnostic and therapeutic needs of patients with rheumatic disease, namely the family practitioner, pediatrician, or internist, the rheumatologist, and the orthopedist. Whether other team members are used—psychiatrist or clinical psychologist, physiatrist or specialized therapist—really depends upon this professional climate, patient need, and clinical/societal environment. Furthermore, the key to the comprehensive, team approach is the *coordination* of professionals and the *communication* between them and with the patient. In fact the professionals' interactions are as important as the team structure *per se*.

The Primary Physician. Most instrumental in initiating a comprehensive care plan is the *family practitioner, pediatrician,* or *internist* who is sensitive to specialized rheumatologic need. The role of this primary physician entails the following activities:

General health maintenance and counseling

Separation of the major from the minor rheumatic syndromes

Appropriate referral to rheumatologist for diagnosis and therapeutic plan

Continuing collaboration in monitoring disease and its therapy

The accepted role of this primary physician determines the entire health care system and team availability to patients not only at the outset but as clinical problems continue to arise in those with chronic disorders. In view of the breadth of rheumatic disease, the initial sorting-out process can be difficult relative to the need for specialized, ongoing care, and it is often helpful and a bona fide basis for referral to elicit the rheumatologist's view as to the diagnostic probabilities. Similarly, with shared continuing care, the question relative to the relationship (or not) of a new clinical problem to the underlying rheumatic disease can best be answered without delay through collaborative effort.

The Rheumatologist.   Pivotal to the coordination of care and its effectiveness is the rheumatologist, not only initially, but throughout a patient's course of disease. This doctor's role entails the following:

Specific diagnosis as early as possible

Design of therapeutic program with immediate and long-term goals

Establishment of an appropriate management team for comprehensive care

Coordination of professionals' efforts

Assurance of effective communication between team members and with patient

Education of patient and family relative to disease process, its therapy, and its implications

The early role of the rheumatologist may relate primarily to clinical diagnosis with the development of the relevant data base and its appropriate interpretation. Sorting out the self-limited from chronic disorders and avoidance of premature, erroneous diagnostic labels is of key importance in the psychological as well as medical management of patients with polyarthritis. Each year a significant number of patients present with impaired function, even invalidism, from a misdiagnosis of rheumatoid arthritis and their perception and anticipation of inevitable crippling.

With diagnosis the immediate and, if appropriate, long-term therapeutic plans can be defined. Necessary consultants and team members are recruited even at this early stage of chronic disorders. The process of educating patients and their families similarly begins now. The key role of the rheumatologist necessarily surfaces with the commitment and opportunity to organize, coordinate, collaborate, and communicate across disciplinary lines. Furthermore, the responsibility for effective synthesis of diagnostic opinions and views on management rests with the rheumatologist, who must assure consistency of information and input transmitted to patients and their primary physicians.

The ideal relationship of the rheumatologist to patients' family practitioners or internists is one of continuing partnership and mutual decision making with shared follow-up of patients. If circumstances dictate otherwise, the rheumatologist must remain available on an intermittent, problem-oriented basis. This relationship (as consultant only) can also be effective if adequate information and education have been communicated to primary physician and patient alike with respect to disease, therapy, and available resources.

The Orthopedist. The involvement of the orthopedist extends well beyond surgical intervention, as shown by the following list of functions performed.

Specific diagnosis of structural defects

Nonoperative management of mechanical abnormalities and dysfunction

Surgical interventions
  Diagnostic biopsy
  Acute treatment
  Reparative procedures
  Joint reconstruction
  Joint replacement

Collaborative planning and staging of procedures

Education of patient and family relative to surgical methods, pre- and postoperative program and surgical implications

The orthopedist's involvement should be solicited early, not late, in the course of chronic inflammatory and degenerative joint disorders as well as certain of their articular and periarticular complications (such as septic arthritis or tendon ruptures or entrapment syndromes in the rheumatoid patient, ischemic bone necrosis in the corticosteroid-treated individual). Nonoperative intervention (splinting, serial casting) for those with potentially reducible structural abnormalities, more often periarticular than intrasynovial in origin, can be vital in restoring optimal function. Occasionally open synovial biopsy can be helpful in early diagnosis (for granulomata or tumors, etc.) when the clinical picture, synovial fluid analysis, and closed needle biopsy are inconclusive. In chronic forms of arthritis, early and recurrent coordinated planning of orthopedic needs and interventions in conjunction with medical therapy can help to forestall the time for major reconstructive and replacement surgery.

No aspect of patient care in rheumatic disease demands more collaborative effort than the issues relating to orthopedic surgery. While acute surgical needs (such as drainage of a refractory septic joint or mechanical repair) are relatively straightforward, the timing and sequencing of reconstructive procedures often represent delicate decisions that must include concern for the disease process as a whole and, even more, patients' readiness and attitudes. The decision-making process appropriately begins well in advance of the anticipated surgical date; and the support of primary physician and rheumatologist should be well integrated with that of the orthopedic surgeon from the outset. In our program almost half the orthopedic referrals are anticipatory and for evaluation when surgery is only a future possibility.

The Physiatrist. Similarly the physiatrist enters the management team effort from the outset when physical limitations and rehabilitative potential are being defined. This physician performs the following functions:

Specific diagnosis of musculoskeletal dysfunction

Electrodiagnosis: nerve conduction times and electromyography

Assessment of management by physical and occupational therapists

Education of patient and family relative to activity program, home adaptations, work simplification, and the like

Establishment of an initial baseline of joint and muscle dysfunction and the capacity for specific activities of daily living is key to the long-term management as the immediate treatment program. Occasionally the identification of specific neuropathies, entrapments, and the character of a myopathy through electrodiagnostic testing becomes a major therapeutic guide. However, the major role of the physical medicine program concerns the management of acute and chronic musculoskeletal disorders.

In this regard the physiatrist may be an anomalous member of the therapeutic team in view of the supervisory role rather than direct patient intervention in many, if not most, clinical settings. Even with the design of individual patient's programs the responsibility of the physiatrist, the implementation of serial assessments and treatments is by the physical and occupational therapists. Furthermore, with the enormous need for but unavailability of physiatrists in many areas, the orthopedist or rheumatologist may interact directly with the therapists in program planning and management. Regardless, the salient issue is the inclusion (or not) of physical medicine in the mainstream of management of patients with rheumatic disorders. This is essential to the comprehensive care program. In no management segment is education of patient and family more crucial if compliance with an exercise program and needed home adaptations is to be achieved; and the educational process may be necessarily shared by all members of the physician team and the involved therapists as well.

The Psychiatrist. Finally, however constructed in membership, the physician team must be sensitive to the psychosocial factors that can so influence patients' acceptance of disease and compliance with therapeutic designs. It becomes unrealistic in most communities and centers to delegate all interventions to the *psychiatrist or clinical psychologist;* and, again, with their limited availability, the direct collaboration of the rheumatologist or orthopedist with the cadre of arthritis health professionals (social worker, vocational counselor, and the like) is effected and can be effective. Selective psychiatric input for those who have organic mental illness as part of the basic disease (as in the psychotic reaction of systemic lupus) or who have serious depression stemming from the impact of their chronic illness may be a major factor in limiting disability. However, there are few patients, if any, with chronic types of rheumatic disease who do not require constant support and positive reinforcement from family physician and rheumatologist who must remain alert and sensitive to the psychological and social aspects of each patient's situation.

SUMMARY

The acute and, even more, the chronic problems of rheumatic disease are legion and require for resolution the appropriate involvement of a multidisciplinary group of physicians and allied health professionals. There is no single formula for design of the professional team that can or should be extended to all patients if optimal use of professional resources and optimal care of patients are to be realized. However, the family physician, internist or pediatrician, and the rheumatologist remain the most consistent physician team members over time, and it is the rheumatologist's responsibility to provide continued, shared care and constantly to define and coordinate the needed multidisciplinary interventions. A diagnostician role alone falls short of assuring the comprehensive patient-and-family care these disorders so often require. However, with flexibility in assumed roles, with sensitivity to total patient care and with effective interprofessional relationships, the physician team can provide the framework for positive outcomes in most patients.

Finally, it must be emphasized that fundamental to the construct is the educational process by which professionals can acquire increased sensitivity to the roles of each other and patients with their families can achieve the necessary understanding of disease and its management to assure compliance and optimal patient function. Quite apart from individual patient care, it is the responsibility of the physician team—especially rheumatologist and orthopedist—with their arthritis health professional colleagues to provide educational forums for other professionals and the public alike with respect to the specialized needs of patients with rheumatic disorders. The educational process is critical to the goal of improved utilization of physicians' services, cost effectiveness, and positive patient outcomes in this area of medical need.

8

The Role of the Podiatrist, Prosthetist, and Orthotist

Martin Snyder, D.P.M.

Podiatry is a profession that focuses upon one area of the body, the lower limb. While the four-year graduate course of instruction in every podiatry college is geared to the foot and leg, the entire body is studied, with special emphasis placed upon various systemic diseases that may be manifest in the foot and leg. The Council on Education of the American Podiatry Association, which certifies the five schools of podiatric medicine, requires that a specific number of the faculty hold the M.D. or the Ph.D. degree.[1] The admission requirements are similar to schools of medicine. Students must have undergraduate degrees in one of the sciences such as chemistry, zoology, bacteriology, or related subjects.[2]

Upon completion of the 4-year graduate course of studies in podiatric colleges, the degree Doctor of Podiatric Medicine (D.P.M.) is granted. In several states podiatric examining boards require at least 1 year of residency in Council on Education approved programs before issuing a license to practice.[3] (See figure 8.1).

All of the podiatry colleges have a working agreement with some major university or medical center in the community. This allows for an interchange in some of the clinics between both medical and podiatric schools and provides the genesis of interaction between medical and podiatric students.

Many medical groups such as prepaid health plans and the health maintenance organizations include podiatrists as an integral part of their staff. This is significant since such medical groups are concerned with the prevention of disability and the early disclosure of medical problems, which is particularly important in caring for the arthritic patient.

The scope of care and various modalities used by the podiatrist includes both conservative and surgical regimens. Physical examination skills, required for prescribing shoe modifications and orthotic design, are stressed in podiatry colleges. Podiatry has been in the forefront of the study of lower limb biomechanics, which has led to many innovative shoe appliances fabricated from a variety

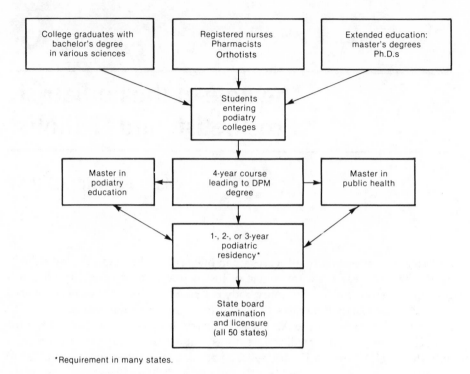

*Requirement in many states.

Figure 8.1. Sources of students entering podiatry colleges: advanced educational opportunities and emergence into related fields.

of materials (see figure 8.2). Since arthritis is often present but unrecognized in the small joints of the feet, careful examination of every patient with rheumatic disease (regardless of the initial site of complaint) is warranted.[4] When an abnormality is discovered, the help of a qualified podiatrist or orthotist may be required.

CONSERVATIVE MANAGEMENT

For conservative management of the arthritic patient, there are many possible regimens of treatment.[5] A pyramid of mechanical and conservative care for the rheumatic patient is presented in figure 8.3 to depict what is available through the specialty of podiatry. The base of the pyramid contains essential elements: biomechanical examination, diagnosis, patient education and advice.[6] The physical

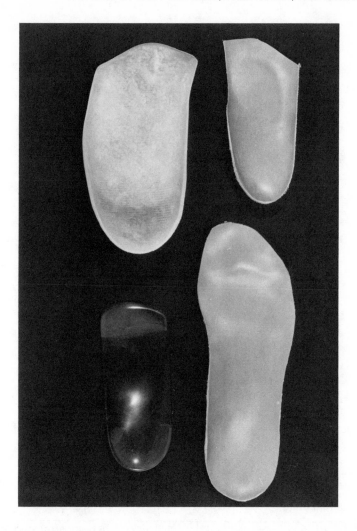

Figure 8.2. Various appliances and orthoses for foot support and control. The upper left is a UCBL (University of California Biomechanics Laboratory) made from polyethylene; next to it is a standard support for long arch and metatarsal.

examination of the lower extremity is paramount. Providing patient education regarding the diagnosis and possible solutions to foot problems is also critical if success is to be achieved. This includes shoe information such as wearing the proper footgear and checking the wear patterns due to pressure and stress. Education regarding the value of cushioning is important at this time. As treatment becomes more complex, one moves up the pyramid. Special materials are employed, internal and external shoe modifications can be prescribed (as shown

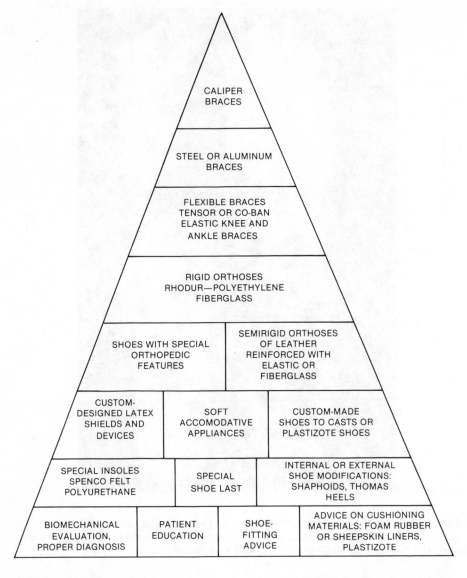

Figure 8.3. A pyramid of mechanical and conservative care for the rheumatic patient. Appliances higher in the pyramid are more complicated and difficult to construct and entail more fitting.

in figures 8.4–8.6. Certain shoe styles may be specified for some foot types. Shoes themselves are not corrective, yet some may be helpful in reducing restrictive pressures.

Further up the pyramid of conservative measures are soft latex shields that

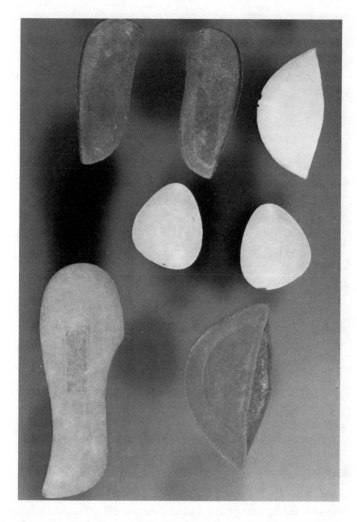

Figure 8.4.   Some internal shoe modification items include clockwise from upper left corner, medium-size rubber scaphoid wedge (superior view); rubber metatarsal pad left (and right first below), large scaphoid wedge (plantar view), leather heel wedge with forward extension, rubber heel wedges, left and right (superior and inferior views).

are fabricated to casts of the feet or toes. These are removable and provide excellent relief of stress areas. Shoes that are made to casts of the feet have extra inlays and conform to unusual contours of the feet or toes (figure 8.5). As more support is required, semirigid orthoses such as leather reinforced with Celastic, metal, or fiberglass are used. Finally at the apex of the pyramid, bracing with elastic bindings, CO-BAN, polyethylene, and other thermoplastics for contoured support are employed. This overview presents only a small portion of orthoses and newer materials that are available to the podiatrist and orthotist or prosthetist.

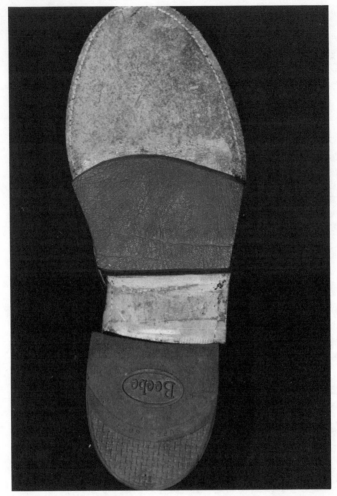

Figure 8.5. External shoe modification—plantar metatarsal bar shown in plantar view.

Certainly, it is the responsibility of the primary care physician to seek out specialists in these fields to make use of their knowledge and skills using these materials. The particular device used depends upon the stage of the disease and the changes in the functioning foot and leg. Early identification of impending deformity will call for simpler devices. Later, as the disease progresses, more definitive, expensive and firmer orthoses will be required.

SURGICAL MANAGEMENT

Surgical care of the arthritis patient has advanced because of new techniques available. The main podiatric contribution to the surgical repair of the rheumatic

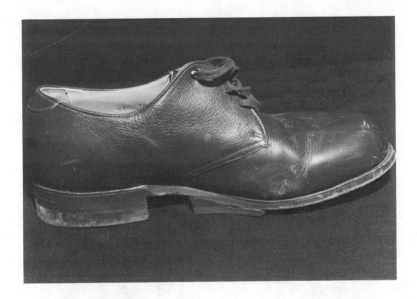

Figure 8.6. Lateral view of metatarsal bar.

patient has been in the correction of painful nails, hammer toes, metatarsal depressions, and bunion deformities. Major foot surgery, including rear foot fusion, total joint replacements of ankles, and large tendon transfer, is within the realm and expertise of the orthopedic surgeon.

ORTHOTIST VERSUS PROSTHETIST

The orthotist and the prosthetist provide a link in the chain of therapy that many people with arthritis require. The prosthetist is concerned with the replacement of limbs. The orthotist is the professional who follows prescriptions and makes orthotic devices or mechanical aids for living parts. Just as the lay person is confused with the role of the various professions in eye care such as the opthalmologist, optometrist, and optician, so do health professionals incorrectly identify the role of the orthotist and prosthetist.

Orthotists have a varied background in many fields. They must follow a 4-year course of study leading to a degree as an associate in the arts and sciences[7,11] and enabling them to produce braces and modify orthoses to the individual needs of patients. The curriculum includes study in anatomy, physiology, principles of mechanics, and the development of some mechanical engineering skills. Candidates must possess an artistic talent and certain deftness.

Many courses are the same for prosthetists. At one point, however, the curriculum diverges since the orthotist fabricates braces, orthoses, and mechanical

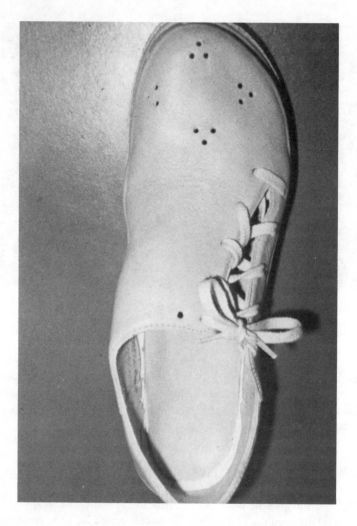

Figure 8.7.   Space-contoured inlay depth shoe made to cast of foot—especially indicated for arthritic toe and rear foot deformities.

aids for the living part,[8,10] whereas the prosthetist creates artificial limbs for missing members of the body.

Since much time is spent creating and fitting various orthoses, the orthotist must have the capacity to relate to the client in understandable terms and with patience. It is very important for the patient to understand that a single fitting of an appliance may not be enough and sometimes adjustment must be made before the particular device serves its purpose in the best fashion. The podiatrist may order some orthoses that may help one part of the body and cause distress in another area. The orthotist who fabricates a poorly designed device may delay the complete relief that the patient requires. Thus the best prescribed and most efficiently designed orthosis becomes an integral part of the treatment that the physician seeks for the patient.

SUMMARY

The treatment and rehabilitation of the arthritis patient encompasses many medical disciplines. A team effort spells success. The podiatrist and orthotist, among many others, enjoy a meaningful role in the total scheme of caring for the arthritis patient.

REFERENCES

1. Council on Education, American Podiatry Association, Procedures for accrediting colleges of podiatric medicine. Con Pod Ed 130. Washington, D.C., August 1979.
2. Catalog for Admission, California College of Podiatric Medicine. San Francisco, 1981–82.
3. Arizona Revised Statutes 32–804, Section R4-25-30. Arizona State Board of Podiatry Examiners. Phoenix, Ariz., 1980.
4. Sbarbaro JL, Katz WA. The feet and ankles in the diagnosis of rheumatic diseases. In: Katz WA, ed., Rheumatic diseases diagnosis and management. Philadelphia: J.B. Lippincott, 1979:177–179.
5. Swezey RL. Guidelines for the physical management and rehabilitation of the arthritic patient. In: Hollander JL, ed., The arthritis handbook. West Point, Pa.: Merck Sharp and Dohme, 1974:85–102.
6. Dagnall JC. Podiatry and arthritis. Bull Rheumatic Dis 1972–73;1:692–694.
7. Personal communication, John Strong, Prosthetist, Veterans Administration Medical Center, Tucson, Ariz., 1982.
8. Holmes DW. Orthotics of the foot and ankle. In: Helfet AJ and Greubel Lee DM, eds., Disorders of the foot. Philadelphia: J.B. Lippincott, 1980:232–243.
9. Meyer PR. Lower limb orthotics. Clinical Orthopedics Related Res 1974;102:88–89.
10. Nickel VL. Orthopedic rehabilitation—challenges and opportunities. Clinical Orthopedics Related Res 1969;63:153–161.
11. Nickel VL. Orthotics in America. Clinical Orthopedics Related Res 1974;102:10–17.

ADDITIONAL READING

Belleau W. Podiatry as a career. Milwaukee, Wis.: Park Publications House, 1966:1–3.
Greenfield HI. Manpower problems in the allied health field. JAMA 1968;206:1542–1544.
Podell RN. Issues in the organization of medical care. New Engl J Med 1971;284-11: 586–589.
Polley HF, Hunder GG. Rheumatological interviewing and physical examination of the joints, 2nd ed. Philadelphia: W.B. Saunders, 1978.

9

The Pharmacist's Contribution to Patient Care

William L. Fritz, R.Ph., M.S.

In the era of the American Revolution, apothecaries, or pharmacists, were trained to compound sometimes exotic potions. In addition to trituration, they applied extraction and maceration techniques using specific parts of various plants either shipped to the colony from Europe, hand grown, or gathered in the wild. These were then made into oral doses such as pills, powders, elixirs, spirits or into topical salves, liniments, plasters, and poultices. Many apothecaries were also scientists, conducting clinical research on the effects of new agents they had discovered. Most important, the colonial American apothecary was a patient-oriented primary care practitioner.

Patients were seen and treated in the apothecary's shop for a variety of common illnesses. Records show that the apothecary made rounds to the homes of patients when they could not come to the shop. Patients with illnesses outside the apothecary's expertise were referred to a physician, or the apothecary consulted with a physician regarding these patients. Physicians then recommended specific medication, which was compounded by the apothecary and given to the patient with explanation of how to use it, what dose to give, what side effects to expect, and other information pertinent to the drug and disease.[1]

The early era of American pharmacy was relatively short. The pharmaceutical manufacturing industry grew and more efficiently prepared the drugs. The division between pharmacy and medicine became more distinct, and the pharmacist became more and more a dispenser of drugs. Today's version of the apothecary's shop bears more resemblance to a department store with emphasis on the business techniques employed in effective marketing, stock turnover, corporate finance, and the like. Typically the pharmacy is placed to the rear of this operation, so that patients must work their way through the household appliances and products, tobacco departments, not to mention jewelry and cosmetics, to present the prescription to the pharmacy clerk. The pharmacist then types, counts, licks, and sticks, as is required by law, and returns the filled prescription to the clerk for sale to the patient.

It is interesting to contrast the training and function of the apothecary of colonial America with that of today. The apothecary was trained by an apprenticeship and then practiced the art and science of a patient-oriented profession. Today's pharmacist has received formal college training in at least a 5-year program with heavy emphasis on both physical and life sciences, as well as pathology and therapeutics. Yet this individual for a variety of economic, legal, and social reasons ends up running a business that deals with customers rather than patients.

Fortunately the pendulum has begun to swing back again. Patient benefits resulting from utilization of the knowledge and skills of the pharmacist are being demonstrated. Colleges of pharmacy have not deemphasized therapeutics in favor of business administration, but rather have intensified clinical training. As was pointed out by the Study Commission on Pharmacy (the Millis Commission), modern pharmacy encompasses not only the development, manufacture, and distribution of drug products but includes the development, organization, and distribution of knowledge and information about drugs.[2] The educational trend is toward a 6-year or longer program leading to a doctor of pharmacy degree that places even heavier emphasis on therapeutics. Postdoctoral residencies and fellowships in specific areas of clinical practice are becoming necessary for entry level positions. The momentum is rapidly gaining for a return of the apothecary, today termed clinical pharmacist.

CLINICAL PHARMACY

Clinical pharmacy is a term applied to patient-oriented drug services. It implies the application of scientific knowledge and clinical training to promote optimal drug therapy. This concept implies a close association between the clinical pharmacist, the patient, physician, and others providing health care services. Clinical pharmacists have not abdicated their concern for manufacturing and distribution aspects of pharmacy but have expanded their practice to emphasize rational therapeutics.

Many services provided by clinical pharmacists are well documented in the literature. Most of these services are of a general nature and may apply to any drug-taking population of patients. There are relatively few references regarding activities specifically related to arthritis patients. Other than supplying the correct, properly labeled drug product and keeping accurate records, pharmacists are involved in patient drug therapy in other more direct or knowledge-based ways. These include taking medication histories; maintaining drug profiles; monitoring for drug interactions and compliance; consulting on therapeutics by pharmacokinetic individualization of drug dosage; detecting and managing drug reactions; consulting on drug selection; providing drug information services; managing stable chronic patients' drug therapy; counseling patients; participating in investigational drug studies; advising patients on over-the-counter drug use; and actually prescribing drugs under specific conditions.

Clinical pharmacists have demonstrated the ability to acquire a more accurate and complete drug history and allergy profile than those obtained by patient questionnaires[3] or by physicians.[4] Pharmacists are taking drug histories as a routine function in many patient care settings. In other settings medication histories are taken in selected patients who are suspected of having drug-related problems, such as blood dyscracies, liver or renal failure, or skin reactions. The pharmacist's involvement may lead to decreased hypersensitivity reactions by advanced identification of drug allergies and knowledge of cross-allergenic agents or may establish this diagnosis retrospectively. An accurate drug history may be useful in avoiding potential drug reactions and in planning future therapy.

A pharmacist-maintained drug-profile monitoring system may improve drug therapy by decreasing or detecting adverse drug reactions, drug interactions, unnecessary drug use, and improper dosing.[5] This has been shown to be particularly useful when a patient is seen by various physicians and specialists, who may prescribe drugs with duplicating or interacting effects. Although the incidence and severity of drug interactions has probably been overstated, pharmacists have been the leaders in documenting this growing body of knowledge. Applying the pharmacist's knowledge of drug-drug, drug-laboratory, and drug-diet interactions may reduce adverse reactions, improve efficacy, aid in laboratory test interpretation, and identify or avoid deviations from expected drug effect due to patient diet.[6] Through monitoring of outpatient drug profiles, the pharmacist can estimate drug compliance. If compliance is poor, the pharmacist can counsel the patient regarding proper drug use, determine if an adverse reaction is causing the patient not to take his medication, and, with the physician, reevaluate response to therapy.

Pharmacists have traditionally acted informally as a therapeutic consultant to patients, physicians, and other health professionals. More recently with increased education and clinical training, pharmacists have formalized consulting services. One area of expertise possessed by the clinical pharmacists and by very few individuals in other disciplines is the knowledge of pharmacokinetics. This is an important tool for proper dosing of many drugs that have a narrow therapeutic index, such as aminoglycosides, anticonvulsants, antiarrhythmics, digitalis glycosides, and theophylline formulations. Although most clinical pharmacists possess these basic skills and informally consult and verify doses, a growing number of pharmacists specialize in this area and have full-time clinical consulting services and their own analytical lab and conduct clinical research in the discipline.

Other specialized pharmacy consulting services also exist. Hyperalimentation consulting services, for instance, have been broadly published.[7,8] Clinical specialty areas of pharmacy practice are almost as numerous as those in medicine. They include oncology, cardiology, nephrology, pulmonology, general surgery and subspecialties, gastroenterology, rheumatology, gynecology, family practice, psychiatry, pediatrics, gerontology, infectious disease, and endocrinology.

In addition to consulting services, many of these clinical pharmacy specialists manage the therapy of patients with chronic disease in their practice site. These activities have been most widely established for hypertensive patients, patients receiving anticoagulant therapy, psychiatric patients, particularly manic depressives receiving lithium, and narcotic addicts in methadone maintenance programs. In most of these programs the pharmacist sees the patients for routine clinic visits and evaluates therapeutic response, orders appropriate laboratory tests if necessary, and adjusts drug doses or changes drug products to optimize therapy. Typically these changes in therapy conform to a local protocol or are made by the authority of a sponsoring physician. In several states laws have been recently changed to permit specially trained clinical pharmacists the authority to prescribe drugs on their own responsibility.

Education of the patient about his disease and its therapy has been one of the weakest links in drug treatment. Pharmacist's involvement in patient-counseling activities has dramatically increased in hospital and clinic settings and in community pharmacies.[9] These activities have been particularly rewarding when the pharmacist has direct access to the patient's medical chart and laboratory reports. This information used in conjunction with the pharmacy-maintained drug and allergy profile allows informed application of this drug knowledge.[10] The pharmacist may easily pick up on adverse drug reactions, non-compliance problems, subtherapeutic or potentially toxic dose, and other drug-related problems at an early stage. Several studies have demonstrated substantial improvement in drug compliance in pharmacist-counseled patients.[11] Other studies have shown patient cost savings.[12] Many pharmacists are now supplying written reinforcement to patients (patient package inserts) in addition to verbal counseling. These documents are written in lay terms and can be reviewed by the patient at home, in a relaxed atmosphere where distractions are less and retention is greater.

The pharmacist's role in the treatment of patients with arthritis ranges from drug dispensing to postdiagnostic management. Monson et al. reported benefits of a clinical pharmacist in their rheumatology clinic.[13] This study demonstrated improved drug documentation, decrease in prescription duplication, and improved compliance. The function of the pharmacist in their setting included an initial patient interview to establish a complete drug history of prior and concurrent drug use, including adverse drug reactions. Patients were counseled regarding proper use, storage, and potential adverse drug effects. Patients specifically requesting to talk with someone about their medications were referred to the pharmacist. In this study, the pharmacist also provided inservice programs for clinic personnel. The pharmacist was a fully interactive member of the team treating this population of arthritis patients who documented his patient-related activities and recommendations in the patient's chart.

Other roles for a pharmacist in the treatment of arthritis patients have been established. Pharmacists have conducted drug utilization reviews in patients receiving nonsteroidal anti-inflammatory agents. Information gathered in such studies has been analyzed and used as a feedback method of education for physicians to promote rational and appropriate drug use.[14]

SUMMARY

Although in the recent past the pharmacist has been thought of as a dispenser of medications, this role appears to be changing to that of a more knowledge-based clinical practitioner. Like the colonial American apothecary, he is directly advising and interacting with patients and other health professionals. Although this is not yet the practice norm, the trend is rapidly gaining momentum.

REFERENCES

1. McKenney JM, Witherspoon JM. Return of the apothecary. Arch Intern Med 1981;141:1417.
2. Pharmacists for the future, the report of the Study Commission on Pharmacy (Millis Commission). Ann Arbor, Mich.: Health Administration Press, 1975.
3. Cradock JC, Withfield GR, Menau JW, Fortner CL. Postadmission drug and allergy histories recorded by a pharmacist. Am J Hosp Pharm 1972;29:249-252.
4. Covington TR, Pfeifer FG. The pharmacist-acquired medication history. Am J Hosp Pharm 1972;29:692-695.
5. Solomon KD, Baumgartner RP, Glascock LM, Glascock SA, Briscoe ME, Billups NF. Use of medication profiles to detect potential therapeutic problems in ambulatory patients. Am J Hosp Pharm 1974;31:348-354.
6. Hansten PD. Drug interactions. 4th ed. Philadelphia: Lea and Febiger, 1979.
7. Skoutakis VA, Martinez DR, Miller WA, Bobbie RP. Team approach to total parenteral nutrition. Am J Hosp Pharm 1975;32:693-697.
8. Powell JR, Cupit GC. Pharmacists' role in monitoring total parenteral nutrition. Drug Intell Clin Pharm 1974;8:576-580.
9. Selle RI, Munice HL. Clinical pharmacists—drug educators. Milit Med 1979;144:249-250.
10. Smith WE. Using the patient profile. Drug Intell Clin Pharm 1974;18:10-15.
11. Cole P, Emmanuel S. Drug consultation—its significance to the discharged hospital patient and its relevance as a role for the pharmacist. Am J Hosp Pharm 1971;28:954-960.
12. Ryan PB, Johnson CA, Rapp RP. Economic justification of pharmacist involvement in patient medication consultation. Am J Hosp Pharm 1975;32:389-392.
13. Monson R, Bond CA, Schura A. Role of the clinical pharmacist in improving drug therapy. Arch Intern Med 1981;141:1411-1444.
14. Fritz WL, Gall EP, Price D. Ibuprofen utilization review in outpatients. Hosp Formulary 1980;15:678-684.

10

Community Resources

Clifford M. Clarke, C.A.E.
Michelle Boutaugh, M.P.H.

People with arthritis can have needs ranging from making their home more accessible to reentering the work force. Many services can be provided by hospital-based health professionals as described in previous chapters. However, hospitals cannot provide all of the services individuals with arthritis may require. This chapter will describe the range of services that can be provided by the Arthritis Foundation and other resources that may be available in the community setting.

THE ARTHRITIS FOUNDATION

The Arthritis Foundation is a national, publicly supported health agency with 71 chapters and divisions across the country. It conducts research, education, and patient-service programs. There are two professional membership sections within the organization; the American Rheumatism Association and the Arthritis Health Professions Association. Members of these associations are physicians, scientists, physical and occupational therapists, nurses, and other health professionals involved in arthritis research and treatment. The Arthritis Foundation also has a special membership section called the American Juvenile Arthritis Organization, which represents the special needs of children with arthritis and their families.

The local chapters and divisions of the Arthritis Foundation vary in the specific types of programs they offer, but their services may include the following:

Information. Literature about the various forms of arthritis is available free of charge. In addition to pamphlets, most chapters offer films, slide presentations, and reference materials. Public forum and health fairs are educational activities conducted by most of the chapters to provide information about arthritis that is of interest to the general public. Many chapters also have a speakers' bureau that provides informational sessions on arthritis to lay and professional groups in the community.

Referral.   Each chapter of the Arthritis Foundation maintains a list of physicians who are board-certified or board-eligible in rheumatology or have taken sufficient postgraduate courses in rheumatology to qualify them to treat arthritis patients. These lists are available to people requesting them.

Counseling.   Many chapters provide one-on-one or group assistance with dealing with problems caused by arthritis. This assistance is provided by professionals or trained volunteers who have arthritis.

Patient Education.   Classes are coordinated by many chapters. These usually are run by local hospitals, under the direction of area arthritis health professionals. In these classes people with arthritis can learn about their illness and how to deal with arthritis on a daily basis.

Arthritis Clubs.   Many chapters of the Arthritis Foundation sponsor Arthritis Clubs. These clubs provide a mechanism for individuals with arthritis to meet together and share mutual problems and successes. The clubs also may provide educational presentations and social activities.

Home Visit Programs.   These programs are usually implemented by trained lay persons, although health professionals are sometimes involved in assessment and therapy. The services may include supportive listening, provision of information about the chapter and community services, assistance with self-help devices, and adaptation of the home environment.

Exercise Programs.   Many chapters, in conjunction with hospitals or agencies such as the YMCA, provide group exercise classes in pools or nonaquatic facilities. Some programs are designed to be therapeutic, but most have a recreational focus.

Clinics.   Some chapters fund clinics at local hospitals or multidisciplinary teams travel to rural sites and provide comprehensive diagnostic and evaluation services.

Miscellaneous Chapter Social Services and Patient Advocacy.   The Arthritis Foundation acts as a community mobilizer and advocate for the needs of individuals with arthritis. Many chapters have individual staff members who serve as advocates for patients who are unable to obtain services for which they are eligible and for health providers who are having difficulty in getting the needs of their arthritis patients met in the health and social service system.

Many chapters maintain loan closets through which self-help devices and medical equipment can be obtained. A few chapters are able to provide transportation services. Indigent persons are sometimes able to obtain financial aid to assist with purchase of medical supplies or therapy. Many chapters offer a drug discount program in cooperation with local drugstores for provision of arthritis-related medications at reduced costs.

To obtain the address of the closest chapter or division consult the list at the end of this chapter (see Appendix A).

MULTIPURPOSE ARTHRITIS CENTERS

Several communities are fortunate enough to have a Multipurpose Arthritis Center (MAC) within a university medical center. These centers are funded by the National Institute of Arthritis, Diabetes, and Digestive and Kidney Diseases (NIADDK).

The purpose of the center is to promote the effective utilization of available knowledge for the treatment of arthritis and to develop new knowledge essential for the control of arthritis and related musculoskeletal diseases. To accomplish these overall goals, the centers have three major operational components: basic and clinical research; professional, patient, and public education; and community-related activities.

A list of the currently funded centers and information about their recent activities can be obtained from the Multipurpose Centers Program Director, National Institute of Arthritis, Diabetes, and Digestive and Kidney Disease, Westwood Building, Room 403, Bethesda, Maryland 20205.

Arthritis Information Clearinghouse

The Arthritis Information Clearinghouse is a service of NIADDK that compiles and disseminates information about arthritis and related musculoskeletal diseases. Information includes print and nonprint materials, programs and resources related to public, patient, and professional education. Materials are reviewed, abstracted, indexed, and added to a retrievable data base. Bibliographies and fact sheets on relevant topics are compiled and distributed. The Arthritis Information Clearinghouse serves professionals. All patient requests are referred to the Arthritis Foundation.

To use the clearinghouse services write to the Arthritis Information Clearinghouse, 1700 North Moore Street, Arlington, Virginia 22209. A direct telephone line to the clearinghouse is (703) 558-8217.

OTHER TYPES OF COMMUNITY RESOURCES

Medical

Nursing. Public health nurses, the Visiting Nurses' Association (VNA), and other health agencies offer treatment and maintenance care in the home. Look in the white pages of the phone book in county government listings to contact the public health department. The VNA may also be located in the county government listings or with other home care agencies under a heading like "Home Health Agencies" in the yellow pages. A physician referral may be required before services can be commenced by these agencies.

Rehabilitation

Occupational Therapy. The services of occupational therapists may be offered at rehabilitation centers or may be available through public or private home health agencies. Rehabilitation centers are listed in the phone book yellow pages. A physician referral is usually required.

Physical Therapy. This service also may be available through the VNA and other home health programs and at most rehabilitation centers. Independent Living Centers (ILC) offering physical therapy services are opening up throughout the country. Those centers offer services that permit individuals to function independently, outside of institutions. Many of the centers are federally funded and provide services at little or no cost to the patient. Contact the state vocational rehabilitation agency for information about ILCs in your area. Again, a physician referral may be required.

Rehabilitation Centers. Outpatient services of physicians, physical and occupational therapists, social workers, counselors, and psychologists are usually offered at these centers. Day services to assist individuals with independent living functions often are available. A physician referral may be required.

Vocational Rehabilitation. A state and federal program is offered through the Division of Vocational Rehabilitation (DVR). Financial assistance is provided with job training or retraining if it is likely that the individual can be gainfully employed. DVR can finance corrective medical or surgical treatment if the individual is declared eligible for services. Counseling, vocational evaluation, training, and placement also are available services. Look in the phone directory under state government listings and contact the nearest office for referral information.

Sheltered Workshops. Goodwill Industries, Salvation Army, and Crippled Children and Adult Societies offer vocational programs for people who cannot participate in competitive employment. A state vocational rehabilitation counselor should be able to provide information about programs like this in the area.

Help with Daily Living

Equipment. Persons requiring wheelchairs, canes, and other types of medical equipment may be able to receive them on loan or receive financial aid for equipment through organizations like the American Red Cross, Easter Seals, and Elks, Lions, Kiwanis, and Rotary Clubs. Contact the local organizations for information about their services. The city Chamber of Commerce may be able to provide a list of these and other service organizations.

Transportation. Public transportation adapted for the handicapped is available through local, county, or city government. Voluntary health organizations, the American Red Cross, and clubs often have free transportation available for the handicapped. The local United Way often has a list of agencies that provide these services.

In many states persons certified by their physicians as being severely disabled can be eligible for special license permits allowing the person to park in handicapped parking zones. Contact your state's department of traffic or transportation for more information.

Public Access. Although federal and usually state legislation exists to promote barrier-free architecture, access to and within many facilities is still a problem for the disabled.

Many communities do have organizations that can assist in the identification of barrier-free facilities and/or can advocate for compliance to legislated standards for barrier-free design. For instance, many communities have "Access Guides" listing accessible buildings, including banks, churches, hotels and motels, libraries, stores, museums, recreational facilities, restaurants, and theaters.

Contact the following types of organizations for information and assistance: chapters of the National Easter Seal Society, your state governor's committee on employment of the handicapped, rehabilitation institutes and centers, and state centers for the handicapped. Look in the phone directory under the state government listings or the yellow pages under social services. Local travel agencies and national motel/hotel chains may also provide information about accessible facilities.

Local rehabilitation centers, vocational rehabilitation agencies, Independent Living Centers, and nonprofit agencies for handicapped may offer assistance in providing architectural modifications in homes, such as bathroom and kitchen alterations.

Special arrangements can be made for air, rail, and bus travel by contacting the airline, train, or bus company in advance. Services can include assistance with transport within the airport or bus or train station; with baggage; with boarding and with accommodations on the carrier.

Home Bound Services.   Home health care services usually offer homemaker assistance, as well as local churches and the local social services department. "Meals on Wheels," community groups, and churches may provide meals to homebound patients. Many of the programs for homebound children with arthritis are provided through a state bureau of crippled children.

Counseling

Vocational, personal, and family psychosocial counseling is available from the following social agencies: family service agencies; family and children's societies; councils on aging; departments of social services; private social service agencies such as Catholic Social Services; community mental health centers and other mental health agencies; and private practitioners such as social workers, family counselors, marriage counselors, clinical psychologists, clergymen, psychiatric nurse specialists, and therapists. Look in the yellow pages under social service organizations, and under the headings counselors, psychologists, and psychiatrists.

FINANCIAL ASSISTANCE

Medicare.   This federal health insurance program is administered by the Social Security Administration for people 65 and older and for some individuals under 65 who are disabled and eligible for Social Security Disability Insurance.

Medicare pays in part for medically necessary inpatient care in a skilled nursing facility and for home care by a home health agency. Medicare also helps pay for medically necessary physician services, outpatient hospital services and therapy, and a number of other medical services and supplies.

Persons apply for Medicare at a Social Security office (listed under "U.S. Government" in the phone directory).

Social Security Disability Benefits.   Eligible for these monthly benefits are persons in the following categories:

1.   Disabled workers under 65 who have worked long enough and recently enough in a job that is covered by Social Security
2.   Persons disabled before the age of 22

3. Children (persons under 21) whose parent covered under Social Security retires, becomes disabled, or dies
4. Widows who become disabled before or within 7 years of the husband's death, or within 7 years after receipt of benefits by a mother caring for minor children stop.

An individual is considered disabled by a condition if the condition is severe enough to keep him or her from working and is expected to last for at least 12 months or to result in death. Individuals who receive monthly Social Security Disability Insurance for two consecutive years are eligible for Medicare. Disability benefits are also obtained through the Social Security office.

Supplemental Security Income (SSI).   SSI is available to the disabled individual who is in financial need, if he or she is unable to engage in substantial gainful activity due to a physical or mental impairment that either can be expected to result in death or has lasted or is expected to last for 12 months or longer. Applications for SSI should be made at a local Social Security office. People receiving SSI are automatically eligible for Medical Assistance (Medicaid).

Medical Assistance (Medicaid).   These health care benefits are for individuals who are identified as categorically or medically needy (which means they earn sufficiently low income to be eligible for free medical services.) Benefits vary from state to state, but minimum benefits are federally determined to be the same as those provided under Medicare. Applications for Medicaid are taken at county welfare offices or social services departments.

Veterans Administration.   Services provided by the Veterans Administration include disability compensation, pension, and medical service to eligible veterans. Outpatient and home care services are available to some persons. For information about eligibility requirements, contact the nearest VA hospital.

FINDING RESOURCES

Since individual health professionals may not be able to meet all of their patients' needs directly, they should be able to inform their patients about other available services and to direct them to the appropriate resource.

One of the simplest ways to discover such resources is to seek help from others who may already have gathered the necessary information. Hospital discharge or home-care coordinators, public health nurses, hospital and county social workers, health planning councils, the United Way, and the local chapters of the Arthritis Foundation are among those who may be of help.

If there is no previously compiled information, try enlisting the help of volunteers through the local Arthritis Foundation chapter or division, local hospital auxiliaries, or a voluntary health agency to identify resources.

The easiest way to collect information about possible resources is to make contact with agencies by telephone. Clearly state your purpose on the telephone, explaining, for example, that you are seeking information to aid people with arthritis. Appropriate questions to ask include requesting the name of a contact person, hours of operation, description of services, eligibility limitations, area served, referral procedure, and availability of any written materials about program.

If it appears that the agency might be frequently utilized, a personal visit is beneficial. Make an appointment with the contact person to help develop a good working relationship and to inspect the facility for accessibility. When inspecting the site, note proximity of the location to public transportation, and existence of architectural barriers at entrances and in restrooms.

The result of a little detective work can provide a fairly comprehensive list of agencies and individuals, complete with addresses, phone numbers, and specific services available from each. This information can be stored on file cards, in a looseleaf notebook, or in file folders. Printed directories containing key information can be developed for distribution to persons requiring information about resources.

FACILITATING RESOURCE UTILIZATION

Once the health professional knows what potential resources exist, the next most important task is to clarify what the person or family wants and the willingness to be referred. Sometimes the client may need to be motivated to utilize a resource. Because of past frustrating experiences, shyness or fear about seeking new services may exist.

Once the person agrees to seek outside services and the specific resource has been chosen, obtain referral, consent, and medical history forms if needed and make arrangements for their completion and distribution to the community resource. If the agency requires that the person make an appointment, explain the procedure. Make arrangements for follow-up of the visit.

The health professional may need to function as an advocate, explaining procedures, accompanying persons through procedures, and acting as a liaison with the community resources. However, persons should be encouraged to participate in this process as actively as possible. Persons may require information, motivation, and training in problem-solving and in the appropriate utilization of resources. Health professionals such as social workers can do some of the busy work for the patient who is unable to get help on his own.

SUMMARY

There are many arthritis support services available. A valuable role of physicians and allied health professionals is not only providing information and referral to community resources, but ensuring that these community resources are effectively utilized by people who have arthritis and by their families.

Appendix 10A

Local Chapters and Divisions of the Arthritis Foundation

ALABAMA
Alabama Chapter
13 Office Park Circle—Room 14
Birmingham, Ala. 35223
Tel: (205) 870-4700

South Alabama Chapter
304 Little Flower Avenue
Mobile, Ala. 36606
Tel: (205) 471-1725

ARIZONA
Central Arizona Chapter
2102 W. Indian School Road
Suite 9
Phoenix, Ariz. 85015
Tel: (602) 264-7679

Southern Arizona Chapter
4520 E. Grant Road
Tucson, Ariz. 85712
Tel: (602) 326-2811

ARKANSAS
Arkansas Chapter
6213 Lee Avenue
Little Rock, Ark. 72205
Tel: (501) 664-7242

CALIFORNIA
Northeastern California Chapter
1722 "J" Street—Suite 321
Sacramento, Calif. 95814
Tel: (916) 446-7246

Northern California Chapter
203 Willow Street—Suite 201
San Francisco, Calif. 94109
Tel. (415) 673-6882

San Diego Area Chapter
6154 Mission Gourge Road—Suite 110
San Diego, Calif. 92123
Tel: (619) 280-0304

Southern California Chapter
4311 Wilshire Boulevard
Los Angeles, Calif. 90010
Tel: (213) 938-6111

COLORADO
Rocky Mountain Chapter
234 Columbine Street—Suite 210
P.O. Box 6919
Denver, Colo. 80206
Tel: (303) 399-5065

CONNECTICUT
Connecticut Chapter
370 Silas Deane Highway
Wethersfield, Conn. 06109
Tel: (203) 563-1177

DELAWARE
Delaware Chapter
234 Philadelphia Pike—Suite 1
Wilmington, Del. 19809
Tel: (302) 764-8254

DISTRICT OF COLUMBIA
Arthritis Foundation
Metropolitan Washington Chapter
1901 Ft. Myer Drive—Suite 507
Arlington, VA 22209
Tel: (703) 276-7555

FLORIDA
Florida Chapter
3205 Manatee Avenue West
Bradenton, Fla. 33505
Tel: (813) 748-1300

GEORGIA
Georgia Chapter
1340 Spring Street—Suite 103
Atlanta, GA 30309
Tel: (404) 873-3240
1-800-282-7023

HAWAII
Hawaii Chapter
200 North Vineyard Boulevard
Suite 503
Honolulu, Hawaii 96817
Tel: (808) 523-7561

IDAHO
Idaho Chapter
700 Robbins Road—Suite 1
Boise, Idaho 83702
Tel: (208) 344-7102

ILLINOIS
Central Illinois Chapter
Allied Agencies Center
320 East Armstrong Avenue
Room 102
Peoria, Ill. 61603
Tel: (309) 672-6337

Illinois Chapter
79 W. Munroe—Suite 1120
Chicago, Ill. 60603
Tel: (312) 782-1367

INDIANA
Indiana Chapter
1010 East 86th Street
Indianapolis, Ind. 46240
Tel: (317) 844-3341

IOWA
Iowa Chapter
1501 Ingersoll Avenue—Suite 101
Des Moines, Iowa 50309
Tel: (515) 243-6259

KANSAS
Kansas Chapter
1602 East Waterman
Wichita, Kansas 67211
Tel: (316) 263-0116

KENTUCKY
Kentucky Chapter
1381 Bardstown Road
Louisville, Ken. 40204
Tel: (502) 459-6460

LOUISIANA
Louisiana Chapter
4700 Dryades
New Orleans, La. 70115
Tel: (504) 897-1338

MAINE
Maine Chapter
37 Mill Street
Brunswick, Me. 04011
Tel: (207) 729-4453

MARYLAND
Maryland Chapter
12 West 25th Street
Baltimore, Md. 21218
Tel: (301) 366-0923

MASSACHUSETTS
Massachusetts Chapter
59 Temple Place
Boston, Mass. 02111
Tel: (617) 542-6535

MICHIGAN
Michigan Chapter
23400 Michigan Avenue
Suite 605
Dearborn, Mich. 48124
Tel: (313) 561-9096

MINNESOTA
Minnesota Chapter
122 West Franklin—Suite 440
Minneapolis, Minn. 55404
Tel: (612) 874-1201

MISSISSIPPI
Mississippi Chapter
6055 Ridgewood Road
Jackson, Miss. 39211
Tel: (601) 956-3371

MISSOURI
Eastern Missouri Chapter
7315 Manchester Boulevard
St. Louis, Mo. 63143
Tel: (314) 644-3488

Western Missouri/Greater Kansas
  City Chapter
8301 State Line, Suite 117
Kansas City, Mo. 64114
Tel: (816) 361-7002

MONTANA
Montana Chapter
2 Polly Drive
P.O. Box 20994
Billings, Mont. 59101
Tel: (406) 657-7961

NEBRASKA
Nebraska Chapter
2229 N. 91st Court, #33
Omaha, Neb. 68134
Tel: (402) 391-8000

NEVADA
Nevada Division
3160 So. Valley View Boulevard
Suite 107A
Las Vegas, Nev. 89102
Tel: (702) 367-1626

NEW HAMPSHIRE
New Hampshire Chapter
P.O. Box 369, 35 Pleasant Street
Concord, N.H. 03301
Tel: (603) 224-9322

NEW JERSEY
New Jersey Chapter
15 Prospect Lane
Colonia, N.J. 07067
Tel: (201) 388-0744

NEW MEXICO
New Mexico Chapter
5112 Grand Avenue, N.E.
Albuquerque, N.M. 87108
Tel: (505) 265-1545

NEW YORK
Central New York Chapter
505 E. Fayette Street, 2nd Floor
Syracuse, N.Y. 13202
Tel: (315) 422-8174

Genesee Valley Chapter
973 East Avenue
Rochester, N.Y. 14607
Tel: (716) 271-3540

Long Island Division
501 Walt Whitman Road
Melville, N.Y. 11747
Tel: (516) 427-8272

New York Chapter
115 East 18th Street
New York, N.Y. 10003
Tel: (212) 477-8310

Northeastern New York Chapter
1237 Central Avenue
Albany, N.Y. 12205
Tel: (518) 459-5082

Western New York Chapter
1370 Niagara Falls Boulevard
Ionawanda, N.Y. 14150
Tel: (716) 837-8600

NORTH CAROLINA
North Carolina Chapter
P.O. Box 2505, 3115 Guess Road
Durham, N.C. 27705
Tel: (919) 477-0286

NORTH DAKOTA AND
SOUTH DAKOTA
Dakota Chapter
1402 N. 39th Street
Fargo, N.D. 58102
Tel: (701) 282-3653

OHIO
Central Ohio Chapter
2501 N. Star Road
Columbus, Ohio 43221
Tel: (614) 488-0777

Northeastern Ohio Chapter
11416 Bellflower Road
Cleveland, Ohio 44106
Tel: (216) 791-1310

Northwestern Ohio Chapter
4447 Talmadge Road
Toledo, Ohio 43623
Tel: (419) 473-3349

Southwestern Ohio Chapter
2400 Reading Road
Cincinnati, Ohio 45202
Tel: (513) 721-1027

OKLAHOMA
Eastern Oklahoma Chapter
2816 E. 51st Street—Suite 120
Tulsa, Okla. 74105
Tel: (918) 743-4526

Oklahoma Chapter
3313 Classen Boulevard—Suite 101
Oklahoma City, Okla. 73118
Tel: (405) 521-0066

OREGON
Oregon Chapter
Barbur Boulevard Plaza
4445 S.W. Barbur Boulevard
Portland, Oregon 97201
Tel: (503) 222-7246

PENNSYLVANIA
Central Pennsylvania Chapter
P.O. Box 668, 2019 Chestnut Street
Camp Hill, Pa. 17011
Tel: (717) 763-0900

Eastern Pennsylvania Chapter
311 S. Juniper Street—Suite 201
Philadelphia, Pa. 19107
Tel: (215) 735-5272

Western Pennsylvania Chapter
2201 Lawyers Building
428 Forbes Avenue
Pittsburgh, Pa. 15219
Tel: (412) 566-1645

RHODE ISLAND
Rhode Island Chapter
850 Waterman Avenue
East Providence, R.I. 02914
Tel: (401) 434-5792

SOUTH CAROLINA
South Carolina Chapter
1802 Sumter Street
Columbia, S.C. 29201
Tel: (803) 254-6702

SOUTH DAKOTA
See North Dakota

TENNESSEE
Middle-East Tennessee Division
210 25th Avenue North—Suite 1202
Nashville, Tenn. 37203
Tel: (615) 329-3431

West Tennessee Chapter
2600 Poplar Avenue—Suite 200
Memphis, Tenn. 38112
Tel: (901) 452-4482

TEXAS
North Texas Chapter
6300 Harry Hines Boulevard
Suite 211
Exchange Park
Treadway Plaza
Dallas, Texas 75235-5207
Tel: (214) 956-7771

Northwest Texas Chapter
3145 McCart Avenue
Fort Worth, Texas 76110
Tel: (817) 926-7733

South Central Texas Chapter
503 South Main Street
San Antonio, Texas 78204
Tel: (512) 224-4857

Texas Gulf Coast Chapter
9111A Katy Freeway—Suite 210
Houston, Texas 77024
Tel: (713) 468-6572

West Texas Chapter
2317 34th Street
Lubbock, Texas 79411
Tel: (806) 793-3273

UTAH
Utah Chapter
Graystone Plaza, #15
1174 E. 2700 South
Salt Lake City, Utah 84106
Tel: (801) 486-4993

VERMONT
Vermont Chapter
Richardson Place—Suite 2E
Church Street
Burlington, Vermont 05402
Tel: (802) 864-4988

VIRGINIA
Virginia Chapter
1900 Byrd Avenue—Suite 100
P.O. Box 6772
Richmond, Va. 23230
Tel: (804) 282-5491

WASHINGTON
Western Washington Chapter
726 Broadway—Suite 103
Seattle, Wash. 98122
Tel: (206) 324-9940

WEST VIRGINIA
West Virginia Chapter
440 4th Avenue   P.O. Box 8473
South Charleston, W.V. 25303
Tel: (304) 744-3042

WISCONSIN
Wisconsin Chapter
1442 N. Farwell Avenue—Suite 508
Milwaukee, Wis. 53202
Tel: (414) 276-0490
1-800-242-9945

WYOMING
Part of Rocky Mountain Chapter
(See Colorado)

Techniques in the Care of Patients with Rheumatic Disease

In the first section of this book we discussed the roles of the various health professionals who care for patients with arthritis. The techniques of care of the rheumatic disease patient may be employed by any or all of these health professionals. Good care techniques are based on an excellent history and physical examination of the patient. While different health professionals may employ different parts of the history and physical examination it is important for all of them to review the data from their own perspective with each patient. It is also important for the health professional to explain the necessity for repeating some of the physical examination that may have been done by the primary care physician, or other health care provider. Things change over time and one health professional may have expertise in examining a certain area that another does not.

Once an adequate history and physical examination is done an assessment and plan is arrived at. The purpose of this section is to discuss various types of rehabilitation techniques that may fit into the assessment and plan. One of the problems in rehabilitation medicine has been that some techniques have not been well accepted by health care providers. Chapters in this section try to examine each of the techniques that are regularly used, point out which of them have been scientifically tested and which of them are used by common agreement. Whether or not a physician or other health care provider is utilizing the techniques described, it is important for them to understand their use, efficacy, and the potential for the interaction with other techniques used in the total management of the patient. While medications are not discussed per se in this section they obviously are important in allowing various rehabilitation techniques to be performed with greater ease and a greater success rate.

11

Techniques in the Care of Patients with Rheumatic Disease

11

Musculoskeletal Examination

Timothy M. Spiegel, M.D., and
Solomon N. Forouzesh, M.D.

A careful examination directs the clinician to the correct diagnosis and to an understanding of the functional impact of the rheumatologic disorder. The joint, the functional unit of the musculoskeletal system, consists of the articular surface, bone, synovial membrane, capsule, ligaments, and muscles and tendons (figure 11.1). The articular surface is composed of cartilage, which has neither blood supply nor nerves. The synovial membrane is a delicate lining tissue, which provides for the nutritional requirements of the cartilage. Capsule, ligaments, and tendons provide support for the joint. Bursae are not integral aspects of joints but decrease friction between two moving components. The bursa can be thought of as a deflated balloon that can conform to glide between two moving components and reduce friction that would lead to heat accumulation and tissue injury. During examination, mental visualization of the anatomy aids in localizing the site of the symptoms. A rapid and complete rheumatologic examination should follow a pattern that includes inspection, palpation, and testing passive range of motion, stability, active range of motion, and muscle strength.

Inspection. A patient's movement, posture, and gait give invaluable aids to diagnosis. Reluctance to grasp firmly during handshake may indicate an inflammatory arthritis of small joints. Visible erythema, swelling, and deformity can establish the pattern of joint involvement. Severity of functional limitations can be observed when the patient enters the room or when he is disrobing for physical examination.

Palpation. Palpation of the joint margin determines whether localized synovial proliferation is present. Knowledge of articular and nonarticular anatomy is vital to correct interpretation. An examiner can rapidly recognize each of these ana-

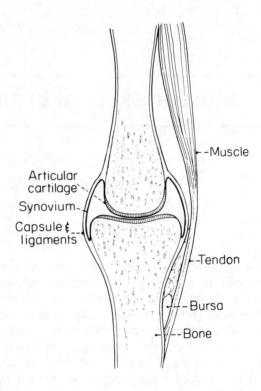

Figure 11.1.   Joint anatomy. Schematic representation of the relationship of structures at the joint.

tomic sites and can thereby focus on the problem. Palpation is of great importance to separate inflammatory arthritis (synovial proliferation) from arthralgia (painful joints).

Passive Range of Motion.   While the patient is relaxed, passive range of motion should be tested by the examiner. Range of motion is often the only clue to separate inflammatory synovitis from arthralgia. When range of motion is limited, the examiner must determine if the limitation is due to effusion, synovitis, joint surface abnormality, loose bodies or capsular or muscular contractures. Measurements of passive range of motion and normal values are available in the suggested reading list at the end of the chapter.

Stability.   To determine whether a pathologic condition of the bone, capsule, ligament, or tendon is causing abnormal movement (instability, subluxation, or dislocation), the joint should be moved under stress in the direction it is not supposed to move by virtue of its contour, ligaments, and capsule. During movement, the joint is normally supported by active muscular contractions. Ruptures in ligaments or laxity of the capsule will result in abnormal mobility of the joint.

Active Range of Motion.   Active range of motion is a measure of the working relationship of the entire musculoskeletal system. If active range of motion is less than passive range of motion, muscular weakness, neurologic damage, or pain should be suspected.

Muscle Strength.   Strength of individual muscles should be tested in a comfortable midposition of the muscle. Grading systems are based on the ability of the muscle to move against force through a complete range of motion. Grade 5 (normal) muscular strength, for example, can move the joint through a full range of motion against full resistance applied by the examiner. Grade 4 (good) can move against gravity with only moderate resistance by the examiner. Grade 3 (fair) means the muscle can move the joint through a full range of motion against gravity only. Grade 2 (poor) strength can move the joint through a full range of motion only when the force of gravity is not acting to resist the motion. Grade 1 (trace) implies muscle contractions but insufficient strength to produce motion even with gravity eliminated. Grade 0 strength is complete paralysis and no visible or palpable contraction.

UPPER EXTREMITY

Shoulder

The shoulder girdle is composed of three joints and one "articulation": the sternoclavicular joint; the acromioclavicular joint; the glenohumeral joint (the true shoulder joint); and the scapulothoracic articulation. All four work together in a rhythmic fashion to permit universal motion. The glenohumeral joint permits two-thirds (120°) and the scapulothoracic articulation contributes one-third (60°) of total abduction (180°). Although considered to be a ball-and-socket joint, the glenohumeral joint is actually a ball-and-flat joint, requiring the rotator cuff for stability.

Range of motion is tested by asking the patient to touch the fingertips to the back of the neck and then to touch between the scapula (figure 11.2a and b). If normal, this can be done, and the shoulder girdle is most likely functioning correctly. However, determination of a limited range of motion requires more care.

First, the pain threshold is estimated by pressure over the coracoid process, which has a periosteal covering. The pressure required to produce threshold pain can be compared to that causing pain in the other important anatomic sites to determine the specific location of the patient's pain. Areas to be palpated are the (1) anterior joint space, (2) biceps tendon, (3) subacromial bursa (supraspinatus

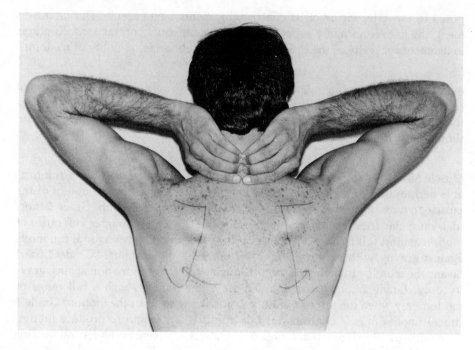

Figure 11.2a. Shoulder range of motion can be observed by having the patient place the fingertips at the base of neck (a) and then between the scapula (b). If this motion is performed without pain, the shoulder is probably normal.

tendon), (4) posterior joint space, and (5) acromioclavicular joint (figure 11.3). None of these regions are painful unless localized disease is present. Pain in the arterior and posterior joint space suggests inflammatory synovitis of the glenohumeral joint. Since the four rotator cuff muscles surround the joint, localized pain may be due to an injury to the rotator cuff.

Pain during active range of motion can be utilized to determine which of the rotator cuff muscles is injured. For instance, since the supraspinatus muscle is responsible for initiating abduction, pain due to supraspinatus tendinitis is most pronounced when the patient actively abducts the arm.

Subacromial bursitis (supraspinatus tendinitis) is palpated between the tip of the acromium and the tuberosity of the humerus. Pain in the acromioclavicular joint is easily detected by palpation of the joint. Prominent bony proliferation can be palpated if degenerative joint disease is present.

Special clinical maneuvers may provide clues to uncover a specific type of pathology and are most helpful when previous portions of the examinations have led one to suspect a specific type of pathology. Two such tests for the shoulder are the Yergason test of the long head of the biceps tendon and the drop-arm test

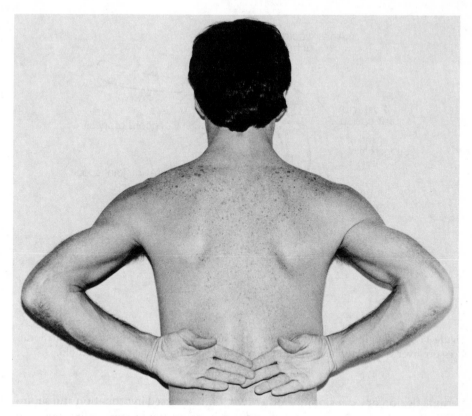

Figure 11.2b. *(continued).*

for rotator cuff tear. The Yergason test measures inflammation of the biceps tendon in the bicipital groove. To conduct this test, the elbow flexed to 90° and the shoulder externally rotated, the wrist is supined against resistance (figure 11.4). This will cause pain in the stretched biceps tendon if tendinitis is present. The drop-arm test is used to detect tears in the rotator cuff. Instruct the patient to abduct the arm fully and then slowly lower the arm to the side. If there are tears in the rotator cuff, especially in the supraspinatus muscle, pain will induce the patient suddenly to drop the arm to the side from a position of about 90° of abduction. Since the shoulder is a classic area of referred pain, a complete examination should include evaluation of the cardiovascular system, cervical spine, soft tissue structures of the thorax, and the gall bladder.

Elbow

The elbow is a hinge joint composed of three articulations: the humeroulnar joint, the humeroradial joint, and the radioulnar joint. The humeroulnar joint

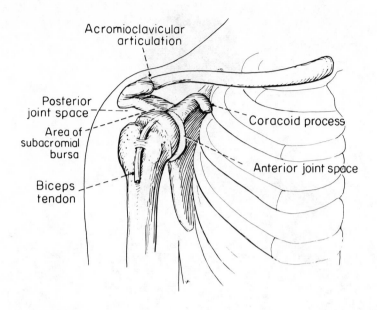

Figure 11.3. Shoulder palpation localizes the site of anatomical pain or inflammation. Pressure over the uninvolved coracoid process can determine the pain threshold.

permits flexion or extension; the other two joints are used in pronation and supination. Synovium may be palpated midway between the humeroradial joint and the tip of the olecranon process (figure 11.5). Since normal extension of the elbow is to 0° in men and an additional 5° of hypertension in women, limitation in joint extension is a sensitive indication of inflammatory synovitis or previous injury. Supination of the forearm is accomplished by both the elbow and the wrist. Lateral epicondylitis (tennis elbow) is inflammation of the wrist extensors at their origin on the humerus (figure 11.6). The diagnosis is established by eliciting localized pain when the extended wrist is forcibly brought to the neutral position by the examiner against resistance by the patient. The patient will experience a sudden, severe pain at the site of the wrist extensors' common origin, the lateral epicondyle. The olecranon bursa is separate from the true elbow joint and should be palpated for the presence of effusion or nodules.

Wrist and Hand

This complex and delicately balanced series of joints is used for almost every act of daily living. The wrist is inspected to determine its alignment and the presence of swelling. Early synovitis can be detected by palpation of the lateral aspect of the ulnar styloid (figure 11.7). The normal range of wrist motion is 90° flexion

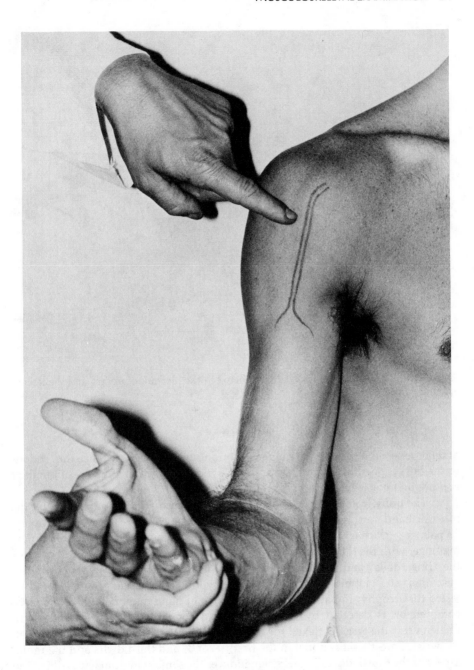

Figure 11.4.   Yergason's sign localizes bicipital tendinitis by producing pain in the area where the examiner is pointing when the forearm is supinated against resistance.

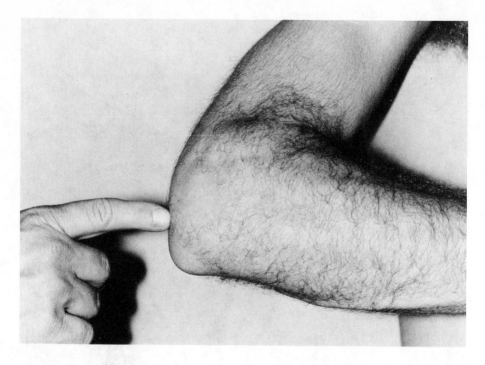

Figure 11.5.   Elbow synovitis is palpated between the olecranon process and the lateral epicondyle of the humerus.

and 85° extension. Decreased range of motion suggests disease. Since the tendons to the fingers pass through the wrist, wrist synovitis or trauma may result in their rupture and consequent immobility of fingers.

The bony framework of the hand is formed into an arch, supported by the intrinsic hand muscles. If the intrinsic muscles of the hand are absent or atrophic, its palmar surface will lose its normal contour. Examine the pinch of each opposing finger with the thumb. In addition, observe the general condition and color of the fingernails and evaluate for sclerodactyly, Raynaud's phenomenon, vasculitis, and clubbing. Both thenar and hypothenar muscle groups should be tested for atrophy. In patients with complaints of hand numbness, median nerve compression is detected by two specific tests for carpal tunnel syndrome. In Phalen's test the wrist is flexed for 60 seconds to attempt to increase pressure in the wrist. Paresthesia is noted in the first, second, and third digits and the radial aspect of the fourth digit. Tinnel's sign induces the same symptoms by striking the median nerve at the wrist with a reflex hammer.

The palmar aspect of the hands should be palpated for nodules in the flexor tendon sheaths, since the nodules in this area can cause disability due to "trigger finger." Other tests of the upper extremity should include the evaluation of vas-

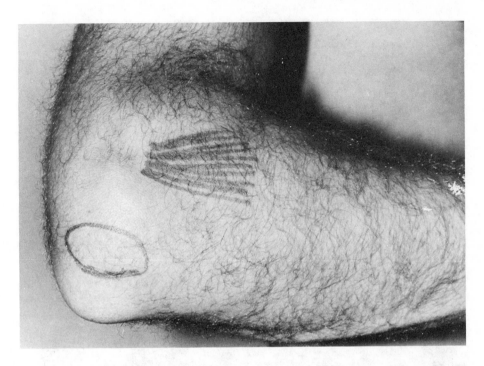

Figure 11.6. Lateral epicondylitis (tennis elbow) is diagnosed by referred pain when the extensor muscles of the wrist are contracted against resistance. The lines represent the origin of the lateral epicondyl and extension musculature. The circle represents localization of elbow synovitis.

cular competence. The radial arteries should be palpated with the extremity in different positions, including full anterior abduction and lateral motion of the head. The Allen test is used to determine whether both radial and ulnar arteries are intact. In this test the arteries in the wrist are compressed digitally after the patient has clenched the hand into a fist to force the blood out, and adequacy of blood flow is determined by releasing one artery at a time. If the blood does not diffuse into the hand when the fist is unclenched, the artery not compressed is occluded.

The metacarpophalangeal and interphalangeal joints are examined by producing slight traction on the digit and then palpating at the joint margin (figure 11.8). The pressure should be sufficient to blanch the nail bed of the examiner. Erythema, synovial hypertrophy, and effusion can be palpated. Examination should include observation for ulnar drift, swan-neck deformity, and boutonniere deformity. The combined range of motion of the metacarpophalangeal and interphalangeal joints should permit the tips of the fingers to touch the hand creases. Even if mild disease is present, the tips of the fingers cannot touch the palmar creases.

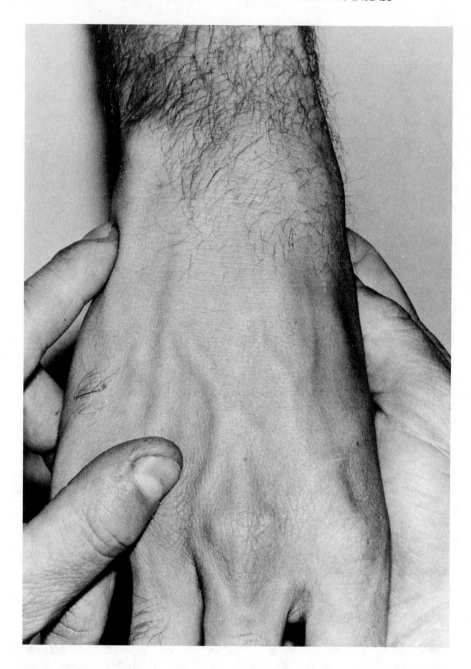

Figure 11.7. Early synovitis of the wrist produces soft tissue swelling at the ulnar styloid region and decreased passive range of motion.

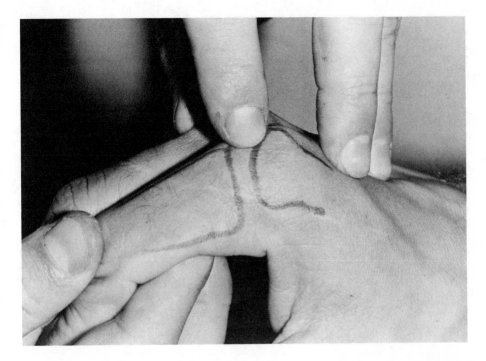

Figure 11.8.   Synovitis of the metacarpophalangeal joints is palpated at the joint margin with slight distraction of the joint.

AXIAL SKELETON

Cervical Spine.   Inspection of the cervical spine will give clues to the alignment of the entire vertebral system. The neck should be palpated with the patient in a supine position to relax the paraspinal muscles and localize the pain or spasm (figure 11.9). Mastoid and spinous processes can be palpated as well. A shift in the normal alignment of the spinous processes may be due to a unilateral dislocation of fracture of a spinal process following trauma.

Cervical spine examination should include the structures of the neck, including the sternocleidomastoid muscle, lymph nodes, thyroid gland, carotid arteries, and parotid glands.

Cervical motion consists of flexion, extension, rotation, and lateral bending. These specific motions are also used in combination to give the head and neck the capacity for a diversified motion. Approximately 50 percent of rotation takes place between C-1 and C-2 (atlas and axis). The remaining 50 percent of rotation is relatively evenly distributed among the other five cervical vertebrae. Lateral bending, a function of all the cervical vertebrae, does not occur as a pure motion but rather functions in conjunction with elements of rotation. Because

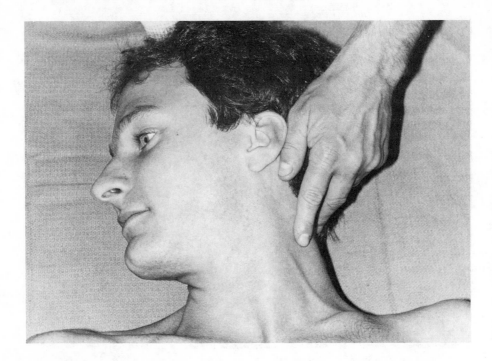

Figure 11.9. The cervical spine is best palpated when the patient is supine and the paracervical muscles are relaxed. Range of motion measurement can distinguish muscle pain from bony changes.

cervical spine disease may be associated with radicular involvement, neurologic testing should include each cervical root, which exits through the foramena above the vertebral body.

Temporal Mandibular Joint. Instruct the patient to open and close the mouth. The mouth normally opens wide enough so that three fingers can be inserted between the incisor teeth, a distance of approximately 3.5 to 4 cm (figure 11.10). The temporomandibular joint, a hinged structure, glides forward and laterally. Symmetry of bite and occlusion is observed. Palpate over the lateral temporomandibular joint and into the external auditory canal to detect clicks and crepitation.

Back. With the patient standing, inspect for kyphoscoliosis in the thoracic and lumbar region. Normally the lumbosacral area has a lumbar lordosis, which can be aggravated or straightened. Palpation of the paravertebral muscles will detect muscular spasm and "trigger points." Pain at the spinous process suggests local-

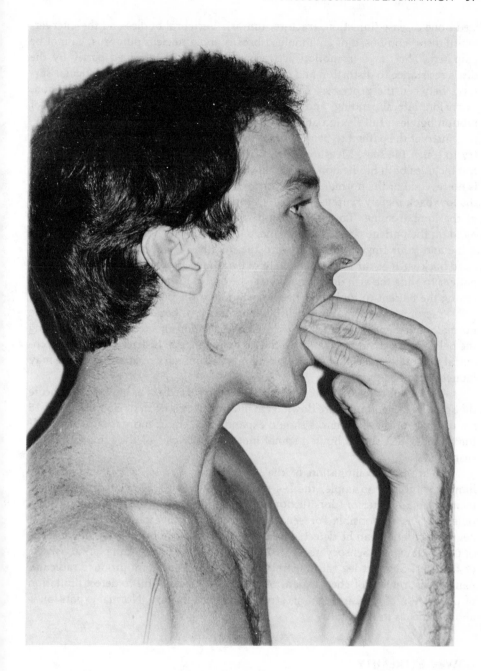

Figure 11.10.   The temporomandibular joint opens the jaw approximately 3 cm, which can be approximated with three fingers of the dominant hand.

ized bone disease (infection, fracture, tumor). Vertebral bodies and the intervertebral discs, composed of an annulus fibrosus and a nucleus pulposus, cannot be palpated. The range of motion between vertebrae is determined partly by the disc's resistance to distortion and partly by the angle and the size of articular surfaces between the processes. The movements of the lumbar spine are: flexion, extension, lateral bending, and rotation. Normally there is approximately 66° of motion between full flexion and full extension of the lumbar spine. To test flexion, instruct the patient to bend as far forward as possible with knees straight and try to touch the toes. Measure the distance from the fingertips to the floor. The test includes both hip flexion and spinal flexion. It is interesting to note that there is no reversal of the normal lumbar lordosis during flexion and that, at the most, the low back merely flattens out. Extension is performed by the intrinsic muscles of the lumbar spine. To test extension, stand beside the patient and place one hand on the patient's back so that your palm rests on the posterior superior iliac spine and your fingers extend toward the midline. Then instruct the patient to bend backward as far as possible. Lateral bending is best measured by asking the patient to slide the arm down the side of the body. Rotation can be measured by asking the patient to look over first one and then the other shoulder.

Sacroiliac joint motion is difficult to measure because the joint has little normal movement. Therefore physical examination is directed toward stabilizing the pelvis and extending one leg to the extreme range in order to provoke mechanical pull on the sacroiliac joint. During rectal examination, lateral pressure may induce sacroiliac pain.

The Schober test determines lumbar flexion regardless of hip flexion. Locate the spine of L-5 and measure down 5 cm and up 10 cm. With flexion the initial 15 cm distance of the skin marks should expand to 20 cm or more (figure 11.11). If the Schober test shows limited spinal motion, ankylosis of the lumbar spine is suspected.

Neurologic examination of the lower extremity assists in evaluating the lumbar spine. For example, the L-4 neurological level is associated with movement of tibialis anterior (dorsiflexion and inversion of the foot) and with the knee reflex. L-5 is responsible for sensation on the dorsal aspect of the foot. S-1 neurologic deficit can be detected by impaired pronation of the foot and absence of the ankle reflex. Sensory nerves from S-1 supply the lateral and plantar aspects of the foot. Straight leg raising stretches the nerves and may produce radicular pain. Measurement of chest expansion at nipple line is useful to detect limitation of the motion of the cartilaginous structures of the thorax. (Normal expansion is about 2 inches in the adult.)

LOWER EXTREMITY

Hip and Pelvis

During inspection of the hip area, five pelvic regions should be observed: the femoral triangle, the greater trochanter, the area of the sciatic nerve, the iliac

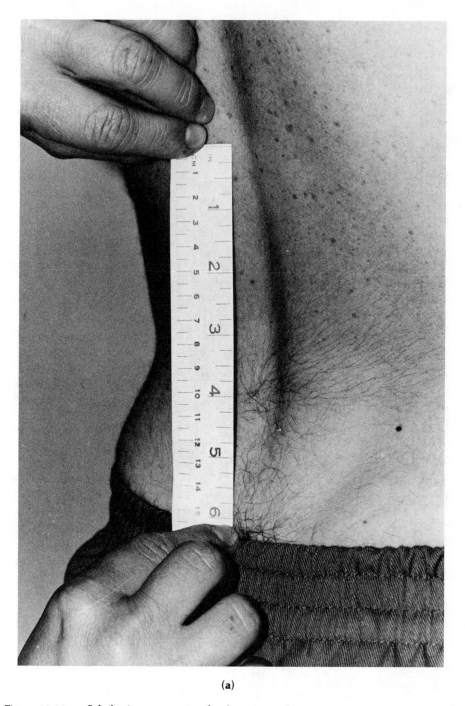

(a)

Figure 11.11a. Schober's test measures lumbar motion by expansion of skin marks from 15 cm (a) to 20 cm (b).

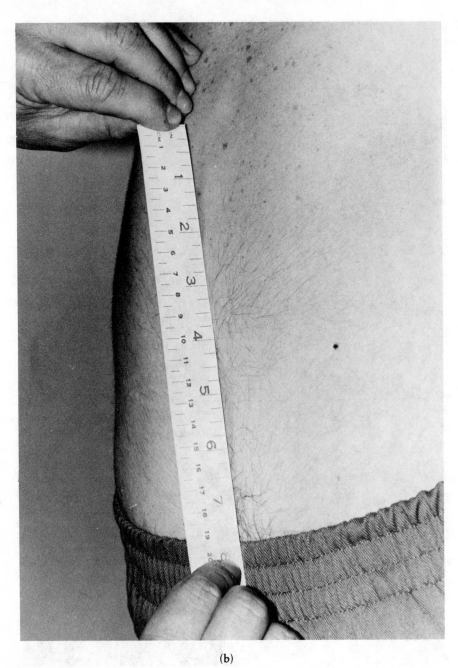

(b)

Figure 1.11b.   *(continued).*

crest, and the hip and pelvic muscles. To palpate the greater trochanter, pressure is applied to the most prominent and superior part of the femoral bone; tenderness is indicative of trochanteric bursitis. Leg length discrepancies should be observed. Also, ischeal bursitis is easily confused with sciatic pain. The sciatic nerve is located halfway between the ischeal tuberosity and the greater trochanter, but the ischeal bursa is medially located.

Hip pain is commonly perceived in the inguinal region. Range of motion of the hip can be tested quickly in abduction and internal rotation. Flexion of the hip is approximately 135° in a normal individual but is limited by the hamstring muscles if the leg is straight. It is important to note that on occasion the patient may substitute motion of the pelvis and lumbar spine to compensate for decreased range of hip motion. To evaluate accurately the range of motion of the hip, such compensatory motion can be prevented by stabilizing the pelvis throughout the examination. For example, examination of hip flexion with stabilization of pelvis is called the *Thomas test*. With the patient in a supine position, the examiner's hand is placed under the pelvic area and then the hip is flexed. At this point the lumbar spine is flattened and the pelvis is stabilized. Further flexion can originate only in the hip joint. Have the patient flex the other hip in a similar fashion; then have him grasp one leg around the knee to hold it close to his chest and let his other leg down until it is flat on the table. If the hip does not extend fully, the patient may have a contracture that prevents full extension.

External rotation of the hip is 45° in a normal subject, and internal rotation is approximately 35°. Examination of the hip should test the function of the various muscle groups as well as being a sensory examination. These groups of muscles are divided as follows:

Primary flexors—iliopsoas and rectus femoris

Primary extensors—gluteus maximus

Secondary extensors—hamstrings

Primary adductor—adductor longus

The Trendelenburg test is designed to evaluate the strength of the gluteus muscle. Stand behind the patient and observe the dimples overlying the posterior superior iliac spine. Then ask the patient to stand on one leg. The gluteus medius muscles on the supported side should contract as soon as the other leg leaves the ground and should elevate the pelvis on the unsupported side (figure 11.12). This elevation indicates that the gluteus medius muscle on the supported side is functioning properly; it is designated a negative Tendelenburg sign. If the pelvis on the unsupported side fails to elevate or actually descends, however, the gluteus medius muscle on the supported side is either weak or nonfunctioning.

Physical Examination of the Knee

Inspection will determine whether the patient is "bowlegged" (genu varus) or "knock kneed" (genu valgus). On the medial aspect of the knee, the medial tibial

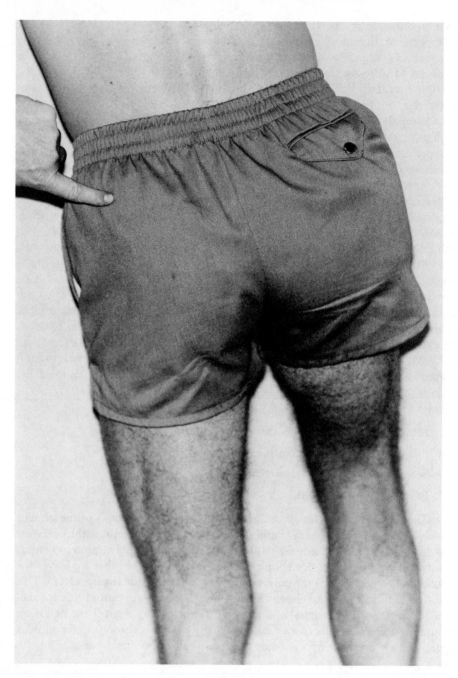

Figure 11.12. The Trendelenburg test evaluates the strength of the gluteus muscle. As the patient raises one leg, the examiner observes the pelvic rotation. With weakness of the gluteus muscles or pain of the gluteus medius bursa, the normal pelvic rotation will not occur.

plateau, tibial tubercle, and medial femoral condyle are palpable. Laterally the lateral tibial plateau, lateral tubercle, and femoral condyle along with femoral epicondyle and head of the fibula are palpable. The active and passive range of motion of the knee should be tested. Manual flexion is 135°, extension is zero, internal rotation 10°, and external rotation is 10°. Stability of the cruciate ligaments is tested by the drawer sign (figure 11.13). Perform this test when the patient is sitting in a flexed-knee position by pulling the knee structures forward with both hands. Ordinarily there is no anterior motion of these structures, but in internal derangement there is an obvious forward movement. Lateral and medial colateral ligaments are tested for instability both with the knees in full extension and in 15° flexion. The suprapatellar bursa is part of the true knee joint, and joint effusions are detected by demonstrating a fluid wave or a balottable patella. The anserine bursa, which is just medial to the tibial plateau, is frequently tender in both inflammatory and noninflammatory disease of the knee joint. Another test to detect meniscal tears is McMurray's test, which is performed with flexed knee and internal or external rotation of the tibia. If there is a palpable or audible click, the test is considered positive for a damaged medial meniscus.

The examiner should test the quadriceps muscles for atrophy and strength. Hamstring muscles are tested in a prone position with knee flexed; the examiner tries to reduce this flexion against the patient's resistance. The popliteal area may develop a Baker's cyst if synovium is trapped and expands through a oneway ball-valve effect. Under pressure this cyst can dissect into the calf muscles and may rupture and mimic thrombophlebitis.

Physical Examination of the Foot and Ankle

Abnormalities of the arch of the foot can be detected by inspection. They include a high arch (pes cavus) and a flat foot deformity (pes planus). Hallux valgus, bunion toe, is a common alignment change due to incorrect shoe wear. Bunions and other callus formations at points of pressure should be noted. The true ankle mortis permits 35° of dorsiflexion and 55° of plantar flexion. Synovitis of the joint is palpated anteriorly between the lateral and medial malleoli. It may be difficult to detect because the synovium lies beneath many soft tissues. Pain threshold and edema may be tested by direct palpation of the medial and lateral malleoli. If the malleoli are unusually tender to palpation, it is difficult to judge the significance of tenderness on the synovium. Similarly edema may cause swelling over the ankle joint.

The subtalar joint is formed by the talus-navicular-calcaneus junction. The subtalar joint permits lateral and medial motion of the hind foot. While walking over irregular surfaces, the subtalar joint corrects these irregularities and provides balance.

The forefoot is composed of the metatarsal bones and the phalanges. Hallux valgus denotes external deviation of the first toe.

Soft tissue problems in the foot are confusing, but a few simple terms will

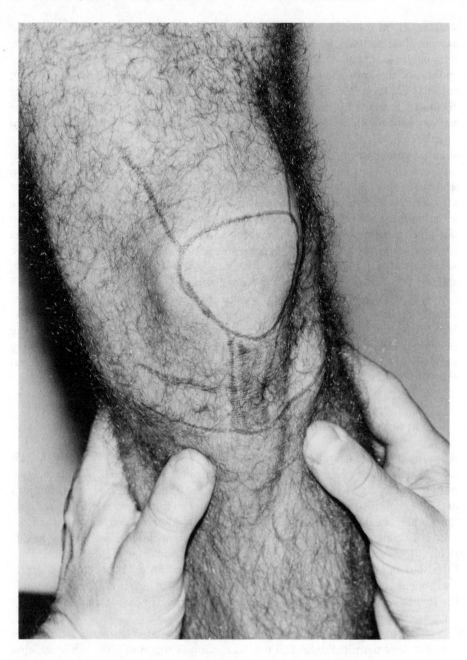

Figure 11.13. The draw sign measures stability of the cruciate ligament by resisting forward motion of the tibia. The lower leg should not be able to be pulled forward by this method.

enable the physician to approach common problems. "Corns" are calluses that result from pressure. Warts appear to be corns, but if gently shaved the normal skin folds will not be present in warts. A bunion is an inflamed bursa that has undergone fibrosis and localized bony proliferation.

ARTICULAR VERSUS NONARTICULAR

A common problem in a musculoskeletal examination is attribution of symptoms related to the true joint or to adjacent structures such as muscles, bursae, or nerves. Muscles may be tender and produce pain when palpated over a localized trigger point. The etiology of the trigger point is disputed, but it is usually located in the midportion of a muscle and may be firm and have a nodular feeling. Fibromyalgia is a clinical term used to describe the condition of the patient who has multiple areas of pain associated with trigger points.

Bursae become inflamed due to misuse. Most bursae are unnamed because they infrequently result in symptoms. Since bursitis has a different therapeutic approach than does arthritis, careful examination should be done to separate articular problems from the common nonarticular, bursal inflammation.

Nerve pain can usually be separated from articular disease because the pain is diffuse, and joint examination does not reveal synovitis, and the range of motion is normal.

SUGGESTED READINGS

Cailliet R. Soft tissue pain and disability. Philadelphia: FA Davis, 1977.

Gall EP, Gooden MA. Examination of the musculoskeletal system. 2nd ed. Department of Biomedical Communications, University of Arizona, 1983.

Hoppenfeld S. Physical examination of the spine and extremities. New York: Appleton-Century-Crofts, 1976.

McRae R. Clinical orthopaedic examination. Edinburgh: Churchill Livingstone, 1976.

VIDEOCASSETTE

Gall EP. Physical Examination of the musculoskeletal system. Obtained through Southwest Arthritis Center, University of Arizona Health Sciences Center, Tucson, Az 85724.

Hahn B. Examination: the patient with arthritis. Obtained through Medical Library 142/JB, VA Medical Center, St. Louis, Mo. 63125.

12

Needs Assessment

Catherine A. Novak, M.S.N.

The primary purpose of a needs assessment is to gather information about patient problems and the needs that must be met to manage those problems. Information gained from the needs assessment provides a foundation for the development of treatment goals and a personalized rehabilitation program.

Since individuals with arthritis are affected differently by the illness, the nature and degree of patient problems will vary. This variability requires a systematic method of assessment to discover specific patient needs. However, individuals with arthritis do share a number of common problems that can be used to construct a well-organized needs assessment.

It is virtually impossible for one person to gather all the information necessary to determine every need of a patient with arthritis. Opinions from different health professionals may contribute valuable information to the assessment process and may in fact be essential to the development of a workable treatment program. Whenever possible, the skills of therapists, nurses, social workers, and other health professionals should be employed to fullest advantage.

An outline for a needs assessment is described in this chapter (see table 12.1). It may be used as an elaboration on one portion of a comprehensive patient evaluation or in a short form to monitor the progress of established patients. The assessment of needs is a continual process requiring periodic revision to keep pace with the changing problems. The outline provides a framework with which to review and revise the rehabilitation program.

Three main categories of needs have been designated in the assessment outline to permit an organized approach. Within each category of need—physical, psychosocial, and environmental—problems and corresponding needs are discussed. The most useful initial approach may be simply to ask the patient to describe his or her main problem and most pressing need.

Table 12.1. Form for Assessing the Needs of the Rheumatic Disease Patient

PATIENT ASSESSMENT

Name:_____   M.D._____   Date Completed:_____

Age:_____   R.N._____

Diagnosis:_____

Area of Need	Extent of Need*			Recommendation/Comments
	Patient	M.D.	R.N.	
I. Physical				
A. Pain				
1. Stiffness/gelling				
2. Tenderness				
3. Swelling				
B. Joint Function				
1. Range of Motion				
2. Capacity for Self-care				
C. Fatigue				
II. Psychosocial				
A. Personal				
1. Counseling				
2. Health Education				
B. Family Relationships				
C. Social Relationships				
D. Occupational Relationships				
III. Environmental				
A. Transportation				
B. Home Modifications				
C. Job Site Modifications				

*Rating Scale:

0

None	= 0
Mild	= 1
Moderate	= 2
Severe	= 3
Incapacitating	= 4

ASSESSMENT OF PHYSICAL NEEDS

Individuals with arthritis experience a variety of physical problems, all of which demand attention. Two major difficulties, pain and loss of function, occur so frequently that patients with arthritis can be expected to have the corresponding two immediate needs: relief of pain and preservation or improvement of function.

Pain

Most patients with arthritis are prompted to seek medical treatment for the relief of pain.[1] It is the most common complaint of the person with arthritis, and consequently its relief is a prime physical need. Stiffness, tenderness, and swelling also contribute to the intensity of pain and together promote lack of mobility and loss of function.

Ideally the discomfort of the patient is addressed within the context of the medical regimen. If inflammation is the source of discomfort, an appropriate medical regimen must first be established to reduce imflammation and thereby reduce discomfort. Restoration of comfort may not be achieved rapidly, despite proper medical therapy. Other measures may be required to ease pain and encourage function. Medication only for the relief of pain is not usually recommended, as analgesic therapy precludes the use of pain as a barometer for the treatment regimen and deprives the patient of an intrinsic protection mechanism. In addition, some chronic pain may always be present, and the use of analgesics may become an undesirable long-term habit.

Pain has different meanings for each individual. It is important for the patient to be able to describe clearly the character and pattern of pain and to distinguish between pain and stiffness. These differences may influence the identification of needs and suggest strategies for relief.

A host of nonpharmacologic measures are available to relieve pain. To reduce the acute pain of inflammation, short-term strategies, such as adjustment of medications, systemic and local rest, and the use of warm moist heat may be indicated. Occupational and physical therapists who are skilled in the use of splints and adaptive devices for local rest, positioning techniques for comfortable systemic rest, and the application of heat may be able to help.

Patients with chronic pain also benefit from the attentions of these therapists, as many strategies used for relief of acute pain can also be adapted for chronic pain. Therapists may recommend additional, long-term measures, such as joint-protection instruction or pacing of activities to manage chronic pain.

Several forms of chronic pain management now enjoying a wave of interest among arthritis health professionals may prove to be valuable for the relief of chronic arthritis pain. Progress in the use of biofeedback and transcutaneous stimulation techniques for the relief of intractable pain suggest potential applications in arthritis. A less complex program composed of techniques for reducing stress, such as meditation and positive imagery, has also been received with enthusiasm and used to decrease muscle tension and ease pain. Descriptions of these measures appear in detail in other chapters of this book and merit consideration for the patient with arthritis.

In some instances pain appears to be influenced by the emotional state and coping resources of the patient.[2] (Psychosocial aspects of arthritis are reviewed in greater depth in subsequent chapters.) Some patients may need only reassurance and support from the physician or health professional to experience an easing of tension and pain.

Significant stiffness or gelling again suggest the need for assistance from the occupational or physical therapist, who can recommend a variety of methods to manage these problems. The patient should be asked how long morning stiffness or rigidity after immobility lasts. Warm showers or baths, local heat packs, and gentle stretching exercises are examples of ways to minimize stiffness.

Swelling and tenderness can intensify the discomfort of a painful joint; therefore measures such as those discussed for relief of inflammation may need to be applied.

Loss of Function

Functional ability is frequently compromised in patients with arthritis and should be assessed carefully. The combination of pain and structural changes caused by inflammation promotes disuse of joints and results in loss of motion and muscle strength. The assessment of functional needs is therefore a critical part of the overall needs assessment.

Absence of joint pain does not rule out the possibility of previous damage from arthritis, and limitations in extremes of motion may be detected in supposedly unaffected joints. If limitation of motion and decreased muscle strength are present on examination, an individualized exercise program developed with the aid of a physical therapist may be required to recover range of motion and strength. Patients with full range and strength can also use a simple program to check regularly range of motion and report change.

The loss of articular motion is a prelude to loss of function and should prompt careful examination for functional impairment. The patient should be asked to discuss activities that have become difficult or impossible and questioned about ability to perform activities of daily living. Loss of motion can limit the ability of the patient to complete basic self-care activities such as bathing, dressing, cooking, eating, or even moving around at home. Patients may be reluctant to mention more personal problems caused by arthritis, such as difficulty with sexual intercourse, and should be offered the opportunity to discuss personal issues.

Interference with activities of daily living requires the expertise of an occupational therapist to assess the extent of limitation and recommend a management program. Adaptive and assistive devices can provide greater independence for some patients, while others may require instruction in simpler or less tiring ways to manage daily activities. Principles of joint protection and energy conservation may be used to reduce joint strain and physical effort during activity. A home visit by a public or visiting nurse or a therapist may be needed to assess self-care abilities and mobilize community resources.

Fatigue.   The fatigue associated with arthritis can also interfere with the completion of daily activities, and though the adoption of regular rest periods may be helpful, pacing of activities and energy-saving techniques offer long-term preventive strategies. Lack of appetite and insufficient nutrition can also exacerbate fatigue and deserves a review of eating habits. A professional nutrition evaluation may yield valuable advice on dietary improvements and food preparation.

ASSESSMENT OF PSYCHOSOCIAL NEEDS

Arthritis can have wide-ranging and disruptive effects on the life of an individual. The extent to which changes occur depends in part on the severity of the illness, but even patients with mild involvement must grapple with the implications of arthritis.

It is generally accepted that psychosocial factors play a role in the management of arthritis. Although these factors have not been shown to affect the course of illness, evidence does suggest that they influence the way patients respond to a treatment program.[3] Psychological factors, then, should be considered during the evaluation and treatment of the patient but unfortunately do not always command immediate respect and can become lost in the concentration on physical data.

Though a detailed psychosocial assessment may be too involved to complete during most initial patient evaluation, information about several key areas should be obtained to assist in the determination of the need for specialized evaluation or treatment. Specialized services, such as counseling, may be obtained from arthritis nurse specialists, social workers, or psychologists, depending on the nature of the patient's problems.

The subject of psychological aspects of arthritis may be approached during the evaluation by asking the patient to describe how his life has changed since the arthritis appeared. The character and extent of the changes, as well as the patient's attitude while describing them, will provide an excellent starting point.

An appreciation should be gained for the effect of arthritis on the patient's self-image, family and home life, social relationships, and career. What is the patient's impression of arthritis—what meaning does it have for this individual? Most patients are concerned about crippling and harbor misconceptions about arthritis. The patient's demeanor while discussing the arthritis may also offer helpful clues. Are there signs of unusually intense anger, anxiety, or depression? Each individual responds differently to arthritis, and a wide range of behaviors, including brief situational depression, can be expected to occur. However, unusually intense or protracted reactions may require professional counseling.

Family Needs. The response of patient's family to the diagnosis of arthritis may also yield important information regarding the adjustment to illness. An understanding and supportive family can buoy and encourage the patient, but unsympathetic or overly protective families interfere with the patient's response to treatment. Relationships in the family may be disrupted by the effects of the illness, especially if the family member with arthritis can no longer fulfill a family role. If the patient and family are distressed by the effects of the disease, involvement in a support group or professional counseling may be necessary.

Social Isolation. Patients with arthritis may become socially isolated as inability to plan ahead or honor commitments discourages social relationships. The fatigue and unpredictability of arthritis frustrates the patient and confuses friends who may not understand the nature of the illness. Opportunities to socialize diminish and if prolonged walking or sitting is involved, the patient may not take advantage of the opportunities offered. An estimate of the number of social encounters the patient can recall from the past month may provide a rough picture of the patient's social activities.

Work. Work performance may be affected by arthritis, and information about the difficulties imposed by the disease can be valuable. Patients with control over the amount and pace of work seem to remain employed longer than patients with little influence on the flow of work.[4] Individuals with physically demanding and rigid jobs may be forced to seek other employment or stop work entirely. Vocational rehabilitation counseling is indicated for patients who must find less physically taxing work and can provide job training as well as assistance in job placement.

Informational Needs. Patients with arthritis will also need to learn how to manage independently some of the problems created by the illness. To do so they will require continuing information about arthritis and its treatment. Education of the patient is a key element of the rehabilitation program and in recent years has become a specialty of many health professionals. Since arthritis patients obtain information from many different sources, both professional and public, one professional should coordinate education efforts and act as a research person. (The implementation and benefits of patient education are discussed in chapter 25.)

ASSESSMENT OF ENVIRONMENTAL NEEDS

Transportation. Obstacles in the environment can pose considerable frustration for patients with arthritis. Lack of access to transportation may limit activity and encourage social isolation. Transportation vehicles may be inadequately prepared for passengers with crutches, walkers, or wheelchairs, and the use of public transportation may require long waits in bad weather.

Barriers.   Obstacles to independence exist in the home or office and are most accurately determined by a thorough home assessment or on-site job evaluation at the office. An occupational or physical therapist usually can provide an initial assessment and suggest simple modifications and more efficient organization of surroundings, but a rehabilitation engineer or others experienced in interior design must be consulted for actual structural changes. (See chapter 24.) Many simple changes, such as increased chair lift, reorganization of shelves, or rearrangement of furniture can be accomplished with minimal effort and justify a referral for environmental assessment.

Information obtained during the assessment of functional needs can reveal potential problems in independence and suggest the need for more specialized assessment. A detailed discussion of the purpose, techniques, and advantages of home or work assessment and modification appear in a later chapter.

ASSESSMENT TOOL

One format for an assessment tool is suggested in table 12.1. It follows the outline of the chapter and includes space for the patient to assess the severity of problems, along with the physician and nurse. The form is intended only to offer a starting point for organizing patient asessment and is in no way comprehensive. Several more detailed assessment tools that have been tested and refined are discussed in the literature,[5] and may provide greater assistance to the reader interested in comprehensive evaluation tools.

SUMMARY

Assessment is a continuing process and must be revised as patient problems and needs change. A variety of health professionals may contribute to the needs assessment.

Major needs of patients with arthritis can be grouped into the categories of: relief of pain, preservation of function, psychological adjustment to illness, and promotion of independence. Psychosocial factors may influence the outcome of the treatment program and warrant support from nurses, social workers, or psychologists. Education of the patient is an essential element of the rehabilitation program and deserves careful planning and review.

The information obtained from a needs assessment forms the basis of an individualized rehabilitation program.

REFERENCES

1.   Polley H, Hunder G. Physical examination of the joints, 2nd ed. Philadelphia: WB Saunders, 1978.

2.   Pigg JS. Nursing care of the hospitalized patient with rheumatic disease. In: Ehrlich GE, ed., Rehabilitation management of rheumatic conditions. Baltimore: Williams and Wilkins, 1980, ch. 5, pp. 76–103.
3.   Baum J, Figley B. Psychological and sexual health in rheumatic disease. In: Kelley et al., eds., Textbook of rheumatology. Philadelphia: WB Saunders, 1981, ch. 34, pp. 501–510.
4.   Yelin E, et al. Work disability in rheumatoid arthritis: effects of disease, social and work factors. Ann Int Med 1980; 93:551–556.
5.   Liang MH, Jette A. Measuring functional ability in chronic arthritis: a critical review. Arth Rheum 1981;24:1.

13

The Exercise Program

Betty A. Wickersham, B.S., R.P.T.

The physical therapy management of arthritis should be individualized according to the patient's response and the extent of the disease. A logical progression of physical therapy (PT) treatment is schematically represented by the pyramid in figure 13.1.

PYRAMID: FIRST LEVEL

The base of the pyramid is the solid foundation needed for treatment and requires accurate diagnosis and adequate referral to a physical therapist from the physician. This consultation should contain information about the patient that will aid in successfully planning, implementing, monitoring, and conducting a physical therapy program. For example, the amount of joint destruction that is known, the presence of subluxation, disc disease, or osteoporosis can all affect the kind of exercise given or stretching techniques used. The therapist also should be aware of the patient's drug therapy since the PT regimen often is built around the use of muscle relaxants and analgesics.

Depending upon information received from the referring physician, the physical therapy evaluation may range from a few questions regarding past treatment experiences and a cursory muscle and joint evaluation to a thorough examination of the patient, especially if the physician's referral includes only a diagnosis and basic treatment order. Regardless of the adequacy of the referral, a brief history should be taken by the therapist to gain insight into the following:

1. Patient's knowledge of disease.
2. Patient's expectations of outcome of treatment. Are they realistic? The therapist may need to help revise the patient's goals.
3. Family or work problems that may take priority over the physical therapy program. The therapist may have to help the patient solve home problems or even adapt the therapy program to fit the patient's life-style.

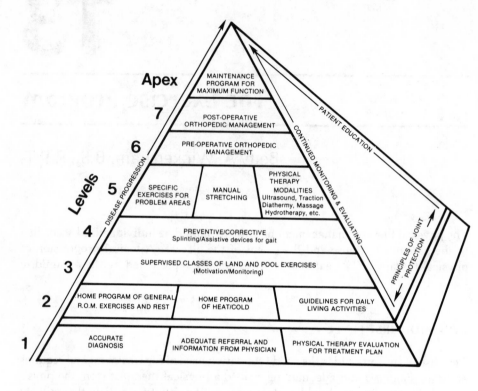

Figure 13.1. Physical therapy treatment pyramid.

4. The patient's past experience with physical therapy treatment. What helped? What did not?

5. Present exercise and activity programs. Were they given by a professional or self-initiated? The patient may be undertaking inappropriate exercise and activities on the advice of friends or family members. However, some self-initiated programs may be good, innovative programs that can be adapted as part of the overall program.

6. What other health care professionals does the patient see? The patient may be seeing an occupational therapist, a counselor, a podiatrist, or even another physical therapist. In order to best serve the patient and avoid confusion, the therapist must know what other treatments the patient is receiving and what is being taught by other members of the team. Lack of communication with other health team members including the physician may cause failure of the team approach.[1]

7. The patient's history of the past and present drug therapy. Osteoporosis with vertebral collapse may follow long years of inactivity or corticosteroid use. In such cases overzealous mobilization of osteoporotic bones can cause fractures. Another example includes knowledge of prescribed analgesic and

muscle relaxants that can then be used to the patient's advantage by timing the stretching and strengthening exercises to profit from the effects of the drugs.

If the physician's referral is not complete, then the therapist must do a thorough evaluation before beginning treatment. Along with the brief history just outlined, the therapist must know the status of all the major joints and related musculoskeletal structures to determine the ratio of exercise and rest, what kind of exercises are indicated, when splinting is necessary, when assistive devices are needed for gait, and what other specific problems need attention. The treatment plan should be flexible to allow for modification as the patient experiences remissions and exacerbations. This necessitates open communication between the physician and the therapist.

PYRAMID: SECOND LEVEL

The actual treatment regimen begins with the second level of the pyramid. Here the patient is taught a home program of range-of-motion exercises and how to schedule periods of rest and exercise. (The remainder of level 2 activities are discussed in other chapters of this book.)

Rest

The persistent, chronic pain of arthritis as well as the systemic effects of the disease itself results in fatigue.[2] In addition the drain on the patient's psychological resources adds to the problem of excessive fatigue.[3] The amount of rest needed for the patient with arthritis has never been agreed upon. In patients with systemic disease, fatigue increases with disease activity and decreases as disease activity subsides.[4] Melvin reports that the consensus of opinion is that patients with active, systemic disease need from 10 to 12 hours of rest per 24-hour period. Some physicians recommend this be broken down to 8 hours at night with two 1-hour rest periods during the day.[5]

Given commonsense guidelines, most patients can judge for themselves how to balance rest with their exercise program and other activities on a daily basis. However, guidelines of any kind should be regularly reinforced by every member of the health team. For the many patients with little flexibility in their daily schedules, taking one or two rest periods may not be possible. Rest periods may have to be altered to fit what the patient is willing or able to do (see chapter 22, on energy conservation).

The benefits of emotional rest have been documented when hospitalized patients improve without change of treatment. Many physicians feel this is due to the psychological rest from the daily emotional stresses the arthritis patient encounters at home and work.[6] Hospitalization for emotional rest may not be feasible, but referral to a family counselor knowledgable in arthritis management can bring about similar improvement.[3]

Inflamed joints may need more rest and protection from stress than bed rest provides. Simple splints worn at night or more complicated functional splints to wear during activity can provide rest and protection (see chapter 16).

Exercise

One of the most important aspects in the treatment of arthritis is the exercise program.[5,7,8] It has often been stated that exercise and rest are the cornerstone in the overall medical management of the disease. Unfortunately education regarding what kind of and how much exercise is frequently overlooked by the busy physician. If it is mentioned to them at all, patients may be given a list of exercises to do without regard to their particular needs or tolerance and without guidelines of any kind. Or they may be told simply to exercise daily for 15 or 20 minutes, with no other information being offered! It may not be until deformities occur and the patient complains of a loss of function that the physical therapist is called upon. Ideally, as soon as the diagnosis is made, the patient begins a supervised program of active range-of-motion exercises to be done at home. Depending upon the predisposing factors, some deformities and loss of range of motion will occur regardless of measures taken. However, many deformities can be prevented if discovered in time and others can be slowed down, minimizing loss of function.[9-11] Preventive measures usually are easier to implement than corrective measures.

Deformities and loss of function in arthritis are caused by changes in articular and periarticular tissues that are directly or indirectly related to the disease process.[12] Early tissue changes cause pain and stiffness that interfere with movement before there is actual, permanent loss of function. For example, accumulation of intraarticular fluid can cause excessive capsular tension resulting in stretch pain.[12] If this occurs, the patient is reluctant to move the joint and will hold it in a flexed position to relieve the capsular stretch, causing both the capsule and muscles to undergo adaptive shortening.[7] Muscle spasm around a painful joint may cause a feeling of stiffness with resulting loss of movement, or there may be reflex blocking of muscle action. If there is prolonged, fixed flexion of a joint, permanent shortening of the muscles occurs with loss of muscle strength. Ligaments and capsules may become stretched due to joint effusions and overgrowth of the synovium. This, along with abnormal alignment secondary to loss of articular cartilage, may cause subluxation leading ultimately to loss of function and deformity.[13]

There is no documentation to indicate that exercise programs can change the course of disease or prevent all deformities. However, by keeping muscle strength and joint range of motion as normal as possible without further damaging diseased intra- and extraarticular tissues, contractures can be prevented, other deformities slowed down, and much loss of function prevented or delayed.[14]

One of the misconceptions held by patients about the purpose of exercise is that the major benefit will be relief of pain. Some relief of muscular pain can be expected as weakened muscles become stronger through exercises. Some relief of pain may result as contracted tissues are stretched out. However, intraarticular pain caused by bone encroachment into soft tissue, stretched ligaments, or the invasion of the disease process into subchondral bone seldom is affected by exercise. Most patients who complain that exercises do not help are referring to pain. Patients need to understand that the primary purpose of an exercise program is not the relief of pain but to keep muscles and joints working as normally as possible, thus keeping the whole person functional.

Passive exercises, in which the therapist brings about the desired movement of the patient while the patient remains passive and relaxed, are seldom used in arthritis since acutely inflamed joints need to be rested. Only after the pain and inflammation have subsided are range-of-motion exercises begun. These may begin as passive joint motion but must then be gradually evolved into isometric and assisted exercises and finally into active exercises as soon as the patient can tolerate them in order to delay muscle atrophy and prevent joint contractures. Exercises are of three types: isometric, assisted, and active. Isometrics are a muscle-setting exercise in which there is no joint movement, but the muscle is tensed or contracted by the patient. Assisted exercises are so called because the joint is moved by the patient with the assistance of the therapist. In active exercise the patient alone moves the joint.

A combination of active range-of-motion exercises and isometric exercises can maintain muscle strength and improve range of motion. Studies have shown the benefits of such exercises. Three to four repetitions a day of moving a joint through its range of motion will usually maintain that range of motion.[14,15] One daily, brief, maximal, isometric contraction lasting from 1 to 10 seconds is sufficient to stimulate an increase in static muscle strength.[16,17] If limitations are present, range-of-motion exercises can increase range-of-joint motion.[5] The purpose of the exercise program is to preserve function by maintaining the present level of muscle strength and preventing disuse atrophy, maintaining the level of the range of motion, minimizing deformity, or increasing and improving the range of motion and muscle strength when necessary. Active range-of-motion exercises will not, however, necessarily relieve pain, develop normal muscle strength, or develop normal endurance.

The patient should be taught to take each major joint through its full range of motion. If possible, this is done as an active exercise. Assisted or passive motion may be used when pain or muscle weakness prevents active motion. Patient education should begin at this point as the patient is taught the rationale for each movement and the guidelines for pain. The uninformed patient may feel that an exercise program is inconsistent with what his joints are telling him.

Guidelines for Pain

The guidelines need to include information on how much pain and soreness are acceptable for the patient during the first few days of regular exercises. For instance, the patient should expect some extra pain and soreness on the first or second day and be aware that exercises may be somewhat painful while they are being done. But this should not cause alarm or stop the patient from doing the exercises. However, pain lasting more than 2 hours after the exercise or increased pain in the same joint the next day indicates the exercises should be decreased. The guidelines for pain are not only appropriate for an exercise program, but also for other types of physical therapy treatment that the patient might be receiving as well as for recreational activities in which he or she is participating.

Guidelines for Exercise

Usually, the patient is arbitrarily asked to perform each exercise ten times, although fewer might suffice. It has been demonstrated that repeated movement in the arthritic joint tends to cause increased inflammation.[7,18,19] Thus the number of repetitions must be balanced with the potential inflammatory response. Using ten repetitions as a general rule allows warm-up motion without undue inflammation before the patient tries for maximal stretching.

Finally, the therapist should teach the patient to change the exercise repetitions according to the way he feels. If it is a good day, the patient is encouraged to try ten repetitions. If it is a bad day with more pain and fatigue than usual, the number of repetitions can be reduced to three or four, which will maintain the joint range of motion. The patient's pain and fatigue level will change from day to day, even within the day itself.

Depending upon the patient's tolerance, the exercise routine is carried out at least once a day and usually no more than twice a day to avoid undue joint stress. The time of day when exercises are done depends upon the individual with best results occurring when he feels least tired and stiff. This is usually a few hours after getting up in the morning or after a warm shower. Some patients use exercises to limber up before getting out of bed while others exercise before retiring at night to get a more restful sleep and to awaken with less morning stiffness. People with degenerative arthritis may have too much pain later in the day, so they perform the routine in the morning.

The exercises should be taught in a logical order beginning with the patient in a supine position and ending in a sitting or standing position. This is generally easier for the patient to remember and to carry out. Movements should be done slowly and smoothly, with the patient concentrating on doing each individual movement precisely and correctly. Distraction by television, radio, or any other activity during the exercise period encourages patients to use poor exercise techniques.

The Patient's Self-test. In the early phase of arthritis there is usually very little limitation of joint range. As the disease progresses, mild tightness of the involved joints may go unnoticed by the patient. The patient who has been well instructed in a personal exercise program and is faithfully following the routine will be immediately aware of a discrepancy in joint range. By teaching the patient to use a gentle stretching force at the end of the range, even though painful, the limitation can usually be overcome. The range-of-motion program thus can be used by the patient as a self-test and monitoring device. Patients who find that they are losing range of motion and not gaining it back in a few days should seek help from either a therapist or a physician.

PYRAMID: THIRD LEVEL

No matter how well patients understand their disease and the importance of complying with a medical and physical program, they always need spot checks over an indefinite period of time to ensure compliance and to ensure that the program is meeting their needs and that the exercise are still being accurately done. The third level of the pyramid represents one method of reinforcing and motivating the patient while also monitoring the physical therapy program. Supervised classes of land or pool exercises on an as needed basis provide reinforcement and furnish the patient with a less expensive way of maintaining contact with members of the medical team. The classes also provide the physical therapist with a cost-effective method of supervising many patients at one time. Patients are encouraged to attend the ongoing classes periodically to check their own progress and technique and to give the therapist the opportunity to observe and help solve any arthritis-related problems. Patients may remain at this third level indefinitely as long as their conditions remain stable.

PYRAMID: FOURTH LEVEL

When a potential problem surfaces, the therapist notifies the physician and a decision is made as to whether the patient should return to a lower level of the pyramid treatment plan for reinforcement or move to the next level for more complex therapy. For example, if the patient complains that wrist and hand pain and weakness prevents performance of daily activities, the therapist may suggest static wrist splints or resting splints to reduce inflammation, to protect the wrist joints, and to improve grip strength.[21] If a weight-bearing joint flares, the use of a cane or crutches may be indicated.

PYRAMID: FIFTH LEVEL

If preventive measures of exercise and joint protection are not effective, and there is loss of range of motion, decreased muscle strength, increased pain, and gradual loss of function, then the fifth level of the pyramid needs to be considered. Here intervention by the therapist on a one-to-one basis with the patient is most important. Complete communication between the referring physician and the therapist as to the status of the patient's disease is essential. Also the physician, therapist, and any other members of the arthritis team who are involved need to discuss and determine possible reasons for the increased impairment.[23,24] The reevaluation of the patient at this point may reveal noncompliance with medications, emotional problems, a change of jobs, a difficult home situation, increased physical activity, or worsening of the underlying disease. One or all of these situations can affect the patient's response to the disease. If further physical therapy is to be effective, there must be at least an attempt made to resolve these problems. The team approach is important at all levels of the pyramid. Two types of interventions at this level are exercises for specific problem areas and manual stretching.

Specific Exercises for Problem Areas

The patient with arthritis often exhibits extra-articular problems such as some low back conditions, tendinitis, bursitis, and faulty posture. Such problems require additional specific exercises in conjunction with the range-of-motion program but must be adapted to the anticipated response of the underlying disease process. For example, low back exercise may be made more difficult by hip or knee involvement from inflammatory arthritis. Involvement of the cervical spine must be considered carefully. Instability of the atlantoaxial articulation should preclude some neck exercises such as rotation (dropping the chin to the chest and rolling the head).[15] The specific exercises for frozen shoulder syndrome must avoid stressing the elbow, wrist, and hand joints. The use of an overhead pulley may cause an inflammatory response in an involved elbow joint.

Considerable skill, foresight, and thought are required on the part of the therapist before recommending strengthening exercises for problem areas. Studies have shown that repeated, resistive, joint motion aggravates joint disease.[7,18,19] Therefore isometric exercise may be the best approach to strengthening. Brief, maximal, isometric exercise against resistance with minimal yielding can strengthen muscles weakened by arthritis and can usually help avoid flare-up of arthritis inflammation.[16,17] Swezey recommends exercise sessions twice daily if the patient is unable to contract muscles maximally.[15] Edstrom demonstrates that isometric contractions at two-thirds maximum capability held for at least 1 to 6 seconds once daily are an optimal physiologic stimulus for static strengthening.[16,17] To what degree muscle strength gained from isometric exercises can affect endurance and active muscle strength has not been fully studied. But isometrics can improve static muscle strength, maintain muscle tone, circulation, and reflex proprioception until the patient can tolerate more vigorous active exercises.[21,22]

There is often a difference of thought among rheumatologists regarding the safety of using repetitive, resistive, active exercises with arthritic joints. Problems with resistive exercise can perhaps be avoided if the guidelines for exercise are carefully followed. If the exercise cannot accomplish its purpose without joint flare-ups, then comprises have to be made. It might be helpful to remember that the person with joint disease does not require normal muscle power and endurance to function within the limits of his disease.

Manual Stretching

When a patient is unable to maintain maximum range of motion through a regular home exercise program, then specialized help on a one-to-one basis with manual stretching is indicated before the patient returns to the supervised class. If the loss of range of motion is due to an exacerbation, exercise of any kind must wait until the inflammation subsides. During this time, as inflammation regresses, gentle passive motion and isometric exercise (to the point of pain) preceded by superficial heat should be instituted. Gradual assisted motion, when tolerated, is started, then progressed to active motion. Loss of motion cannot always be regained depending on the underlying cause. (See table 13.1.)

Before stretching to increase joint range, the therapist must know the condition of the joint and periarticular tissues (See table 13.1.) Where there is joint capsule contracture or muscle shortening due to spasm or fibrosis, passive stretching by the therapist is necessary. Some investigators advocate heat to improve the stretchability of tissue,[25] although preceding passive stretching maneuvers with heat are not always necessary.[26] The analgesic effect and muscle-relaxing properties of heat may cause the therapist to overstretch sensitive tissue producing more pain and inflammation a few hours later.[26]

The sooner passive stretching is begun, the greater is the chance of success. Gentle stretching is often all that is needed to restore muscle length and release soft tissue adhesions. Passive stretching must not aggravate joint pain and inflammation. Many therapists try to do too much too quickly.[15] The evidence that repeated joint motion aggravates joint disease necessitates that passive stretching sessions must be kept short. A few painless warm-up motions and three or four *gentle* stretching maneuvers for each joint are about the maximum amount of stretching most patients can tolerate. To increase joint range, these stretching sessions are best done daily, but are not always possible for the outpatient. An every-other-day program, tapering off gradually while the patient supplements the stretching with a home exercise program, seems to work rather well.[19]

Forceful stretching can cause tendon rupture, joint subluxation, or fracture of osteoporotic bones.[19] If the patient resists the stretching pressure, the therapist should relax the pressure somewhat, wait, then try again. There are many techniques for stretching painful joint tissue, and therapists all have their own special methods, such as the hold-relax technique, the rhythmic-stabilization technique, or having the patient practice deep breathing with stretching on the exhalation phase. Not all patients respond to the same techniques.

Table 13.1. Predisposing Factors Leading to Loss of Range of Motion

Problem or Condition	Results in Loss of Range of Motion	Suggested Physical Therapy Procedures
Joint effusion or overgrowth of synovium	Pain from stretching of ligaments and filling of capsule joint space (effusion or overgrowth of synovium)	Static splinting to reduce swelling and inflammation
		Mild superficial heat to reduce swelling
	Pain sensitive synovium pinched between articulating surfaces	Passive range-of-motion (ROM) exercises with gentle manual traction to prevent pinching effect
Ligamentous laxity with joint subluxation	Pain from overstretched ligaments and capsule	Strengthen weaker muscles around the unstable joint *before* subluxation occurs
	Joint destruction resulting in malalignment with soft tissue stress pain	Splint joint during stress activities
	Prolonged pull of stronger muscles against weaker ones	Teach principles of joint protection
Joint capsule contracture	Loss of elasticity due to tissue changes caused by inflammation	Persistent gentle manual stretching
	Joint capsule is pain sensitive to stretch	Traction may help
	Synovial adhesions from inflammation	Ultrasound before, during, after stretching
	Faulty posture habits	Correct postural faults
		Severe contractures may be corrected by surgery

Changes in the articulating surfaces	Loss of normal articulating surfaces causing malalignment and stressing pain sensitive tissues Friction of bone on bone causing heat leading to pain	Passive ROM exercises with manual traction to maintain ROM Active ROM exercises to maintain muscle strength Functional splinting (see chapter 16) Joint-protection techniques
Loose bodies in the joint (joint mice)	If loose body is caught between articulating surfaces, movement may be blocked mechanically or by pain from pressure on subchondral bone	Passive motion with manual traction to pull articulating surfaces apart and perhaps displace obstruction
Bony spurs (osteophytes)	May block normal articulating range and impinge on pain sensitive soft tissue or on the nerve itself	Temporary splinting; cervical collar when cervical spine is involved Exercises in painless ROM to maintain strength Traction
Muscle spasm from pain syndrome of bursitis, tenosynovitis, and tendinitis	Long-standing muscle spasm or tension leading to changes in tissue elasticity resulting in muscle shortening	Heat, relaxation techniques, passive ROM graduating to active range in painless arc Muscle strengthening after acute stage
Muscle fibrosis or atrophy	Loss of muscle elasticity Loss of muscle strength Stretch pain	Gentle stretching and strengthening exercise Use of deep heat or ultrasound to facilitate stretching

Table 13.1. (continued).

Problem or Condition	Results in Loss of Range of Motion	Suggested Physical Therapy Procedures
Tendon displacement or rupture	Loss of normal muscle power due to abnormal change in angle of pull	Splint during stressful activities to preserve joint integrity
	Loss of muscle function due to tendon rupture	Principles of joint protection
	Development of contractures with resulting stretch pain	
Fearfulness of pain, moving, creaking joints, abnormal feeling of joints	Apprehension—patient does not know that it is all right to move a painful or creaking joint, or he may not be aware that he is not moving the involved joint	Patient education in regard to joint anatomy and coping with pain
		Assisted range of motion graduating to active range

Sources: This table was derived from information found in *Arthritis and Allied Conditions,* 8th ed., by JL Hollander and DJ McCarty. Philadelphia: Lea and Febiger, 1972; *Textbook of Rheumatology,* WN Kelley, ED Harris, S. Ruddy, and CB Sledge, eds. Philadelphia: WB Saunders, 1981; *Arthritis and Physical Medicine* by S. Licht; and *Clinical Rheumatology,* M Mason and HLF Currey, eds. Philadelphia: JB Lippincott, 1973.

PYRAMID: SIXTH AND SEVENTH LEVELS

When specific joint problems cannot be solved conservatively and surgery is indicated, presurgical patient education by the therapist can help improve patient participation and cooperation.[14,26] The postsurgical physical therapy routine is explained and exercises are taught a few days before surgery. Most physical therapy departments have routine pre- and postoperative procedures they implement depending upon the kind of surgery and the surgeon's preference. If a weight-bearing joint is involved, a preoperative gait analysis helps the therapist train the patient to use a more normal gait after surgery.

PYRAMID: APEX

Whenever the patient's condition stabilizes and his specific needs have been met to the best of the health team's ability, the physician may consider putting the patient on a physical therapy maintenance program. This should be a mutually agreed upon regimen between physician, therapist, and patient. Pool and land exercise classes may need to be continued indefinitely but with regular reevaluation by the therapist. If the patient is faithful about following home exercises, only periodic reevaluation may be necessary. Because the therapist spends more time, more frequently with the patients, problems are often brought to the therapist's attention more quickly than to the physician's. With the patient on a monitored maintenance program, the physician can be assured that the patient will be encouraged to adhere to an exercise regimen and be referred back to the physician if a problem arises.

SUMMARY

Therapeutic exercises cannot change the course of rheumatic disease, nor can any exercise routine prevent all deformity. However, with pertinent information from the physician regarding the patient's history and physical examination, the physical therapist can plan, implement, and monitor an exercise program designed to keep the patient, within the limits of the disease, as functional as possible. To be successful, the exercise regimen must be planned with the full participation of the referring physician, the therapist, and the patient.

Once started, the physical therapy program must be monitored to assure patient compliance and periodically reevaluated for needed changes in management. Patient education begins with the patient learning the guidelines for pain and exercise, what exercises are appropriate and how to do them, and how much and what kind of rest is needed. With an ongoing program of proper physical therapy, the patient may be maintained at this maximum level of function indefinitely.

REFERENCES

1. Epstein C. Breaking the barriers to communication on the health team. Nursing 1974;4(9):65–68.
2. Melvin JL. Rheumatic disease: occupational therapy and rehabilitation. Philadelphia: FA Davis, 1980.
3. Ziebell B. Wellness: an arthritis reality. Dubuque, Iowa: Kendall/Hunt, 1981.
4. McCarty DJ. Clinical assessment of arthritis. In: McCarty DJ, ed., Arthritis and related conditions, 9th ed. Philadelphia: Lea and Febiger, 1979.
5. Fred DM. Rest versus activity in arthritis and physical medicine. In: Licht S, ed. Arthritis and physical medicine. Baltimore: Waverly Press, 1969.
6. Engelman EP. Conservative management of rheumatoid arthritis. In: Hollander JL, McCarty DJ, eds., Arthritis and allied conditions, 8th ed. Philadelphia: Lea and Febiger, 1972.
7. Swezey R. Essentials of physical management and rehabilitation in arthritis. Arthritis Rheum 1974;3(4):349–368.
8. Calabro JJ, Wykert J. The truth about arthritis care. New York: David McKay, 1977.
9. Ehrlich CE. Total management of the arthritis patient. Philadelphia: JB Lippincott, 1973.
10. Rodnan GP. Primer on the rheumatic diseases. Atlanta: Arthritis Foundation, 1973.
11. Flatt AD. Correction of arthritic deformities in the lower extremity and spine. In: Hollander JL, McCarty DJ, eds., Arthritis and allied conditions, 8th ed. Philadelphia: Lea and Febiger, 1972.
12. Freeman MAR. Operative surgery in the rheumatic diseases. In: Mason M, Currey HLF, eds., Clinical rheumatology. Philadelphia: JB Lippincott, 1970.
13. Insall J. Reconstructive surgery and rehabilitation of the knee. In: Kelley WN, Harris ED, Ruddy S, Sledge CB, eds. Textbook of rheumatology. Philadelphia: WB Saunders, 1981.
14. Gerber LH. Principles and their application in rehabilitation of patients with rheumatic diseases. In: Kelley WN, Harris ED, Ruddy S, Sledge CB, eds. Textbook of rheumatology. Philadelphia: WB Saunders, 1981.
15. Swezey RL. Rehabilitation aspects in arthritis. In: McCarty DJ, ed., Arthritis and related disorders, 9th ed. Philadelphia: Lea and Febiger, 1979.
16. Liberson WT, Asa MM. Further studies of brief isometric exercise. Arch Phys Med Rehab 1959;40:330–336.
17. Machover S, Sapecky HJ. Effect of isometric exercise on the quadriceps muscle in patients with rheumatoid arthritis. Arch Phys Med Rehab 1966;47(11):737–741.
18. Ehrlich CE. Rest and splinting. In: Total management of the arthritis patient. Philadelphia: JB Lippincott, 1973.
19. Swaim LT. The orthopedic and physical therapeutic treatment of chronic arthritis. JAMA 1934;103(21):1589–1592.
20. Kamenetz HL. Massage, manipulation and traction. In: Licht S, ed., Arthritis and physical medicine. Baltimore: Waverly Press, 1969.
21. Brewerton DA, Lettin AWF. The rheumatoid hand and its management. In: Parry CBW. Rehabilitation of the hand, 3rd ed. London: Butterworth, 1973.
22. Edstrom L. Selective changes in the size of red and white muscle fibres in upper motor lesions and parkinsonism. J Neurol Sci 1970;11:537–554.

23. Fordyce WE. Behavioral methods in chronic pain and illness. St. Louis: CV Mosby, 1976.
24. Ziebell E, Wickersham EA, Boyer JT. Team arthritis consultation. Phys Ther 1981;61(4):519–522.
25. Swezey R. Arthritis: rational therapy and rehabilitation. Philadelphia: WB Saunders, 1978.
26. Kottke FJ, Pauley DL, Ptak RA. The rationale for prolonged stretching for correction of shortening of connective tissue. Arch Phys Med Rehab 1966;47(6):345–352.
27. Wickersham EA, Schweidler H, Clay C. Arthritis: a self-study manual for physical and occupational therapists. Unpublished paper. Southwest Arthritis Center, Tucson, Ariz., 1982.

14

Hydrotherapy

Betty A. Wickersham, B.S., R.P.T.

Hydrotherapy is the use of water, more particularly warm water, in the treatment of disease. The total body or any of its parts may be treated with water. It is not known how long water has been used as a therapeutic agent. Perhaps it originated when our prehistoric ancestors bathed their sore and aching bodies in a thermal spring and discovered the soothing effect of the heated water. Certainly the ancient Romans popularized it with their public baths. Today the increasing number of swimming pools and hot tubs provides more opportunity than ever for water therapy.

HEAT

Heat is probably the most widely used physical agent for the relief of pain. Lehmann and DeLateur have stated that muscle spasm and pain can be relieved by heat through the reduction of spindle sensitivity to stretch.[1] This effect may be only temporary. In some cases, perhaps due to the interruption of a vicious cycle of pain, spasm, and more pain, the relief of pain and stiffness may last long enough to permit the patient to begin an exercise program that will eventually alleviate the cause(s) of the muscle spasm and pain.[1] Backlund and Tiselius also found that heat application reduces joint stiffness by producing changes in the viscoelastic properties of joints, whereas cold increases stiffness.[2] (The use of heat and cold are discussed in detail in chapter 15.)

Heat and Water

Innumerable arthritis patients have reported that heated baths have helped them cope with their stiffness and pain. Health professionals frequently encourage patients to take warm baths or showers, use warm hand soaks, and apply towels rung out in hot water to enable them to better carry out activities of daily living, particularly their prescribed exercises.

Even though subjective responses are impressive, the use of heated water has not been found to have any significant effect on the progression of joint destruction,[3] nor is there much scientific evidence to support the enthusiastic claims of hydrotherapy, even though much has been written about the history of water therapy, the geochemistry of water, the physiology of body water, the psychology of water therapy, and the penetration of mineral water and general properties of water. One study found that although the body's response to immersion in up to 40°C of heated water has an initial stimulating effect, there is a general muscular relaxation as the body adapts to the temperature.[4]

The range of painless movement increases more rapidly in warm water than with any form of dry heat treatment. This is attributed to the conductivity and thermal capacity of water; that is, heat moves more rapidly from warm water to objects in it or surrounding it than from any other substance and water absorbs or gives off more heat for each degree of resultant change in its own temperature than any other known substance.[4]

Besides its conductivity and thermal capacity, water has two other properties that make it helpful in treating the arthritis patient—buoyancy and viscosity.[4] Buoyancy is the upthrust action of water acting at right angles to the surface. Viscosity is the resistance offered by a fluid to a change of its form. Both buoyancy and viscosity can be used in exercises of the following types:

1. Passive motion. Body buoyancy produces movement while muscles relax.
2. Assisted motion. Motion through gentle contraction of the muscles caused by the upthrust action of water.
3. Supported motion. Moving a body member in the horizontal plane will have the support of the water.
4. Controlled resistance. The faster a body member moves through the water, the greater is the tension the muscle must develop. The patient can control the force of the resistance by increasing or decreasing the speed of this movement. This kind of controlled resistance is less likely to cause a flare-up of the joint disease.[5-7]

HYDROTHERAPY EQUIPMENT

In medium-size physical therapy departments, whirlpool baths of two or three designs may be found. A small tank, raised to table height off the floor is used to immerse the elbow, wrist, and hand (figure 14.1). A large, deeper tank is used to treat the foot, ankle, and knee. If a tank is large enough, a seat may be placed in it and the patient can be immersed up to the shoulders in a somewhat cramped sitting position (figure 14.2). A long, shallow tank that is only a few inches off the floor will accommodate a patient sitting with legs extended (figure 14.3).

The larger physical therapy department may have a Hubbard tank in which

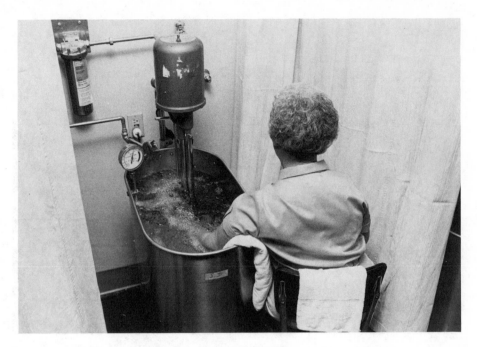

Figure 14.1.   Whirlpool bath for hydrotherapy of elbow, wrist, and hand.

the patient can be fully immersed in a supine position (figure 14.4). This tank is shaped to allow underwater movement of the extremities in all ranges and is equipped with overhead cranes that lift the patient on a stretcher from the bed or litter into the water. Whirlpool baths and usually Hubbard tanks have underwater mechanisms that force a mixture of air and water into the bath, creating the effect of an underwater massage. Both water temperature and the force of the agitators can be regulated.

The choice of water temperature and treatment time is determined partly by trial and error and depends primarily on patient tolerance and comfort. Treatment time is usually 20 minutes although there is no documented evidence that that is the most effective treatment duration. It has been demonstrated that the systemic temperature of some people will rise rapidly when the body is immersed in heated water. The usual temperature of the whirlpool bath is 43.3 °C if only an extremity is treated. If the whole body is immersed in either the whirlpool or Hubbard tank, the temperature must be lowered to 38 °C or less depending upon the patient's response to hot water. With total immersion, body temperature may be raised if the water is 40 °C or higher.[1] Caution is advised when setting the water temperature because some patients have poor heat tolerance and complain of dizziness and nausea after being in heated water a short time. Moreover, for reasons that are not fully understood, some patients demonstrate more joint and

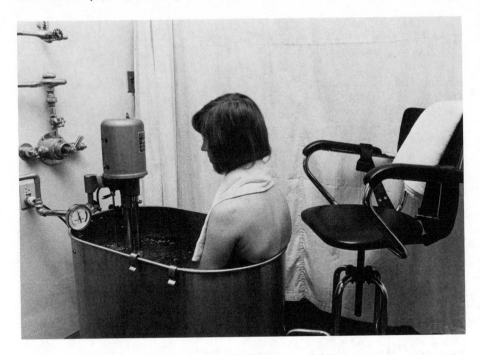

Figure 14.2.   Whirlpool bath, with seat, for treatment of foot, ankle, and knee.

muscle stiffness and pain the day after such treatment. Patients with compromised cardiovascular states may actually develop coronary insufficiency or congestive heart failure if body temperature is raised, increasing cardiac work. Keeping the water at body temperature may prevent these problems and, although the heating effect is negated with the lowered temperature, the patient will still benefit from the underwater exercise.

Whirlpool baths primarily provide temporary relief from pain and stiffness of involved joints and muscles in order that specific out-of-water exercises may be tolerated more easily (see chapter 13). It is important to remind the patient that the use of these treatments is only a means to an end. Whirlpool baths will not ensure maintenance or improvement of function, although they will make exercising easier. The heat and gentle massage action of the underwater agitators in the whirlpool or the Hubbard tanks helps to relax muscles and relieve pain. This effect encourages the patient to move the joints through a greater range of motion.

The therapeutic pool is becoming more popular in large rehabilitation facilities (see figure 14.5). Resembling an ordinary indoor swimming pool, it has various depths and is constructed to accommodate stretcher, wheelchair, and ambulatory patients by means of lifts, ramps, and steps. Depending upon the size of the pool, a number of patients may be in the water at the same time. Thus the

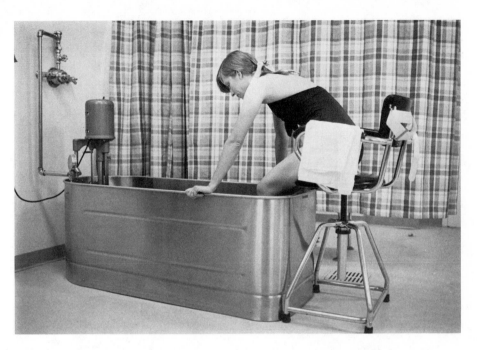

Figure 14.3.   LoBoy whirlpool bath for patient seated with legs extended.

water temperature cannot be regulated for the individual but is set to meet the needs of the majority of the patients being treated. This may be as low as 35.5°C or as high as 38°C.

The therapeutic pool incorporates the benefits of the whirlpool and the Hubbard tank (heat, massage, and limited underwater exercise) with the advantage of more space and depth for unlimited underwater exercises plus numerous activities, including gait training and swimming. For the arthritis patient, traditional range-of-motion exercises must be carried out regardless of pool exercises given for other specific problems. Supplemental pool exercises, such as coordination and balance exercises with various movements performed on vertical, horizontal, and rotary planes, may be gradually added to the traditional range-of-motion program. Recreational therapeutic activities can be adapted to the water for the arthritis patient. Playing volleyball with a soft beach ball or watery versions of badminton, basketball, and ring toss encourages patients to increase their range of motion with little joint stress. Sudden or strenuous efforts should be avoided though. Jogging in shoulder deep water places only minimal stress on weight-bearing joints and uses muscles and coordinated movements that otherwise cannot be experienced by the severely involved patient on dry land. One exercise physiologist has observed that water jogging may also be a means of providing cardiopulmonary exercise for some arthritis patients.[8] Gait training also

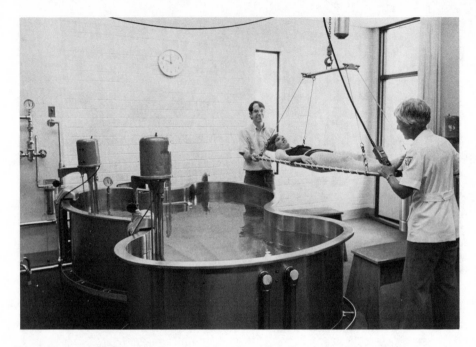

Figure 14.4.   A Hubbard tank equipped with overhead cranes to lift patient from bed or litter into the whirlpool.

can be started early in water without fear of stressing joints because of the buoyancy of the water. This is important, especially in postsurgical patients who have had orthopedic procedures on weight-bearing joints.

Psychological factors of pool therapy should not be overlooked. Pool therapy may help restore confidence to the postsurgical patient who may ambulate without fear of falling, give the patient the stimulation of social contact, provide the opportunity to compete (on the same level as others) in recreational activities that are forbidden on land, and help the patient to release pent-up emotion through physical activity.

PRESCRIPTION FOR HYDROTHERAPY

In addition to the area to be treated, the prescription for hydrotherapy should include:

The type of hydrotherapy
Whirlpool

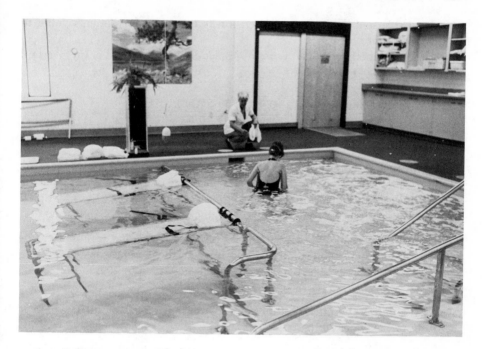

Figure 14.5.   The therapeutic pool.

Hubbard tank
Pool

Water temperature

Treatment duration

Treatment frequency

The kind of exercise or activity to be done during or after the treatment

Precautions and special considerations. For example, cardiac conditions, diabetes, open wounds, age of patient, phase of disease, and degree of inflammation.

POOL THERAPY GUIDELINES

For the chronically ill or disabled patient, underwater exercise is one of the most practical means of maintaining activity and preventing further physical deterioration if used in conjunction with prescribed dry land exercises.[4] Pool therapy needs to be closely supervised, however, to prevent patients from overexercising and becoming exhausted. This same supervision is necessary for patients going to health spas and hot tubs.

Although there are few written procedures for pool therapy, certain guidelines should be observed.[7]

Pool temperature should range from 35.5°C to 38°C.

Depending upon the problem, each patient is seen two or three times weekly (daily is too exhausting).

At the first session, the patient stays in the water 15 to 20 minutes. There are no formal exercises, but the patient is encouraged to move about and use the hydrojets. Patients are cautioned that letting the force of the water play directly on a painful joint may cause an increase in stiffness and pain.

During the second session the patient's response to the first session is evaluated. If no undesirable effects were produced, the patient is instructed in a few basic exercises. The patient stays in the water about 20 minutes.

At the third session the response to the second session is evaluated. If there are no undesirable effects, a full exercise program is carried out. The patient stays in the water 20 to 30 minutes.

At the fourth and all following sessions, patient reaction is always used as a guide as the exercise program increases in complexity. One hour is usually the maximum length of stay in the water.

Unfavorable reactions to pool therapy may be caused by heat sensitivity; overexercise, leading to an increase in joint and muscle pain and stiffness; an increase of extremity volume due to heating, which may produce joint stiffness; and overheating, which may increase fatigue and lower blood pressure.

As the patient reaches a plateau in improvement of joint range, muscle strength, and endurance, the number of sessions per week may be reduced to twice weekly, once weekly and finally on an as needed schedule to ensure that the maximum level of improvement is being maintained. (See table 14.1 for a list of water exercises.)

Using the Backyard or Neighborhood Pool

For some people with joint involvement, swimming even in an unheated pool can be beneficial. With jogging, walking, or bicycling excluded from the exercise program of many people with arthritis, a pool can be a resource for maintenance of aerobics as well as strengthening and stretching exercises. The arthritis patient should be cautioned to avoid excessive chilling and fatigue while in the unheated pool.

Table 14.1. Water Exercises[a]

Exercise (Instructions to the Patient)	Benefit
1. Walk across the pool	
a. Trying to kick the toe out of the water at each step (the goose step).	This stretches the hamstring muscle and improves balance.
b. Sideways taking wide steps.	This stretches hip adductors and strengthens hip abductors.
c. Backward, looking over the left shoulder at the bottom of the left foot, then over the right shoulder at the bottom of the right foot.	This stretches the neck rotators, hip flexors, quadriceps, dorsiflexors of the foot and strengthens the gluteus maximus and hamstrings. It also improves balance and coordination.
d. Backward, looking over the left shoulder at the bottom of the right foot, then over the right shoulder at the bottom of the left foot.	This stretches and strengthens the same muscles as the above exercise. It also strengthens trunk rotation and improves balance and coordination.
2. With the back against the wall of the pool, clasp the hands around one knee and pull it to the chest. Repeat with the other knee.	This stretches the low back and gluteal muscles and stretches the hip into flexion.
3. With hands under the water	These exercises stretch and strengthen the intrinsic muscles of the hands and improve range of motion and coordination of the hands.
a. Try to touch fingertips to the base of the fingers.	
b. Try to touch fingertips to the heel of the palm.	
c. Make a fist.	
d. Stretch the fingers straight.	
e. Spread the fingers apart.	
f. Make an "O" with the thumb and each finger.	
4. Circle the wrists in one direction then the other.	This improves wrist range of motion.
5. Bring the fingertips to the shoulder; then straighten the arms all the way out.	This improves elbow range of motion.
6. Rotate the shoulders forward, upward, and back; then reverse.	This improves scapula range of motion.
7. Arms at the sides, palms facing hips (water is shoulder deep).	These exercises increase shoulder range of motion in abduction and forward flexion.

Table 14.1. *(continued).*

Exercise (Instructions to the patient)	Benefit
a. Raise arms sideways to shoulder height.	—
b. Leading with thumb, raise arms forward, up, and overhead. Stretch tall.	—
8. With the right arm across the chest, take the right elbow in the left hand and pull it across the chest as far as possible, stretching the shoulder. Repeat the process with the left arm in a similar fashion.	This improves shoulder forward flexion, horizontal adduction, and internal rotation.
9. Hands clasped behind neck, or if unable, hands in front of ears. Attempt to touch elbows together in front of face; then pull elbows apart as far as possible.	This exercise improves shoulder abduction, internal and external rotation, and elbow flexion.
10. Clasping hands behind back, pinch shoulder blades together; then keeping elbows straight, push hands away from body. Hold for count of five; then relax.	This exercise helps to strengthen the upper back and improves the range of motion of the shoulder into extension and strengthens the tricep muscles.
11. Hold one foot forward with knee straight and curl toes under; then pull the foot way back. Repeat with the other foot.	This improves range of motion of the toes into flexion and extension and stretches the gastroc muscle.
12. Rotate one ankle through a complete circle in one direction, then the other direction. Repeat with the other ankle.	This improves the range of motion of the ankle.
13. Grasp one ankle from behind with hand and try to touch that heel to the buttocks. Repeat with opposite heel.	This improves the knee flexion and stretches hip flexors.
14. Walk across the pool	
a. Forward on tip toes.	This strengthens plantar flexors.
b. Backward on the heels.	This strengthens the dorsiflexors.

Table 14.1.   *(continued).*

Exercise (Instructions to the Patient)	Benefit
15. Stand with back against the wall and hands on hips. Tucking chin under, slowly turn your head and look over right shoulder, then left shoulder.	This improves neck rotation.
16. Keeping chin tucked under, tilt head to the side as if to pour water out of ear. Repeat, tilting head to the opposite side. (Do not forcibly bend the head backward or forward.	This improves lateral bending.
17. Crouch down in the water so shoulders are underwater. In slow motion, using arms and legs as normally as possible, jog across the pool.	This improves overall coordination and balance.

[a]In general, water exercises are designed to improve the range of motion of the major joints, strengthen the muscles around these joints, and improve balance and coordination. For additional information see chapter 13 for guidelines on prescribing exercises for the arthritis patient.

SUMMARY

The compatibility of the properties of heat and water make hydrotherapy an effective tool for the temporary relief of arthritis joint and muscle pain and stiffness. Hydrotherapy treatment preceding exercise encourages a greater range of motion. Used in the form of warm baths or showers in the home, hydrotherapy will help the patient better cope with the activities of daily living. The whirlpool bath, Hubbard tank, or therapeutic pool should be considered when the area to be treated involves several joints or the entire body. Pool therapy uses the physical properties of water not only to relieve pain and stiffness but also to provide a variety of exercise possibilities without stressing joints.

REFERENCES

1.   Lehmann JR, DeLateur B. Heat and cold. In: Licht S, ed., Arthritis and physical medicine. Baltimore: Waverly Press, 1969.
2.   Backlund L, Tiselius P. Objective measurements of joint stiffness in rheumatoid arthritis. Acta Rheum Scand 1967;13:275.
3.   Mainardi CL, Walter JM, Spiegel PK, Goldkamp OG, Harris ED. Rheumatoid

arthritis: failure of daily heat therapy to effect its progression. Arch Phys Med Rehab 1979;60:390–392.

4. Chepesvik MW. Underwater exercises in neurologic lesions. In: Licht S, ed. Medical hydrology. New Haven, Conn.: E. Licht, 1963.

5. Lowman EN. Physical medicine and rehabilitation. In: Steinberg CL, ed., Arthritis and rheumatism: the diseases and their treatment. New York: Springer, 1954.

6. Harris R. Hydrotherapy in arthritis. Practitioner 1972;208:132–135.

7. Wickersham EA. Guidelines for pool therapy. Unpublished paper. Southern Arizona Chapter, Arthritis Foundation, Tuscon, Ariz., 1974.

8. Wilmore J. Living easier and better. Paper presented at the Arizona Academy of Arthritis Health Professionals annual meeting in Tucson, Ariz., January 1982.

15

Therapeutic Heat and Cold

Barbara Figley Banwell, P.T., M.A.

The use of heat and cold as curative or palliative modalities can be viewed as almost instinctual to man and other animals. Licht[1] has reviewed an extensive and fascinating literature describing the history of thermal therapy as it has evolved from simple snow and radiant sunlight to the more modern artificial sources. Although the first use of heat and cold cannot be documented, it is easy to imagine primitive man seeking comfort for injuries from cool streams or warm sand. The earliest sources of warmth included radiant heat of sunlight, hot mineral springs, and fire. Cold sources were plentiful in cool climates with snow and ice, but even in warm climates such as Rome, snow was compacted and brought from the mountains to be stored in caves for later use. Practical sources of artificial heat and cold were developed only after the discovery and development of electricity in the mid 1800s.

The history of the use of heat and cold therapy for arthritis is well described. The terms that translate to "rheumatism" and "joint pain" occur in many accounts of early medicine. Hippocrates[2] discussed the use of hot water bottles for sciatica and Aurelianus[3] recommended hot water baths for the same ailment. Pliny[4] recommended hot air treatments for arthritic joints, although van der Heyden[5] preferred cold baths. Presumably because of the frequency of rheumatic disorders throughout time, the number and variation of heat and cold modalities for arthritis has flourished. Looking back through the years one cannot ignore the persistent theme of man seeking relief by the use of natural thermal modalities.

THE BASIS OF TREATMENT

The sources of pain in arthritis should be identified in order to understand the use of heat and cold. In the joint itself, free nerve ending pain receptors are found in the capsule and synovium and are stimulated by pressure and chemical substances. Subchondral bone contains pain receptors thought to be responsible for much of the early pain in osteoarthritis. The cartilage itself has no nerve supply, and therefore, although a prime site of pathology, it is not a source of pain. The ligaments, tendons, and muscles have numerous types of receptors, many of which transmit pain impulses and are responsive to stretch. Pain is primarily transmitted by two nerve fiber systems: small myelinated A-delta fibers (sharp, localized pain) and unmyelinated C fibers (dull, aching pain). Deep aching pain is more likely to result in reflex contraction and spasm of nearby skeletal muscles.[6] The pain experienced in arthritis doubtless arises from many different sources that cannot be singled out but may well vary with specific pathologies. The pain of rheumatoid arthritis, for instance, may be due to chemical and pressure stimulation of pain receptors as a result of inflammation; the pain of osteoarthritis may result from changes in the subchondral bone and pressure on nerve branches by osteophytes.

HEAT

Temperature Changes Due to Heat Therapy

Few correlations have been established between the degree of comfort or relaxation achieved and the actual change in tissue temperatures. No "critical temperature" has been established for relief of muscle spasm or pain, although Clarke found an optimum muscle temperature of 27°C for maintenance of sustained muscle contraction.[7] However, the question of intra-articular temperature (IAT) in the management of joint diseases is important to investigate. The relationship of intra-articular temperature to joint inflammation was introduced when Horvath and Hollander demonstrated a positive correlation between IAT and clinical activity in rheumatoid arthritis.[8] They determined the temperature of the normal knee joint at rest to be 32°C, where the rheumatoid arthritis inflamed joint rose to 36°C. Hollander and Horvath measured temperature changes in normal and arthritic knee joints produced by several common heat therapy treatments.[9] Temperature rises ranged from 0.6°C (infrared) to 4.8°C (shortwave diathermy) and varied with different joint diseases. These studies have not been repeated comprehensively on other joints. Harris and McCroskery demonstrated that the 3° increase from 33°C to 36°C in the reaction temperature of an in vitro preparation produced a threefold to fourfold increase in the rate of collagen fibril lysis by rheumatoid synovial collagenase.[10] It was then suggested by Feibel and Fast that thermal therapy that increases the intra-articular temperature of inflamed joints might enhance joint destruction.[11]

Mainardi et al. studied the effect of daily heat therapy over 2 years for patients with rheumatoid arthritis.[12] Seventeen patients with classic or definite rheumatoid arthritis and symmetrical hand and wrist involvement applied heat to the randomly selected experimental hand twice daily for 30 minutes with an electric mitt at 40°C. The other hand served as the control. Intra-articular temperature (IAT) of the metacarpophalangeal joint in a normal individual was measured at almost 40°C 22 minutes after the mitt was applied. IAT was not measured on the rheumatoid arthritis patients. The parameters measured included joint tenderness, swelling, and grip strength. Progression of proliferative lesions was assessed by x-ray analysis at entry, 1 year, and 2 years. The differences between values for the experimental and control hand were calculated for all measures. Differences in tenderness, swelling, and strength were not statistically significant. Lesions observable by x-ray were not observed to progress. Most (16 of 17) patients liked the heat therapy, and nearly as many (11 of 17) felt it was helpful on a day-to-day basis. However, the majority (9 of 17) felt it neither alleviated morning stiffness nor had long-term benefit.

SUPERFICIAL HEAT MODALITIES

Superficial heat modalities primarily produce temperature rises at the skin and subcutaneous tissues, although electric mitts at 40°C have raised the intra-articular temperatures at the MCP joint to almost 40°C within 30 minutes.[12] Most superficial heat modalities require only simple equipment and can be used in the home. Among the most commonly used in arthritis are moist heat packs, paraffin, incandescent bakers or lamps, and electric heating pads or mitts. Most studies of effectiveness conclude that the relief provided is temporary, but if not expensive or used excessively, the modalities are not harmful.

Moist heat packs (Hydrocollator packs) are silica-gel filled canvas packs heated in a hot water bath at 170°F (77°C).[13] They are wrapped in towels for application and stay warm about 30 minutes. Four to six areas can be treated at once. The packs may be removed for observation during treatment. The affected area is accessible for exercise following treatment. Hot packs are practical and economical in home or clinical settings.

Incandescent bakers or infrared lamps provide dry, noncontact heat. These lamps can be set up in a variety of positions and observation during treatment is possible. With care, this luminous heat source may be used in the home.

Paraffin wax baths were first introduced in the English hospital of Colonel Littlewood in 1918, after he heard of tannery workers immersing their hands and feet in vats of wax for relief of pain.[14] The technique spread quickly and has had continued popularity as an arthritis treatment.

Present techniques use paraffin wax that is melted, mixed with mineral oil, and kept in a heated container at about 51°C. The hot liquified wax is applied directly to the skin either by brushing it on or dipping the body part in and out until several layers accumulate. The part is then either immersed in the wax bath for 20–30 minutes or wrapped in towels. Abramson studied the temperature effects of three techniques.[15] Procedure A was 12 dips, a 30-minute wrap, then removal; procedure B was 7 dips, a 30-minute immersion, then removal; procedure C was 7 dips, 30-minute immersion, 30-minute wrap, then removal. The temperature increases in skin and muscle (4 centimeters deep) differed with each technique. Procedure C was most effective in producing and maintaining temperature rise, yielding a 2.4°C rise in muscle at 30 minutes with some increase maintained until 90 minutes after the initial dip. This procedure is lengthy, cumbersome, and limited in the number of joints that can be treated per session. Procedure A, the most common clinical technique, produced at 30 minutes a 4.4°C rise in skin temperature with a 1.0°C rise in muscle temperature, which returned to baseline at 90 minutes. Intra-articular temperatures, clinical effects, and subjective responses were not measured. Neither Abramson nor Stimson correlate temperature changes or treatment techniques with clinical effectiveness.[16]

Many patients and therapists feel that paraffin treatment provides a good preparation for exercise. Gallagher et al., however, found that preexercise paraffin treatments made no significant differences in the range of motion, flexibility, strength, or pain relief achieved in a group of twenty subjects.[17] It is doubtful that this one study is adequate to discount a traditional treatment that is regarded positively and has no documented detrimental effects in the majority of rheumatic disorders. In systemic sclerosis (scleroderma) the significant basic microvascular pathology may well contraindicate paraffin treatments since the mechanism to dissipate heat is impaired and impaired oxygen delivery to tissues increases the possibility of tissue necrosis.

DEEP HEAT (DIATHERMY)

Deep heat or diathermy modalities produce temperature rises in the deeper tissues (4 centimeters and more) by conversion of various forms of energy to heat within the body. Three types of diathermy are shortwave, microwave, and ultrasound. With musculoskeletal disorders shortwave and microwave are used primarily to achieve muscle comfort and relaxation whereas ultrasound is also used over fibrous areas to facilitate extensibility in preparation for stretching. However, the ability of diathermy to raise intra-articular temperature must signal some caution in its use with joint disease.[10] Ultrasound can elevate intra-articular temperatures to as much as 43.5°C.[18] Many reports of successful use in rheumatoid arthritis and ankylosing spondylitis were made before the questions of inflammation and temperature were raised. Diathermy is indicated for secondary muscle spasm in arthritis but should probably be limited to areas where diseased joints will not be heated. All diathermy modalities require special equipment and trained personnel so they are not suitable for home use. Long-term studies on the effect of various diathermy modalities on joint structures would be helpful in clarifying the many questions about these treatments.

COLD

Effects

Cold is defined as being the abstraction of cold, the process by which cold is abstracted, and the sensation that occurs when cold is abstracted.[2] Although its early use is described in medical literature, most of the scientific study of its effects occurred after 1930 when its military and economic consequences were recognized. Lewis observed three stages of superficial vasoconstriction that occur after exposure to cold.[19] He also described the "hunting reaction," a vasodilatation that follows the initial vasoconstriction and occurs when the skin temperature reaches 10°C. Cubbold described a similar vascular response in the intra-articular tissues when they were cooled.[20] The primary physiologic effects of local cooling are alternating vasoconstriction and vasodilatation, reduction of local metabolic rate, and alteration in nerve condition and nerve receptor firing rates.[21]

Cold has been used effectively to reduce both pain and muscle spasm in arthritis patients. Various forms for treatment such as ice, ice and water mixtures, commercial chemical cold packs, and ethyl chloride spray are available. Most people with arthritis can carry out treatment in the home while observing safety precautions.

Cold produces an initial sensation of pain followed by numbness. If the joint itself is to be cooled, the packs should be placed directly over it, avoiding areas where major nerves such as peroneal or ulnar are close to the surface.[22] Bierman and Friedlander found that tissues 4 centimeters deep were cooled about 2°C in 30 minutes.[23] Most recommendations indicate that cold should be applied until numbness occurs but discontinued if severe discomfort occurs. Hypersensitivity to cold has been observed in a few patients, so careful observations should be made during the first few treatments. Exposure to or treatment with cold is clearly contraindicated in patients with Raynaud's phenomenon or other vascular pathology.

Unfortunately there are few well-designed studies to provide guidelines for cryotherapy in rheumatology patients. Hogan et al. demonstrated positive outcomes from the use of ice packs on rheumatoid knees and Rembe found positive trends from the use of ice water baths in the postsurgery rheumatoid hand.[24,25] There are also many opinions regarding the relative clinical superiority of heat and cold modalities. The patient's acceptance of one treatment over another will be an important determinant of the mode selected.

EVALUATION OF HEAT AND COLD

The scientific evaluation of heat and cold modalities has not been carried out with the same enthusiasm as their production and distribution. There is not sufficient information at this point to make definitive statements about the consequences of heat or cold therapy in arthritis. More information is needed about several factors: the baseline intra-articular temperature of all joints, normal and arthritic, at rest and activity, the effect of various thermal modalities upon the intra-articular temperature of normal and arthritic joints, the relationships of intra-articular temperature to perceived sensation of pain and comfort, and the long-term effects of therapy. The serious evaluation of heat and cold modalities in well-designed studies continues to present a challenge to even the best investigator. This evaluation becomes more of a professional obligation to those in the field of rheumatology when the enormous utilization by patients is recognized. The evaluation of minimum cost for maximum effectiveness should be a prevailing activity for health professionals who recommend these modalities.

SUMMARY

Heat and cold modalities are used in the management of arthritis to relieve pain and decrease muscle spasm. Both modalities act directly and indirectly on local nerve and vascular supplies but do not appear to affect the basic joint pathologies. Although information is available on temperature changes of skin, subcutaneous tissue, and muscle during heat and cold treatments, little is known of the intra-articular temperature changes of arthritic joints. Few well-designed studies of the clinical effects of heat or cold that exist indicate that the modalities provide temporary comfort of sufficient merit to justify use. In chronic conditions techniques should be chosen that can be eventually used in the home without professional supervision, although initial treatment should be with professional guidance.

REFERENCES

1. Licht S. History of therapeutic heat. In: Therapeutic heat and cold. Baltimore: Waverly Press, 1965.
2. Bierman W. Therapeutic use of cold. JAMA 1955;157:1189–1192.
3. Aurelianus C. On acute and chronic disease. Translation by IE Drabkin. Chicago: 1950.
4. Severin MA. De la Medecine efficace. Geneva: 1668.
5. Mac-Auliffe L. La Therapeutique physique d'autrefois. Paris: 1904.
6. Lenman JAR. Clinical neurophysiology. Oxford, England: Blackwell Scientific Publications, 1975, p. 83.
7. Clarke R, Helton R, Lind A. The duration of sustained contractions of the human forearm at different muscle temperatures. J Physiol 1958;143:454–473.
8. Horvath SM, Hollander JL. Intra-articular temperature as a measure of joint reaction. J Clin Invest 1949;28:469–473.
9. Hollander JL, Horvath SM. The influence of physical therapy procedures on the intra-articular temperature of normal and arthritis subjects. Am J Med Sci 1949;218:543–548.
10. Harris ED Jr, McCroskery JA. Influence of temperature and fibril stability on degradation of cartilage collagen by rheumatoid synovial collagenase. New Eng J Med 1974;290:1.
11. Feibel A, Fast A. Deep heating of joints: A reconsideration. Arch Phys Med Rehab 1976;57:513.
12. Mainardi C, Walter J, Spiegel P, Goldkamp O, Harris ED. Rheumatoid arthritis: failure of daily heat therapy to affect its progression. Arch Phys Med Rehab 1979;60:390–392.

13. Hydrocollator. Chattanooga Corp. Chattanooga, Tenn.

14. Humphris FH. Melted paraffin bath. Brit Med J 1920;2:397–399.

15. Abramson DJ, Tuck S, Chu LS, Agustin C. Effect of paraffin bath and hot fomentations on local tissue temperatures. Arch Phys Med Rehab 1964;45:87–94.

16. Stimson CW, Rose GG, Nelson PA. Paraffin bath as a thermotherapy: an evaluation. Arch Phys Med Rehab 1958;39:219.

17. Gallagher L, Eshleman J, Schumaker HR. A controlled study of the effects of paraffin baths on the rheumatoid hand. Presented at 1980 Annual Scientific Meetings, Arthritis Foundation, Arthritis Health Professions Section, Atlanta, 1980.

18. Lehmann JR, DeLateur B. Therapeutic heat and cold in arthritis. In: Licht S., ed. Arthritis and physical medicine, vol. 2. Physical Medicine Library. New Haven, Conn: Elizabeth Licht Publisher, 1969.

19. Lewis T. Observations on some normal and injurious effects of cold upon skin and underlying tissues. Brit Med J 1941;2:795–797.

20. Cubbold AF, Lewis OJ. Blood flow to the knee joint of the dog: effect of heating, cooling and adrenaline. J Physiol 1956;132:379–383.

21. Fox RH. Local cooling in man. Brit Med Bull 1961;17:14–18.

22. Drez D, Faust D, Evans JP. Cryotherapy and nerve palsy. Am J Sport Med 1981;9:256–257.

23. Bierman W, Friedlander M. The penetration effect of cold. Arch Phys Ther 1940;21:585–592.

24. Hogan N, Lockard J, Utsinger P. Cryotherapy in the treatment of intractable knee pain in patients with rheumatoid arthritis. Presented at 1981 Annual Scientific Meetings, Arthritis Foundation, Arthritis Health Professions Association, Boston, June 1981.

25. Rembe EC. Use of cryotherapy on the post-surgical rheumatoid hand. Phys Ther 1970;50:19–23.

16

Splints, Braces, and Casts

Melinda S. Seeger, B.S., O.T.R.

The orthotic management of the rheumatic disease patient is one of the most rewarding and yet frustrating experiences occupational therapists encounter in their careers. Because of the complexities of the rheumatic diseases the number of therapeutic absolutes is limited. There continues to abound a large amount of subjective information on the efficacy of various therapeutic measures. Some border on folklore old wives tales and need to be dispelled.

RESULTS OF REST AND IMMOBILIZATION

The use of rest, both systemic and local, has traditionally been advocated in the treatment of rheumatic disease patients. The efficacy of the use of this technique has been substantiated by a variety of basic research and clinical studies.

The effect of a rest program of 13 hours a day with sedentary activity for the remaining time on hospitalized rheumatoid arthritis patients was compared with a control group of patients treated on an outpatient basis on whom there were no physical restrictions.[1] At the end of the 4-week period the hospital in-patient group showed significant lessening of pain severity, severity and duration of morning stiffness, joint tenderness, and increase in grip strength, while in the out-patient group no significant improvement was observed in any of the parameters measured.

In another hospitalization rest program for rheumatoid arthritis patients two groups were compared.[2] In the first there was a minimum of 22 hours of bed rest per day for 4 weeks followed by at least 18 hours in bed during an additional 6-week period. This regimen was compared with the control group of patients who had 8 hours of bed rest at night and were permitted ad lib activity within the hospital. Although the active group was allowed ad lib privileges, their activity level was significantly less than that possible in an unrestricted out-of-hospital environment. The two patient groups were matched for size, age range and mean, sex, and duration of rheumatoid arthritis. This study reported no significant difference in the amount of improvement in the two groups after 10 weeks' time. However, improvement in grip strength, sedimentation rate, walking time, ring size, and number of tender joints occurred in both groups. In the majority, improvement was gradual and punctuated by occasional exacerbations. In the active group of 22 patients, 11 patients were better, 7 unchanged, and 1 worse. By contrast, in the rest group of 20 patients (2 patients were dropped from the study, one for medical reasons and one for noncompliance), 10 improved and 10 were unchanged when evaluated for grip strength, walking time, and joint range of motion. Any deterioration of a significant level occurred in the physically active group.

The use of bed rest with immobilization has also been compared with the use of bed rest alone on 68 rheumatoid patients over a 4-week period.[3] At the end of 4 weeks, complete immobilization was ended in the rest group and thereafter both groups were treated similarly. As in the previous study, the range of movement and functional capacity improved in both groups. Also the disease activity (as defined by changes in sedimentation rate, hemoglobin, joint and systemic involvement) diminished more in the group with the most immobilization or restriction in activity. Following this study no joint ankylosis was seen in either group. The final assessment of these patients done 6 months after admission to the study showed that in the areas of functional capacity, disease activity, and strength of grip, the patients who had the 4 weeks' immobilization were doing better than the control group.

Additional clinical studies on the immobilization of rheumatoid patients' wrists and hands[4] and bilateral knee joints[5] in plaster casts resulted in similar conclusions. Effective pain relief and control of disease activity were obtained in both instances and a full range of motion was rapidly regained in the immobilized joints. It is interesting to note that the patients whose hands were immobilized experienced flares in other joints during the period of the study; however, the immobilized joint never flared even when moderate flares were occurring in other parts of the body.

Evaluation of 8 rheumatoid arthritis patients in a study of the efficacy of the use of the Futuro wrist brace showed 87.5 percent noted improved activity and decrease in day pain, and 75 percent noted relief of night pain. There was an average of 48.9 percent increase in grip strength in these patients.[6]

Further evaluation of patients with traumatic nerve lesions,[7] hemiplegia,[8,9] and polio[10] who subsequently developed rheumatoid arthritis indicates that the paralyzed extremity was unilaterally spared the sequelae of the arthritis, again indicating the effect of imposed rest or immobilization on the development of the rheumatoid deformities.

Additional activity produces synovial fluid volume increases and in the instance of one rheumatoid arthritis patient this correlated positively with the production of blood-stained fluid when walking.[11] This may be a factor in "synovial loading," which has been postulated to increase the incidence of tendon and bone damage.[12] Studies concerning the mechanical influence of activity on the joints of rheumatoid arthritis patients found a definite correlation between the degree of physical activity and development of cystic erosions, probably occurring as a result of raised intra-articular pressure forcing synovial fluid or granulation into the substance of the medulary bone.[13-15]

Intra-articular temperature increases of up to 2.1°F have been shown as a result of simple passive non-weight-bearing exercises.[16,17] This increased temperature may accelerate cartilage destruction and bony erosions.[18]

In recent animal studies immobilization of an extremity from 6 days to 6 weeks resulted in proteoglycan aggregation defects that were not improved by the addition of active or passive range-of-motion exercises without joint loading during the immobilized period. The defect was reversible within 2 weeks; however, it is possible that the use of the involved joint before the reversal of the biochemical changes could lead to cartilage damage.[19,20] A subsequent study suggests that this defect occurs in human joint cartilage as well as canine cartilage.[21]

Thus prolonged complete immobilization of a joint may not be advisable from a biochemical standpoint; however, the previously quoted studies indicate that this is not necessary to obtain the desired alteration in disease activity. Additionally, partial weight-bearing may be indicated if the lower extremity is immobilized.

MECHANICAL FACTORS—ANATOMICAL AND PATHOLOGIC CONSIDERATIONS

To a great extent successful orthotic management of the rheumatic disease patient is dependent upon a clear understanding of the pathological basis of deformity and of the passive and dynamic forces that effect joint position. In rheumatic diseases where synovitis is a factor, the synovitis undermines the stability of the joint. The effusions and synovial proliferation stretch the capsule and loosen ligamentous attachments. The erosion of cartilage results in laxity of the joint capsule as the joint space narrows. The muscle forces are no longer restricted, and their alignment may shift. Their altered pull may lead to abnormal positioning of the joint. Once a deformity develops due to joint laxity, it tends to progress and is probably irreversible. Studies of the incidence and of the anatomy and pathomechanics of joint involvement in rheumatic diseases are dealt with in detail in a number of publications.[22-37]

Preventive Trouble Shooting

Multiple factors are responsible for the success or failure of an orthotic program with the rheumatic disease patient. Awareness of these factors by the physician and the therapist and attention to the ones that are alterable or controllable can greatly increase the chance of the program's success.

The very nature of the rheumatic diseases frequently makes the establishment of a definitive diagnosis a slow process. Even within a defined disease entity, the onset of symptoms may be insidious or abrupt, the disease course may vary from mild and limited to severe and chronic, and the physical and psychosocial functional abilities of the patient may vary widely. To that extent within the area of physical functioning obvious deformity may not correlate positively with the patient's degree of discomfort or functional level; conversely, minimal deformity or physical changes may be the precursor of far greater involvement if not treated.

In addition to the disease-specific peculiarities within the rheumatic diseases, a multiplicity of instructional deterrents may complicate therapy and affect the patient's compliance with a splinting program. Uncertainty regarding the course of the disease, chronic pain, and the side effects of the pharmacological agents are but a few of the factors that may interfere with the patient's program.

Because of the potential physical, psychologic, and socioeconomic consequences of chronic rheumatic diseases, it is imperative that both the physician and the occupational therapist involve the patient and the patient's family or significant others (the "patient group") in all stages of treatment planning. The goal is to provide the necessary input and receive feedback and also make sure the patient group fully understands and concurs with the objectives, scope, and duration of the splinting proposed.[38,39]

This is but the beginning of the education of the patient group, which should be an ongoing part of any splinting program. Throughout the splinting program it is important that the physician and the therapist share mutual goals and objectives as this agreement can be a source of support and reassurance that are a key to patient compliance.

Evaluation and reevaluation of the patient forms the basic framework for the formulation of the orthotic treatment plan. This baseline information must also be acquired if there is to be any objective evaluation of the results of the splinting program. Although not discussed in detail in this chapter, it is assumed that this evaluation is an integral component in all phases of the splinting process and that immedite, intermediate, and long-range goals are set.[40] Due to the fluctuating physical sequelae of the diseases it is important that the evaluations be consistent and appropriate. They should be consistent in the time of day in which they are administered. For example, many patients feel stiff in the morning but may have much better motion in the early afternoon. Thus measurements done on the same patient at varying times of the day may yield very different results and therefore be useless in the evaluation of the efficacy of the splinting program. Additionally, evaluations must be appropriate to the activity required of the patient or the function being tested. There is no benefit of doing a midday evaluation of a functional splint to be used when dressing in the morning as this may not represent the patient's actual functional ability earlier in the day. Consistency and appropriateness are also necessary for effective timing of a patient's treatment sessions.

Awareness of the patient's overall functional status in addition to specific range-of-motion considerations is also important to the success of a splinting program. Immobilization of a joint or joints in a patient with a systemic problem or already compromised activity may impair the patient's functioning to the extent that he or she will not comply with the splinting program. A screening form or evaluation quickly establishes functional deficits or problems and assists in determining the need and appropriateness of the orthotic program. Table 16.1 lists some factors very likely to affect the success of a splinting program for a rheumatic disease patient.

MATERIALS AVAILABLE—THE PROS AND CONS

Unless working with splinting materials routinely, the wide variety of choices available can be confusing to therapists and physicians alike. Luckily a number of publications and references available deal with this subject in great detail.[41-43]

It would be ideal if one material could be adapted to all situations and functions. This is not yet the case, however, and may never be so due to the scope of the splinting needs. Thus a wide range of materials is available for both commercially made and individually fabricated orthotics (see table 16.2). Each has its own advantages and disadvantages as well as proponents and opponents.

Ultimately the choice of a preferred material is subjective and varies according to multiple factors. Table 16.3 describes some of the routine factors one may want to consider when choosing a material. Low-temperature thermoplastic materials are probably the most frequently used type of material in occupational therapy clinics. They have a number of advantages and some disadvantages. Among the advantages are ease of fabrication, ease of adjustment (they are remoldable), light weight, ease of cleaning, and gas autoclavability. Moreover, the thermoplastics are cosmetically acceptable, usually nontoxic, radiolucent, and some may be worn in water. Disadvantages are fewer: these materials are more expensive than some others; they can deform with heat; they are less resistant than some other materials; and they require some prior experience on the part of the fabricator.

Table 16.1. Components of Screening Form or Evaluation

Activities that are difficult
Fatigue factor (end of day)
Pain. Where?
Range-of-motion limitations. Where?
Accommodation. Substitution patterns?
Sleep patterns. How many hours per night? Naps?
Vocation; avocation
Responsibilities
Potential physical assistance—"patient group"
Assistive equipment used—past or present (splints, adaptive equipment, canes, etc.)
Previous treatment by a therapist
Cognitive status

Table 16.2.   Splinting Materials

Splint Materials
  Light forming
  Metal and thermoplastic
  Metal (rigid or dynamic)
  Cloth, elastic, vinyl
  Plaster
  Thermoplastics
    High-temperature (250°–350°F)
    Moderate-temperature (175°–250°F)
    Low-temperature (140°–160°F)
Pressure-distributing Materials—Padding
  Foam (open and closed cell)
  Moleskin—minimal thickness
  Elastomere
Strapping
  Velcro/Duravel
  Webbing
    Cotton
    Nylon

Table 16.3.   Considerations in the Choice of a Splinting Material or Splint

Use situation (vocation/avocation)—heat, water, contraindications, etc.
Resiliency or flexibility required for splints—resting, functional, or corrective
Location and extent of problem area—status of skin, sensation, etc.
Duration of use
Setting in which the orthosis is applied or fabricated. Equipment available—clinic or office
Technical skills of the occupational therapist or physician
Immediacy of need
Cost
Need for splint modification or adjustment
Cosmesis
Ability or need of patient to apply and remove splint independently
Allergies or sensitivity to materials

SPLINTING TYPES

The most common terms used to describe the types of splints, braces, and casts also define their purpose. The three main groups are the resting, the functional, and the corrective orthoses. These splints are defined and their purpose and specific considerations outlined in table 16.4. These categories of splints are by no means exclusive; thus a resting splint might in certain instances serve very well as a functional splint and vice versa.

Table 16.4.   Categories of Splints

Type	Definition	Purpose	Specific Considerations
Resting	Applied during periods of *inactivity* to *immobilize* the involved joint or joints.	Relieve pain Decrease inflammation Prevent development of contractures Maintain proper hand position Decrease or alleviate symptoms of nerve entrapment Support ligaments and joint capsules stretched by the disease process	Acutely position the joint or joints in a pain-free position with the least intra-articular pressure[50] Modify as patient's physical status changes
Functional ("working")	Applied during periods of *activity* to *immobilize* or *protect* the involved joint or joints and the surrounding muscles.	Relieve pain Support unstable joints Accommodate for muscle weakness or atrophy Compensate for/or position deformities that limit function Protect from further damage Assist in controlling inflammation Protect against nerve entrapment or tenosynovitis	Splint only joint/joints involved without limiting mobility of others Consider effect of splinting on other joints in the body—stress transmitted to other joints may aggravate symptoms, because these splints are usually worn in public

Table 16.4. (continued).

Type	Definition	Purpose	Specific Considerations
Corrective ("dynamic")	Applied during periods of *inactivity* to *mobilize* involved joint or joints.	Modify soft tissue contractures (realign or correct)	Apply early for best results Small joints most amenable (elbows traditionally very difficult) Gentle prolonged pressure most effective[45-49] Potential for harm to patient great if not well monitored Should see significant results within 3 weeks if it is going to be successful

SPLINTING PRINCIPLES

The potential to do damage exists with any type of orthosis, although it is probably greater with dynamic splints. Hence a splinting program should be carefully monitored and undertaken only under the direction of a qualified occupational therapist who has experience in orthotics. The wearing schedule for the orthosis should be individually determined for each patient and this should be based on both general and patient-specific principles.

Because each patient responds differently, it is a general principle that splints or braces be applied for a limited period of time initially and then checked and rechecked by the patient and therapist during this period for undesirable side effects. Patient-specific considerations to be aware of when determining the wearing schedule for an orthosis should include patient's orthopedic, vascular, neurological, and cognitive status.

The number of hours a splint should be worn also depends, upon both the stage of the patient's disease and the type of splint prescribed. In general a *resting* splint applied during the acute phase of disease activity is worn continuously except for brief periods of exercise or essential functional activities such as eating or personal hygiene. As the patient's physical activity increases during the subacute phase, resting splints continue to be worn in areas where disease activity has not diminished significantly. Resting splinting in the chronic stage of rheumatic disease is used primarily as a protective and preventive measure, as in splinting wrists with carpal tunnel syndrome or joints where there is subluxation or dislocation.

A recent study has shown surprisingly high patient compliance in wearing full-hand bilateral resting splints (62 percent).[44] The patients appeared to self-regulate their splint wearing appropriately, using the splints more during exacerbations or persistent inflammation and less when their symptoms remitted. Their primary reason for wearing these splints was pain relief. Stiffness and range of motion were not affected by the use or nonuse of hand splints during the period of this study.

By definition *functional* splinting would not be used in the acute phase of the disease process, but during activity in the subacute and chronic phases of rheumatic diseases. The duration of the functional splinting depends upon the severity and duration of the pain the patient experiences during activity, and the potential for further deformity if the joint is left unprotected.

In *corrective* splinting, actual realignment or elongation of the collagen tissue is facilitated. This has been found to be most effective when the splint is worn at less than maximum tension over a prolonged period of time (1 hour or more) and must be individually adjusted to the patient's tolerance and the severity of the condition one is attempting to correct.[45-49] The corrective splint may be applied at any stage of disease activity; however, this splinting is most effective in correcting or modifying soft tissue problems when applied soon after the onset of the deformity. Effective corrective splinting should show significant results within 3 weeks' time. If improvement is not achieved within this period, continued splinting is usually not productive.

When determining the positioning of joints in splints in the presence of synovitis or acute inflammation, it is important that the occupational therapist consider the possible side effects of positioning on intra-articular pressure and formation of deformities. The position of minimum discomfort for patients appears also to be the position of minimum intra-articular pressure on the patient's joint:

Wrist	=	0° flexion/extension and 0° ulnar/radial deviation
Elbow	=	30°–75° flexion
Shoulder	=	0° flexion/extension and rotation and 30°–65° abduction
Ankle	=	15° plantar flexion with subtalar joint in midposition
Knee	=	25°–60° flexion
Hip	=	30°–65° flexion, 15° abduction, and 15° external rotation[50,51]

Thus awareness of these positions of least intra-articular pressure is of use to the therapist in determining not only the position of minimum pain for the patient but also the position in which the least damage is being done to the joint capsule and supporting structures during the *inflammatory* phase of a disease.[12-15] The positioning of the wrist is additionally complicated by the fact that placing it in extension above zero degrees may create a subluxating force.[52] This must be weighed against the potential for the development of ankylosis in an undesirable position in a couple of the rheumatic diseases (psoriatic arthritis and ankylosing spondylitis).

In the instance when joint ankylosis is inevitable, consideration must be given to placing the patient in the optimal functional position. This varies with individuals according to their particular life-style, although there are general rules; for example, in the hand, wrist dorsiflexion is essential for power grasp and conversely some degree of wrist flexion is required for fine prehension activities. Thus if both wrists are involved, the dominant is usually positioned for prehension and the nondominant for power grasp.

EXAMPLES OF SPLINTS SUCCESSFULLY USED

As preferences in splinting materials change so does the preference for specific splints and techniques. Extensive descriptions of the most commonly used splints and braces are available to physicians and therapists.[53-55] The traditionally used splints deserve continued consideration as do the newer materials and techniques.

Hand

Resting splints for the hands are now commercially available in styles which are easily adjustable without special equipment. (See appendix 16.1 for a list of suppliers.) When the whole hand is involved, a functional position resting splint may be utilized. However, it is seldom that a patient should be fitted with bilateral functional-position resting splints, because these have the effect of incapacitating the patient for even the most basic functional activities (figures 16.1, 16.2). Instead one may wish to leave the thumb and/or fingers free in the least involved hand to manage call lights and the like (figures 16.3, 16.4) or alternate the use of the splint to the most symptomatic hand. Resting splints may also be fabricated for individual digits (figure 16.5).

Although very lightweight and comfortable, the volar wire-foam splints may not be durable enough for *functional* purposes. The Futuro splint (figure 16.6) and the Currie Medical splint (figure 16.7) are very practical. The latter splint, of metal-braced vinyl with acrylic lining, is very well accepted by the patients and provides excellent support. Individually fabricated thermoplastic splints are advisable when more support is required or in cases difficult to fit (figures 16.8, 16.9). The ulnar deviation splint in figure 16.9 is useful in acute through chronic rheumatic disease stages.

Individually fabricated thumb splints provide pain relief when CMC

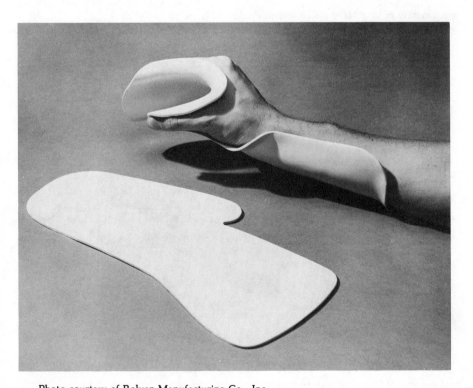

Photo courtesy of Rolyan Manufacturing Co., Inc.
Figure 16.1.   Functional-position resting splint.

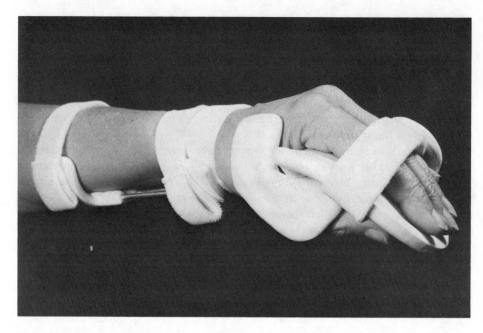

Photo courtesy of LMB Hand Rehabilitation Products, Inc.
Figure 16.2. Functional-position resting splint Volar wire-foam wrist and finger orthosis.

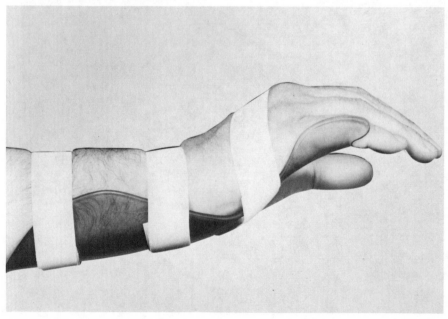

Photo courtesy of Camp International, Inc.
Figure 16.3. Camp-Koch metacarpophalangeal-type splint.

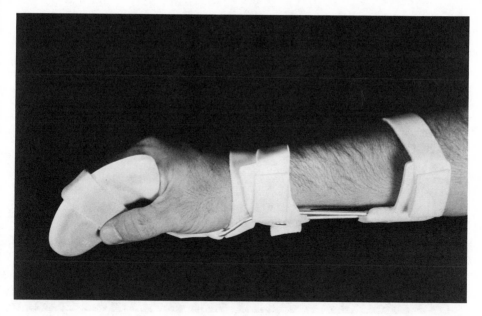

Photo courtesy of LMB Hand Rehabilitation Products, Inc.
Figure 16.4.   Volar wrist and finger orthosis.

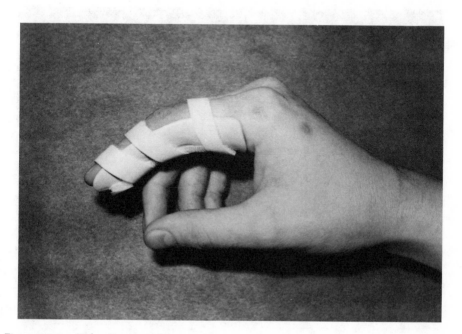

Figure 16.5.   Volar finger trough.

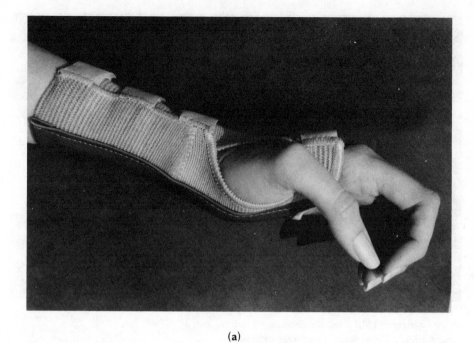

(a)

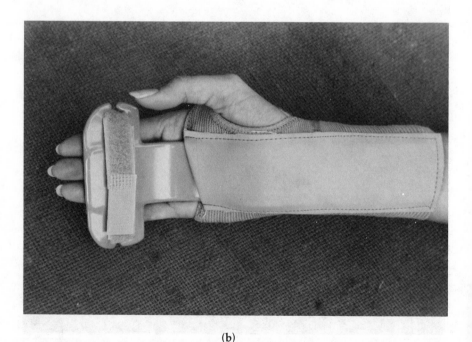

(b)

Figure 16.6. Futuro wrist splint. Volar view shows removable finger supports.

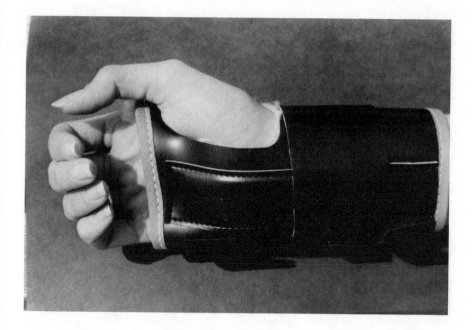

(a)

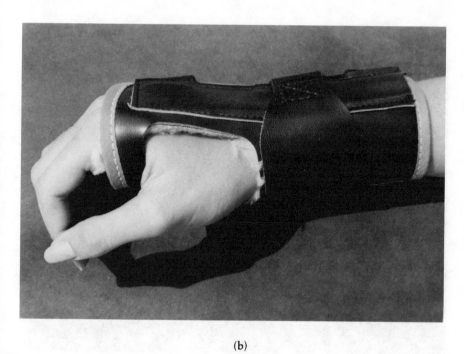

(b)

Figure 16.7.   Currie wrist splint.

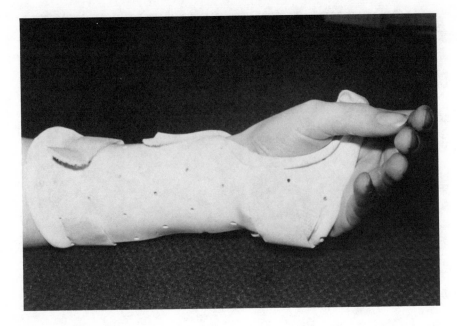

Figure 16.8.   Volar wrist splint.

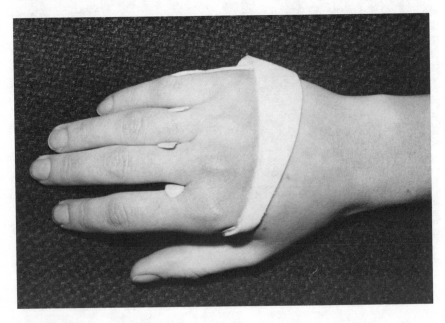

Figure 16.9a.   Ulnar deviation splint.

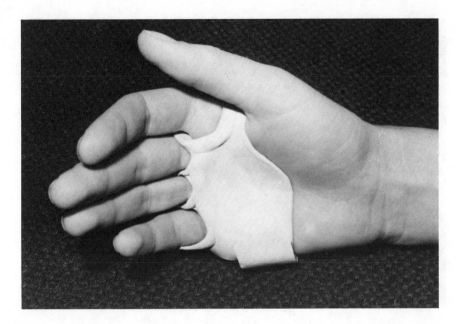

Figure 16.9b. *(continued)*

and/or metacarpophalangeal joints are involved, and they also usually provide symptomatic relief of de Quervain's stenosing tenosynovitis without the addition of wrist immobilization (figure 16.10).

Corrective splints for early swan-neck (figure 16.11) and boutonniere deformities (figures 16.12, 16.13) and proximal interphalangeal and distal interphalangeal tightness (figure 16.14) are also lightweight and easy to apply and remove. The finger splints traditionally used for traumatic finger injuries may also be used with rheumatic disease patients (figures 16.15, 16.16). The more difficult contractures may need to be treated with serial plaster casting.[56]

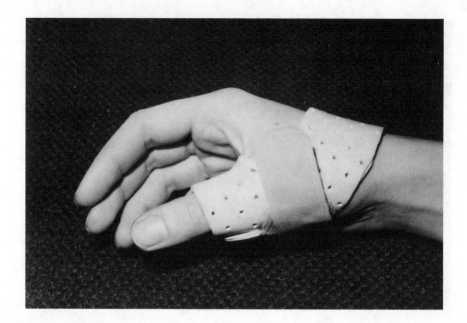

Figure 16.10.   Thumb splint.

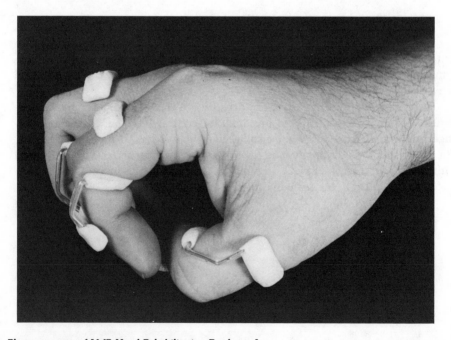

Photo courtesy of LMB Hand Rehabilitation Products, Inc.
Figure 16.11a.   Finger flexion splint.

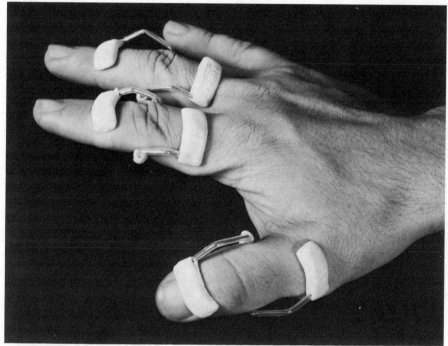

Figure 16.11b. *(continued).*

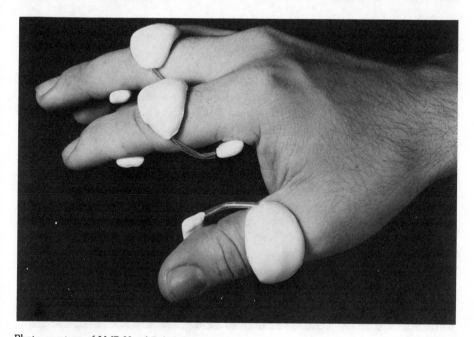

Figure 16.12a.   Extension finger splint.

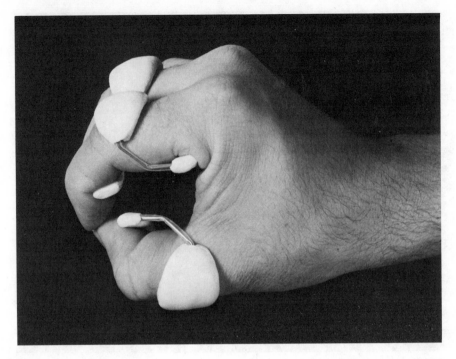

Figure 16.12b. *(continued).*

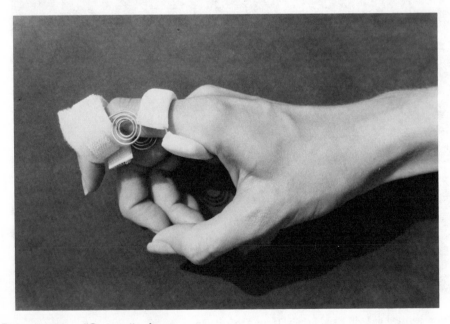

Figure 16.13a. "Capener" splint.

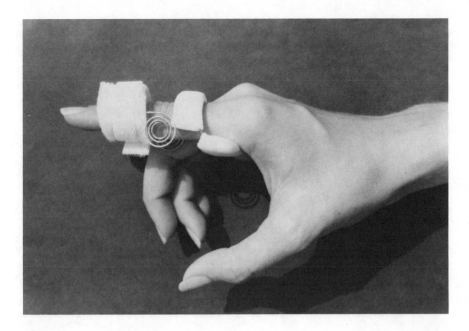

Figure 16.13b.   *(continued).*

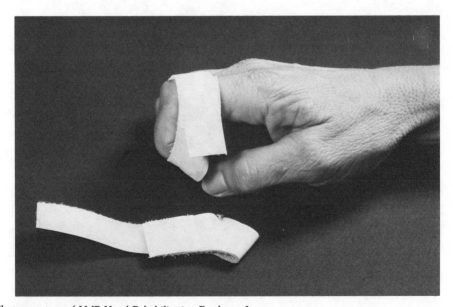

Photo courtesy of LMB Hand Rehabilitation Products, Inc.
Figure 16.14.   Proximal interphalangeal, distal interphalangeal splints.

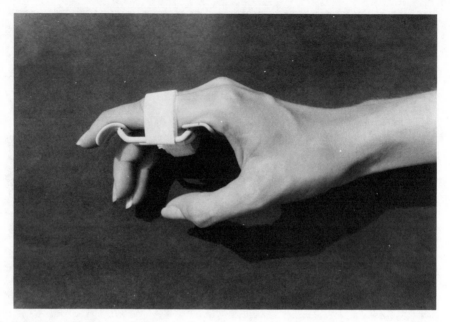

Figure 16.15.   "Safety-pin" splint.

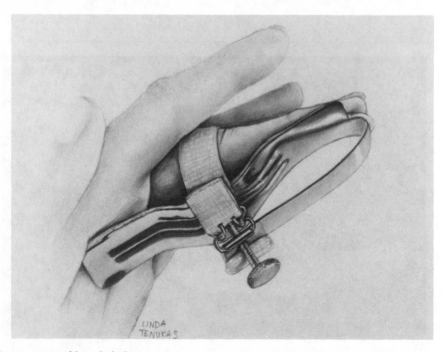

Photo courtesy of Joint-Jack Co.
Figure 16.16.   Joint-Jack splint.

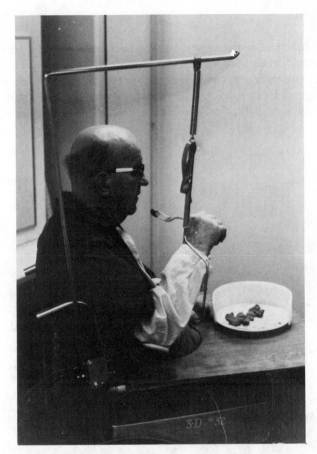

Figure 16.17.   Overhead suspension sling.

Elbow and Shoulder Splints

Acutely involved elbow and shoulder joints frequently benefit from resting splinting in the positions of the least intra-articular pressure. There is no standard splint for this purpose; however, it is usually advisable to use as lightweight and comfortable a material as possible. Elbow involvement usually limits extension that is not functionally significant, and shoulder range-of-motion limitations can frequently be accommodated through mobility in other joints and ADL (aids to daily living) modifications. Thus functional and corrective splinting for these areas is seldom done, because it is usually not identified by the patient as a primary problem. If pain and decreased function is severe enough surgical intervention is usually indicated. An overhead suspension sling may be of functional use in the patient in whom muscle weakness and instability without pain are a factor (polymyositis) (figure 16.17).

Spinal Splinting

One primary function of the cervical collar in the rheumatic disease patient is pain relief through restriction of cervical motion without complete immobilization. Thus patients may experience relief of symptoms with the use of a soft cervical collar (figures 16.18, 16.19). Other, more severely involved patients may require greater degrees of cervical stabilization for relief of their symptoms, and

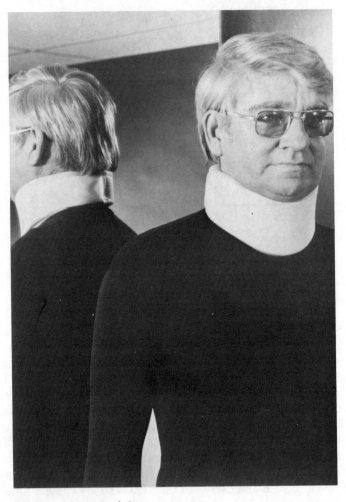

Photo courtesy of Camp International, Inc.

Figure 16.18. Cervical collar.

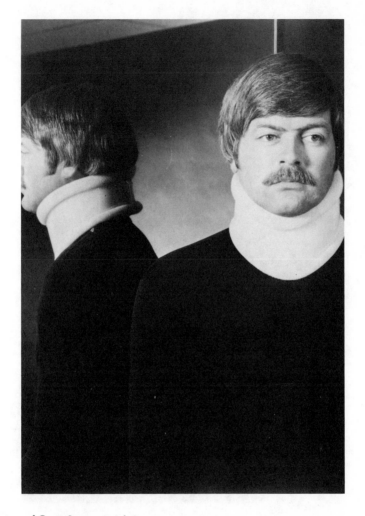

Photo courtesy of Camp International, Inc.
Figure 16.19.   Cervical collar with polyethylene overlay.

there are various cervical devices available for this (figures 16.20–16.22).[57,58] Severe cervical involvement, particularly with atlanto-axial subluxation and/or neurologic compression, should be carefully evaluated and splinted in rigid custom orthosis by specialists.

Effective splinting of the thoracic through lumbar spine is usually more dependent upon motion control than realignment,[59] and these require evaluation and fitting by an orthotist with experience in rheumatic diseases.

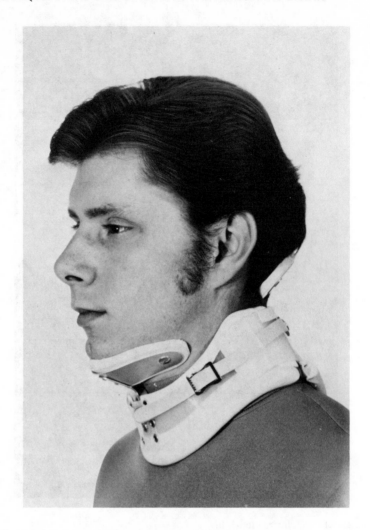

Photo courtesy of Camp International, Inc.
Figure 16.20.   Adjustable two-part polyethylene foam collar.

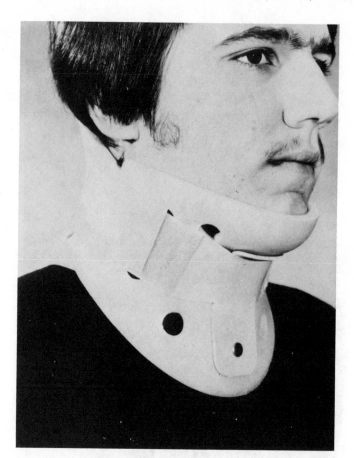

Photo courtesy of Camp International, Inc.
Figure 16.21.   Thomas collar.

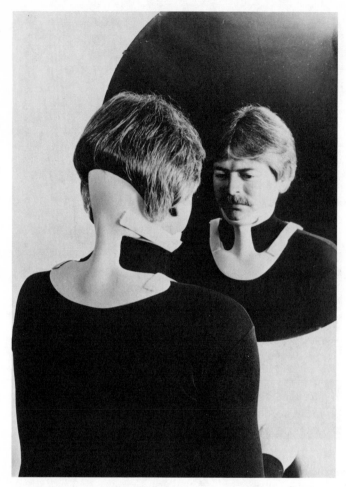

Photo courtesy of Camp International, Inc.
Figure 16.22.   Two-part Cervalite collar.

Lower Extremity

Lower extremity orthotics run the gamut from plaster resting splints to ishial weight-bearing braces.[60] Often in the less severe cases of knee involvement a stock knee brace (figures 16.23, 16.24) or the use of an ambulation aid will be sufficient to decrease pain and increase function. For severe, chronic cases of lower extremity joint involvement, joint arthroplasty is usually the procedure of choice. Thus the more cumbersome braces that reduce weight bearing and correct alignment on the lower extremity are now used primarily for patients for whom joint

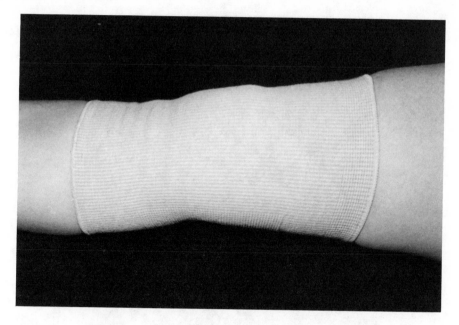

Figure 16.23.   Elastic knee support.

replacement arthroplasty surgery is not possible or in instances of a failed surgical result.

Ankle and foot problems in rheumatic disease patients are frequently the result of involvement in the proximal extremity joints and must be evaluated and treated very carefully, as discussed in chapter 35. Resting splinting may be useful to the patient for positioning and pain relief (figure 16.25).

SUMMARY

The utilization of splinting with the rheumatic disease patient is of proven efficacy. However, for optimal results each procedure should only be undertaken by persons skilled in the use of the various materials and splints and knowledgeable in rheumatic diseases. Overzealous and ill-considered application of splints, braces, and casts will not produce satisfactory results and may cause further damage.

The suggested splinting protocol (table 16.5) summarizes the steps necessary in establishing an effective splinting program. These devices must be only a part of an overall therapeutic program involving the physician, the patient, and trained therapists to relieve pain, maintain and improve muscle strength and function, and control the activity of the rheumatoid process.

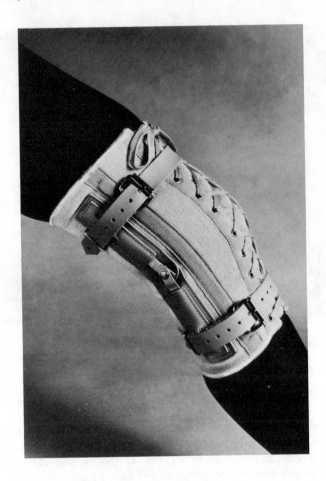

Figure 16.24. Lace-up knee support with lateral bars.

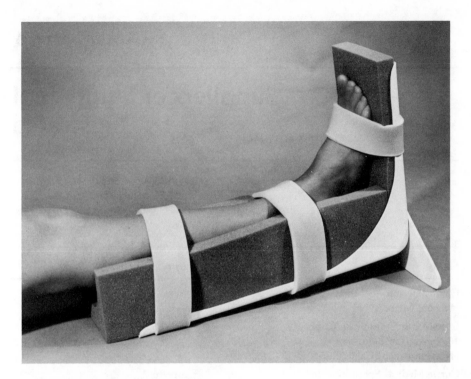

Photo courtesy of Rolyan Manufacturing Co., Inc.
Figure 16.25.   Drop-foot resting splint.

Table 16.5.   Suggested Splinting Protocol

1a.	Evaluate specific area to be splinted—test range of motion, strength/grasp, sensation, pain, swelling, specific deformities, etc.
b.	Complete screening of appropriate (table 16.1) patient.
2.	Determine specific goals and objectives (based on 1a and 1b).
3.	Determine type of splint and material to be used.
4.	Fabricate splint.
5a.	Thoroughly explain use and precautions for splint. Use written instructions and involve the patient's family if possible.
b.	Have patient repeat instructions and apply and remove splint.
6.	Combine with exercise program and other therapeutic techniques.
7.	Do periodic recheck and reevaluation and modify as indicated.

Appendix 16A

Suppliers of Equipment Illustrated

Source	Illustrated in
Camp International Inc. Jackson, Mich. 49201	figures 16.3, 16.8–16.24
Christensen Orthopedic Company 1097 Aviation Blvd. Hermosa Beach, Calif. 90254	figure 16.15
Currie Medical Specialties, Inc. 416 East Live Oak Avenue Arcadia, Calif. 91006	figure 16.7
Joint-Jack Company 198 Millstone Road Glastonbury, Conn. 06033	figure 16.16
Jung Products, Inc. P.O. Box 1337 Cincinnati, Ohio 45201	figure 16.6
LMB Hand Rehabilitation Products, Inc. P.O. Box 1181 San Luis Obispo, Calif. 93406	figures 16.2, 16.4, 16.11–16.14
Rolyan Manufacturing Co., Inc. P.O. Box 555 Menomonee Falls, Wisc. 53051	figures 16.1, 16.25

REFERENCES

1. Lee P, Kennedy AC, Anderson J, Buchanan WW. Benefits of hospitalization in rheumatoid arthritis. Quart J Med 1974;43:205-214.

2. Mills JA, Pinals RS, Ropes MW, Short CL, Sutcliffe J. Value of bed rest in patients with rheumatoid arthritis. New Engl J Med 1971;284:453-458.

3. Partridge REH, Duthie JJR. Controlled trial of the effects of complete immobilization of the joint in rheumatoid arthritis. Ann Rheum Dis 1963;22:91-99.

4. Gault SJ, Spyker JM. Beneficial effect of immobilization of joints in rheumatoid and related arthritis: a splint study using sequential analysis. Arth Rheum 1969;12:34-44.

5. Harris R, Copp EP. Immobilization of the knee joint in rheumatoid arthritis. Ann Rheum Dis 1962;21:353-359.

6. Biddulph, SL. The effect of the Futuro wrist brace in painful conditions of the wrists. S Afr Med J Sept. 5, 1981;60:389-391.

7. Kamermann JS. Protective effect of traumatic lesions on rheumatoid arthritis. Ann Rheum Dis 1966;25:361-363.

8. Bland JH, Eddy WM. Hemiplegia and rheumatoid hemiarthritis. Arth Rheum 1968;11:72-78.

9. Thompson M, Bywaters EGL. Unilateral rheumatoid arthritis following hemiplegia. Ann Rheum Dis 1962;21:370-377.

10. Glick EN. Asymetrical rheumatoid arthritis after poliomyelitis. Brit Med J 1967;3:26-28.

11. Bennett RM, Hughes GRV, Bywaters EGL, Holt PJL. Studies of popliteal synovial fistula. Ann Rheum Dis 1972;31:482-486.

12. Backhouse KM, Kay AGL, Coomes EN, Kates A. Tendon involvement in the rheumatoid hand. Ann Rheum Dis 1971;30:236-242.

13. Jayson MIV, Dixon AStJ. Intra-articular pressure in rheumatoid arthritis of the knee. Ann Rheum Dis 1970;29:401-408.

14. Jayson MIV, Dixon AStJ, Yeoman P. Unusual geodes ("bone cysts") in rheumatoid arthritis. Ann Rheum Dis 1972;31:174-178.

15. Castillo BA, El Sallabe RA, Scott JT. Physical activity, cystic erosions and osteoporosis in rheumatoid arthritis. Ann Rheum Dis 1965;24:522-526.

16. Horvath SM, Hollander JL. Intra-articular temperature as a measure of joint reaction. J Clin Invest 1949;28:469-473.

17. Hollander JL, Horvath SM. The influence of physical therapy procedures on the intra-articular temperature of normal and arthritis subjects. Am J Med Sci 1949;218:543-548.

18. Harris ED, Krane SM. Collagenases (second of three parts). New Engl J Med 1974;284:605-609.

19. Palmonski M, Perricone E, Brandt KD. Development and reversal of a proteoglycan aggregation defect in normal canine knee cartilage after immobilization. Arth Rheum 1979;22:508-517.

20. Palmonski MJ, Colyer RA, Brandt KD. Joint motion in the absence of normal loading does not maintain articular cartilage. Arth Rheum 1980;23:325-333.

21. Perricone E, Brandt K, Palmonski M. Reduced joint usage leads to reduced proteoglycan aggregation in human articular cartilage. Arth Rheum 1980;23:626.

22. Brewerton DA. Hand deformities in rheumatoid disease. Ann Rheum Dis 1957;16:183-197.

23. Swanson AB. Pathomechanics of deformities in hand and wrist. In: Hunter JM, et al., eds. Rehabilitation of the hand, St. Louis: CV Mosby, 1978, pp. 453–467.
24. Swezey RL. Dynamic factors in deformity of the rheumatoid arthritis hand. Bull Rheum Dis 1971–72;22:649–656.
25. Smith EM, Juvinall RC, Bender LF, Pearson JR. Role of the finger flexors in rheumatoid deformities of the metacarpo-phalangeal joints. Arth Rheum 1964;7:467–480.
26. Smith RJ. Balance and kinetics of the fingers under normal and pathological conditions. Clin Orthop 1974;104:92–111.
27. Thomas WH. Reconstructive surgery and rehabilitation of the ankle and foot. In: Kelly WN, et al., eds. Textbook of rheumatology, 1st ed. Philadelphia: WB Saunders, 1981, pp. 1999–2007.
28. Backhouse KM. The mechanics of normal digital control in the hand and an analysis of the ulnar drift of rheumatoid arthritis. Ann Roy College Surgeons Engl 1968;43:154–173.
29. Wise KS. The anatomy of the metacarpo-phalangeal joints, with observations of the aetiology of ulnar drift. J Bone Joint Surg 1975;57B:485–490.
30. Shapiro JS, Heijna W, Nasatir S, Ray RD. The relationship of wrist motion to ulnar phalangeal drift in the rheumatoid patient. Hand 1971;3(1):68–75.
31. Hastings, DE, Evans JA. Rheumatoid wrist deformities and their relation to ulnar drift. J Bone Joint Surg 1975;57(7):930–934.
32. Stack HG, Vaughan-Jackson OH. The zig-zag deformity in the rheumatoid hand. Hand 1971;3(1):62–67.
33. Smith RJ, Kaplan EB. Rheumatoid deformities in the metacarpo-phalangeal joints of the fingers. J Bone Joint Surg 1967;49A(1):31–47.
34. Smith EM, Juvinall RC, Bender LF, Pearson JR. Flexor forces and rheumatoid metacarpo-phalangeal deformity. JAMA 1966;198(2):150–154.
35. Ketchum LD, Thompson D, Pock G, Wallingford D. A clinical study of forces generated by the intrinsic muscles of the index finger and the extrinsic flexor and extensor muscles of the hand. J Hand Surg 1978;3(6):571–578.
36. Swezey RL, Fiegenberg DS. Inappropriate intrinsic muscle action in the rheumatoid hand. Ann Rheum Dis 1971;30:619–625.
37. deAndrade JR, Grant C, Dixon AStJ. Joint distention and reflex muscle inhibition in the knee. J Bone Joint Surg 1965;47A(2):313–322.
38. Oakes TW, Ward JR, Gray RM, Klauber MR, Moody PM. Family expectations and arthritis patient compliance to a hand resting splint regimen. J Chron Dis 1970;22:757–764.
39. Davis MS. Variations in patients' compliance with doctors' orders: analysis of congruence between survey responses and results of empirical investigations. J Med Ed 1966;41:1037–1048.
40. Rizzo F, Hamilton BB, Keagy RD. Orthotics research evaluation framework. Arch Phys Med Rehab 1975;56:304–308.
41. Melvin JL. Rheumatic disease: occupational therapy and rehabilitation. Philadelphia: FA Davis, 1977, pp. 170–171.
42. Malick M. Manual on static hand splinting. Harmarville Rehabilitation Center, Ridge Road, Pittsburgh, Pa. 15238, 1972.
43. Malick M. Manual of dynamic hand splinting with thermoplastic materials. Harmarville Rehabilitation Center, Ridge Road, Pittsburgh, Pa. 15238, 1974.
44. Feinberg J, Brandt KD. Use of resting splints by patients with rheumatoid arthritis. Am J Occup Ther 1981;35(3):173–178.

45. Smith JW. Elastic properties of the anterior cruciate ligament of the rabbit. J Anat 1954;88:369–380.

46. LaBan MM. Collagen tissue: implications of its response in vitro. Arch Phys Med Rehab Sept. 1962;13:461–466.

47. VanBrocklin JD, Ellis DG. A study of the mechanical behavior of toe extensor tendons under applied stress. Arch Phys Med Rehab May 1965;46:369–373.

48. Kottke FJ, Pauley DL, Ptak RA. Rationale for prolonged stretching for correction of shortening of connective tissues. Arch Phys Med Rehab June 1966;47:345–352.

49. Brand PW. The forces of dynamic splinting: ten questions before applying a dynamic splint to the hand. In: Hunter JM, et al.,eds., Rehabilitation of the hand. St. Louis: CV Mosby Company, 1978, pp. 591–598.

50. Eyring EJ, Murray WR. The effect of joint position on the pressure of intra-articular effusion. J Bone Joint Surg 1964;47A:1235–1241.

51. Favreau JC, Laurin CA. Joint effusions and flexion deformities. Canad Med Assoc J March 16, 1963;88:575–576.

52. MacConaill MA, Basmajian JV. Muscles and movements: a basis for human kinesiology, 2nd ed. Huntington, N.Y.: Robert RE Krieger, 1977, pp. 46, 60, 79.

53. Melvin JL. Rheumatic disease: occupational therapy and rehabilitation. Philadelphia: FA Davis Company, 1977, pp. 174–182.

54. Seeger, MS. The roles of splinting and rest. In Bluestone et al., eds., Rheumatology. Boston: Houghton Mifflin Professional Publishers, 1980, pp. 170–183.

55. Swezey, RI. Arthritis: rational therapy and rehabilitation. Philadelphia: WB Saunders, 1978, pp. 83–92.

56. Bell, JA. Plaster cylinder casting of contractures of the interphalangeal joints. In: Hunter JM, et al., eds., Rehabilitation of the hand. St. Louis: CV Mosby, 1978, pp. 644–651.

57. Fisher SV, Bowar JF, Award EA, Gullickson G. Cervical orthoses effect on cervical spine motion: roentgenographic and goniometric method of study. Arch Phys Med Rehab 1977;58:109–115.

58. Johnson RM, Hart DL, Simmons EF, Ramsby GR, Southwick WO. Cervical orthoses. J Bone Joint Surg 1977;59A(3):332–339.

59. Luskin R, Berger N. Prescription principles. In: American Academy of Orthopaedic Surgeons, Atlas of orthotics: biomechanical principles and application. St. Louis: CV Mosby, 1975, ch. 20, pp. 364–372.

60. Staros A, LeBlanc M. Orthotic components and systems. In: American Academy of Orthopaedic Surgeons, Atlas of orthotics: biomechanical principles and application. St. Louis: CV Mosby, 1975, ch. 10, pp. 184–234.

17

Manual Mobilization and Traction

Robert L. Swezey, M.D., F.A.C.P.

Rubbing, squeezing, and licking wounds are instinctive responses to pain. Comfort, consolation, and love typically are accompanied by caressing and stroking. The discovery of endorphins and enkephalins has permitted modern medicine to find a rational physiological basis for some of the instinctive comfort-seeking behaviors in the animal kingdom and in its multicultural manifestations in the human species. Massage as a therapy is widely practiced in primitive cultures and therapeutic use of massage can be traced through written treatises to China, Egypt, India, and Greece.[1-3]

Traction, mobilization, and massage techniques have also been employed for reductions of fractures and dislocations since antiquity. The need to find prompt resolutions of athletic and battlefield casualties provided a stimulus for their development and perfection.[1-5] Massage and traction therapies are widely used and, if not enthusiastically endorsed by the medical profession, they are well recognized as palliative measures. Manipulation of subluxed or dislocated peripheral joints is an accepted part of orthopedic treatment. The use of manipulation for the reduction of shoulder dislocations and knee meniscal derangements as in times past has been considered a part of first aid. These manipulative procedures having proved themselves over time and therefore have not seemed to require other justification.

But manipulation of the spine is another matter! Spinal manipulation has been largely excluded from contemporary medical practice and is often perceived as a relatively recent intrusion by "quacks" into the otherwise orderly development of medical and surgical therapies of spinal disorders. Although it was known to the ancient Chinese, Greeks, and Romans,[1-10] spinal manipulation emerged about 100 years ago[4] as a result of the development of osteopathy and chiropractic. Solid pathophysiologic foundations for treatment of disease at that time were often lacking and empirical and quack therapies were rampant.[1] Thus the advocates of spinal manipulation in the last century can perhaps be forgiven for theoretical misconceptions. [7-9]

MASSAGE

The controversial issue in massage therapy relates to its applications for pain control (acupressure), postural integration (rolfing)[11] and specific therapy for tendinitis (deep friction massage). For many years the focus on massage effects has been on a circulatory phenomena. The autonomic nervous system may be affected and if edema is mobilized, lymphatic and venous return are involved.[12,13] What is at issue, vis-a-vis circulatory and autonomic alterations is the premise that autonomic dysfunction in visceral tissues via viscerocutaneous reflexes cause musculoskeletal dysfunction (such as arm pain or shoulder-hand syndrome following myocardial infarction). The inverse is the rationale for the most controversial aspect of chiropractic and osteopathic adjustment—to relieve pressure on spinal nerves in order to improve functioning of visceral organs.[6–10,13]

Recognition of specific skeletal foci for modulation of pain (acupuncture) and the frequent identity of specific trigger points[15] has provided a basis for scientific investigation of such therapies as local anesthesia,[16] acupuncture,[16] transcutaneous nerve stimulation (TNS), vibration massage[17] and acupressure.[14] From the standpoint of Western medicine, focal deep pressure and massage over trigger points can be presumed to stimulate proprioceptive nerve endings facilitating enkephalin release[14] and to stretch (kneading) musculotendinous structures to implement reflex muscle relaxation via Golgi tendon organ and spindle receptors.[15]

Massage techniques, like all manual therapies—indeed like all hand skills (sewing, potting, carpentry, surgery), require dexterity, training in precise methods and practice in order to be effective. The description of the various massage techniques is left to others.[19,20]

Connective tissue massage is a deep musculosfascial mobilizing technique that attempts to relieve pain as a consequence of traumatic or postural contractures by deep mobilizing massage.[13] This technique is used as a method for pain relief (massage analgesia) and is advocated by many as a specific therapy for tendinitis.[21–23] Precisely located deep transverse frictions are applied for a few minutes to attempt to forcibly break interfibrillary musculofascial adhesions or tenovaginal and tenopereosteal and ligamentous adhesions.[21,22] The principal applications of this method are as a preparation for therapeutic exercise, to facilitate manual articular mobilizations, and to restore pain-free motion of tendons and at tendinous attachments. Unfortunately no study can be cited to document the efficacy of what appears to be a useful treatment modality.

TRACTION

No one seriously questions the essential role of traction in overcoming muscle contracture secondary to arthritis, fracture, or dislocation. The soothing analgesic effects attributed to massage may well augment the relaxation of muscles that occurs when a painful articulated skeletal part is supported and stretched by manual or mechanical traction.[16,17] More to the point, manual as well as mechanical tractions are used as preparations for and often in lieu of other mobilization and manipulative procedures for both peripheral and axial articulations.[10,21-28] The concept that traction in these instances facilitates subsequent mobilizations by relaxing muscles and minimizing pain[29] in a manner analogous to massage is difficult to refute, but what the consequences of capsule and ligamentous or intervertebral distraction may be can create tension (pun intended) between clinical investigators.[29,30]

Traction for peripheral joints is usually administered manually as a static transient pull or a brief series of tractions of a few seconds to 2 or 3 minutes depending on the intended purpose,[21-23] the amount of pain, muscle tension, and the bulk of soft tissue surrounding the joint.[10,21-24,27] In selected cases (infection, trauma) where large proximal joints (shoulders, hips, knees) are involved, pain relief or facilitation of reduction of subluxations may be enhanced by sustained mild mechanical traction.[30]

In traction therapy for cervical, dorsal, and lumbar spine disorders the difficult question is whether or not discs can be separated or indeed must be separated for a reduction of disc herniation to effect pain relief or cure. Studies have shown both partial[29] and complete[21] separation of discs in normal controls after using traction forces much greater than customarily applied, but convincing evidence of vertebral separation in pathologic disc disorders is still not forthcoming.[29-31]

If we in fact cannot effect a reduction of a disc protrusion with traction, why bother? Pain control by the mechanisms previously mentioned may provide an ample answer if safety and costs are acceptable. The cost of traction is clearly controllable and in the case of home cervical or home hanging-traction apparatus, economical equipment can be provided. The safety of traction is not ordinarily a serious matter. The general contraindications are avoidance of spinal traction in inflammatory disorders; tumor (except when used in reduction of pathological fracture); bleeding diathesis; and fear. Specific contraindications are cervical rotation during the course of traction in the presence of vertebral artery insufficiency; cervical traction with temporomandibular joint dysfunction (a mouth guard or forehead-occiput halter rather than mandibular-occiput halter may resolve the problem); and where the chest strap interferes excessively with cardiopulmonary function during pelvic and lumbar traction.[21,28-30] Occasional patients feel weak or have increased pain after vigorous traction, perhaps due to downward traction on a nerve root against a protruding disc; the initial treatment should therefore be done conservatively.[28,29]

What if traction does create significant intervertebral disc separation? Can a few minutes of vertebral separation significantly alter or permanently replace a herniating disc? The question of whether or not a disc herniation can be reduced at all by traction remains in doubt, but there is some objective supporting evidence for this assertion.[29-31] It is conceivable that annular fibers and/or the posterior longitudinal ligament could be pulled taut by traction. At the same time intervertebral separation, however slight, would create a lower intradiscal pressure and exert a force sufficient to reduce a herniation of a still contained nuclear protrusion or a hard dessicated disc fragment. It would further require that the reduced nuclear material or annular fragments then become contained by intact annular fibers and ultimately undergo cicatrization so as to be less predisposed to reherniation,[21,22,32,33] This explanation, well supported by Farfan's[34] pathologic studies,[32] provides much of the basis for manual therapies in spinal derangements.

Nonetheless, bulging discs have been shown in vivo to recede with traction[31] and by clinical criteria have appeared to remain so.[35] If the discs themselves do not actually distract with traction, the adjacent ligaments do stretch. In the case of the cervical spine under gentle traction in flexion, the capsular ligaments elongate as the facets separate. This will occur with any appropriate motion; for example, forward flexion separates facets posteriorly and stretches posterior capsular fibers.[35,36] This tractional movement of ligamentous and osseous structures may permit improved local nutrition to compressed and injured neural and ligamentous structures,[12,21] or simply alter pain perception and modify pain response by stimulation of stretch receptors.[16,17,21]

Manual traction for relief of neck pain and as a preparatory stretch prior to mobilization is widely employed.[29,30] Prolonged horizontal static traction for severe discogenic pain and radiculopathy is occasionally found useful where adequate immobilization and intermittent traction have not been helpful or not feasible.[30] The efficacy of traction for relief of cervical-disc-related disorders has not been established.[30,37] A variety of techniques using various cervical traction time and weight schedules are advocated, but a regimen of seated static traction using the weight of the upper trunk for 5-minute sessions once or more daily has proven efficient and apparently effective.[30] Traction with manipulation of the neck carries the risks associated with manipulation—cerebral vascular occlusion, trauma, fracture—and is both strongly endorsed and decried.[21-23,26,29,30] Cervical traction can also be applied to treat upper dorsal discogenic derangements and is reported to be effective.[21,23]

The lumbar spine requires greater forces for distraction of vertebrae (if indeed distraction is required) and 25–50 percent of body weight in friction-free horizontal table is necessary to achieve an intervertebral distraction.[29] Prolonged pelvic traction in bed using low weights accomplishes little if anything other than enforced bed rest (a not unworthy therapy in most cases of back pain).[29,30] For acute and subacute disc-related disorders, marked temporary relief of pain is achieved with only a few sessions (from two to ten) of brief (10–15 minutes) sustained or intermittent mechanical tractions.[21,29,30]

Some patients with recurrent or chronic disc-related and postural strain problems seem to benefit from short periods of traction once or twice daily. For the patient with cervical discogenic disorders this usually poses no great problem because simple home traction can be used.[30] For patients with dorsal and lumbar disc and facetal derangement the problem is more complex. There are now available several kinds of hanging apparatus that utilize body weight as the tractive force (there is no extrinsic friction to overcome).[38-40] The combination of forceful traction and manipulation requires either two therapists,[21,22] or special equipment [22,40] in many instances.

MOBILIZATION AND MANIPULATION

In a sense, all passive exercises are mobilization procedures. It is when the passive maneuvers deviate from the normal joint range of motion and passively stretch articular structures into those patterns of passive joint movement that are normally present but not elicitable by active muscular contraction (called "joint play" by Mennell)[23] that we begin to shake foundations of credibility.

With mobilization techniques one attempts (after careful assessment) to control pain by careful and precise application of repeated short-excursion, short-duration, manual manipulations (and/or tractions) well within the permissible range of motion of the treated joint.[22,23,27,28] The mobilization excursions are typically increased in depth and scope incorporating greater ranges of joint play in successive treatment sessions depending upon the success in previous sessions of gaining pain control or increasing joint mobility.[21-28] Mobilizations may be given daily when pain control is best achieved by this method.[27,28] For increasing joint range of motion, one to three sessions per week for 2–6 weeks should be adequate to achieve the goals of restoring as pain-free joint mobility as possible.[21,22,27,28]

Controlling Factors in Manual Therapy

The assessment of the indications for manual therapy depends on the answers to the following questions: (1) Is the pathology amenable to manual therapy by virtue of a treatable contracture, subluxation, or painful soft tissue focus? (2) Does the manual therapy selected provide an advantage in safety over alternative therapies? and (3), Is the manual therapy chosen apt to expedite either relief of pain or restoration of joint mobility?

Two clinical problems illustrating these three points are the "frozen" shoulder and the "locked" knee. In a mild noninflammatory adhesive shoulder capsulitis, exercise alone may suffice to restore motion. In cases associated with biceps tendinitis, medication, local steroid injection or tendon friction massage plus mobilization and active therapy may be considered. In a chronic refractory frozen shoulder, manipulation (sometimes forcibly under anesthesia) may be required. The "locked" knee associated with an acutely torn meniscus will be released only by a mobilizing manipulative procedure.

Manipulation

With the exception of the foregoing examples and the treatment of peripheral joint subluxation, the place of manipulation therapy is quite obscure. Although not in the mainstream of medicine, the mainstay of manipulation therapists is spinal manipulation, the thrust of the controversy.[6–10,21–28,32,41]

If the thrust activates the bone of contention regarding manipulation, certainly its loud accompanying audible "pop" or "crack" can be relied upon to give manipulation a further hearing. What is the pathologic lesion that we are thrusting against, popping, and "adjusting?"[7,8] What is the thrust? It is a very rapid motion by the manipulator performed so quickly that the patient cannot inhibit it, nor can the manipulator stop it once he has initiated it. It is this uncontrolled component of the thrust that distinguishes manipulation from mobilization.

The interspinal joints consist basically of the discs and their bilateral facet joints. Movement of any one of these three structures must cause motion in the other two. In the neck the anterior intervertebral joints of Von Luschka and in the dorsal spine the rib articulations can be added to the triad of interdependent articulations. It is obvious and reasonable to infer that pathological alterations of motion in the discs or their facet joints can affect one another and adjacent articulations in a manner similar to the stress on a hip from derangement of a knee. A shrinking, dessicated, aging disc will lead to facet motion or facet weight-bearing stresses and secondary facet joint osteoarthritis.[34] Irritation of these pathologic articular structures stimulates adjacent somatic and autonomic nerves.[34,45] Capsular contractures, bony proliferations, disc herniations, and local edema can impact on spinal nerve roots and less commonly on the spinal cord itself.

Patellae sublux with varying degrees of trauma depending on the ligamentous laxity, the shape of the patella, the shape of the femoral condyles, the position of the body, and the force of the trauma. Shoulders, jaws, and even hips commonly sublux. Why cannot the facet joints do likewise? We know that the facet joints are commonly congenitally malaligned and osteoarthritic.[34] We know that the lumbar paraspinal muscles are inactive and therefore not protective during extreme flexion.[42] Twisting torques produce great stress on the discs and their facet joints.[34] The problem is that we cannot yet arthroscope the facet joints, and whereas the pathology and anatomy of these articulations lends them to credible similes with other small joints, verification is lacking.

The therapeutic dilemma of facet-joint manipulations is similar. Because we can distract and harmlessly audibly click or crack normal peripheral joints[43,44] or manipulate and audibly crack contractured or "seized" joints, it would help if we understood rather than surmised a similar basis for the "crack" in spinal manipulation. But is the facet joint necessarily the seat of the problem? Many authorities, most notably osteopaths,[10,26] say yes, but there are persuasive arguments for the disc as the major locus of pathology requiring and responding to manipulation.[9,10,21–28,32–34]

Extension Therapy

Is an audible sound, however gratifying, necessary to achieve a successful result from manipulation? Clearly it is not in all cases of successful mobilization without thrusting. This is particularly impressive in those cases where an acute or even chronic antalgic sciatic scoliosis (lateral "shift")[32] can be restored without sound or thrust to normal alignment. This takes from 20 to 30 seconds up to a few minutes by gentle pressure.[21,32] The manipulator's shoulder presses against the standing patient's elbow on the shifted side and pushes the rib cage back to midline while the patient's pelvis is drawn toward the manipulator and back under the laterally shifted thorax.[21,23,32]

Anyone who has performed this maneuver has great difficulty in not subscribing to the concept espoused first by Cyriax,[21] documented pathologically by Farfan,[34] and supported strongly by McKenzie[32] that viscus nuclear material that is herniated posterior laterally through intra-annular crevices is being oozed toward a more central intra-annular location. This is then squeezed even more anteriorly (away from the dura and nerve roots) by a repetitive slow extension compression exercise—much like squeezing toothpaste out of a tube.

This extension exercise treatment regimen is then maintained by an exaggerated lordotic posture designed to keep the intradiscal nuclear material located anteriorly until the annular tear heals sealing the nuclear material more centrally in the disc.[32] The frequency of acute discal herniations on assuming an upright posture after prolonged flexion is indirect evidence of the impact of postural shifts (in this case from anterior to posterior) on the nucleus pulposus.[32]

One of the most shocking aspects of manipulation therapy is the assertion that if manipulation to one side does not work you can "turn 'em over and do it on the other—whatever works!" If stretching tight muscles to relieve painful reflex muscle spasm is all we demand from manipulation, perhaps one can beg the question as to the efficacy of these maneuvers. But if gapping facets, freeing adhesions, or reducing an annular herniation is the essential task of manipulation, this hit-or-miss approach needs explanation. The fact of the structural linkage of the facets to the vertebral body makes it obvious that if you tilt one vertebral body (over its inferior disc) you gap the facets on one side and overlap and/or imbricate those on the opposite side. In either case the facet joints are forced rapidly into either extreme of their range during the manipulative thrust and presumably regain normal joint alignment after gapping one side or prying on the opposite (like a reduction of a torn knee cartilage) when the thrust is completed.

If one must affect the annulus to reduce herniation, then tension on its outer fibers will bring some of the oblique annular fibers and the posterior longitudinal ligament under sufficient tension during the torque of a rotary or anterior posterior (flexion-extension) manipulative thrust to push an extruded fragment away from the periphery of the annulus.[33,34,45] In either the instance of facet or annular discal pathology, both the annulus and adjacent facets must be moved in unison during a vertebral manipulation.

Techniques of manipulation of spinal structures are well described and differ in their specificity, forcefulness, the presence of a supplementary traction, and the point of application of the thrust. When the techniques are understood, most manipulations are fairly easily performed.[21-29,33]

Testimony of many patients, bone setters, chiropractors, osteopaths, and physicians aside, the documented evidence for efficacy of manipulative therapy is sparce. In essence what can be said based on three recent careful studies of the effect of manipulation on patients with low back pain without radiculopathy is that a few patients obtained immediate relief.[47] Some patients had more pain during the first week of manipulations, possibly by a sprain. Most patients manipulated recovered somewhat quickly.[48] The ultimate outcome of manipulated and control patients was similar, however.[46-48] But if manipulation can shorten the duration of symptoms for some patients in terms of suffering, economic productivity, and the reduction of cost of medical treatment, this is no mean accomplishment.

Safety of Manipulation Therapy

The safety of manipulation therapy, once obvious factors such as bone tumors, severe osteoporosis, hemorrhage, and sepsis are excluded, is primarily a function of the vulnerability of the vertebral artery and spinal cord. Documentation of cerebral vascular accidents and death from cervical manipulation exists. These instances would appear rare and to the largest extent avoidable by careful pupillary monitoring for central nervous system signs during prepositioning and mobilization and employment of gentle precise techniques that use a minimal thrust.[23-28,49-53] The danger of frequent repeated manipulations lies in the potential for overstretching ligamentous structures and possibly traumatizing facet joints.

Who Should Manipulate?

So who should perform manipulations? For manual therapies to succeed, the manipulator must have skill in both diagnosis and treatment. A well-executed appendectomy in a patient with a renal calculus is of negative value, as is a botched appendectomy in a case of appendicitis. It follows that persons trained in appropriate diagnosis and treatment should apply their skills. In a traditional sense this would exclude all but physicians, but in a practical sense at this writing, with the exception of osteopaths, the vast majority of physicians have excluded themselves from this role. The bulk of manipulative therapy today is literally in the hands of chiropractors. The allopathic physician (M.D.) has the diagnostic skill and a working relationship with physical therapists, many of whom have some manual therapy expertise. But the physician really does not have the knowledge and skills required for an appropriate decision regarding manual therapies. Therapists generally are lacking in sophistication in this area and are not permitted to perform and thereby gain experience in the evaluation for an execution of manipulative procedures. Leaving manipulative therapy to chiropractors and their unscientific traditions is not a solution. Most physicians in the foreseeable future are unlikely to develop an interest in this area. Therefore it seems that an interprofessional specialty of manual therapy that can set standards so that physical therapists, as well as osteopaths, can be guided should be developed to meet the overall needs of manual therapies including manipulation.

SUMMARY

Mobilization therapies include massage, traction, and manipulations with and without a thrust. They play an adjunctive role in management of arthritis and related rheumatic and soft tissue disorders. They have in common a stimulation effect on proprioceptive neural pathways and presumably on complex reflex pathways impacting on pain. They probably have an impact in many instances specifically on pathologic structural derangements.

They are in general safe therapies but require knowledge, experience, and judgment for proper application. They must compete effectively with no therapy or placebos from the standpoint of cost, medical manpower resources, and above all efficacy to justify their clinical applications. At this writing it appears that all classes of mobilizing therapies including manipulations have a place in medical practice. Clearly much research is needed to better define that place, and a concerted effort is needed to determine what medical management manpower resources should be utilized in the application of mobilization therapies.

REFERENCES

1. Bettman O. A pictorial history of medicine. Springfield, Ill.: Charles C Thomas, 1956.
2. Kamenetz HL. History of massage. In: Licht S, ed. Massage, manipulation and traction. New Haven, Conn.: Elizabeth Licht, 1960, pp. 3–37.
3. Lyons AS, Petrucelli RJ II. Medicine: an illustrated history. New York: Henry N Abrams.
4. Licht S. Massage, manipulation and traction. New Haven, Conn.: Elizabeth Licht, 1960, pp. 142–144.
5. Licht S. Massage, manipulation and traction. New Haven, Conn.: Elizabeth Licht, 1960, pp. 220–222.
6. Encyclopedia Britannica, 1969, vol. 16, pp. 1145–1146.
7. Chiropractors: healers or quacks? Part 1. Consumer Reports, September 1975:542–547.
8. Chiropractors: healers or quacks? Part 1. Consumer Reports, October 1975:606–610.
9. Luce JM. Chiropractic—its history and challenge to medicine. Pharos, April 1978:12–17.
10. Hoag, JM, Cole WV, Bradford SG. Osteopathic medicine. New York: Blakiston Div., McGraw-Hill, 1969.
11. Rolfe IP. Rolfing: the integration of human structure. New York: Harper & Row, 1977.
12. Licht S. Massage, manipulation and traction. New Haven, Conn.: Elizabeth Licht, 1960:42.

13. Bischoff I, Elminger G. Connective tissue massage. In: Licht S. ed. Massage, manipulation and traction. New Haven, Conn.: Elizabeth Licht, 1960:57–85.

14. Sjolund B, Terenius L, Eriksson M. Increased cerebrospinal fluid levels of endorphins after electroacupuncture. Acta Physio Scand 1977;100:382–384.

15. Simons DG. Myofascial trigger points: a need for understanding. Arch Phys Med Rehab 1981;62:97–99.

16. Wolf SL. Perspectives on central nervous system responsiveness to transcutaneous electrical nerve stimulation. Phys Ther 1978;58:1443–1449.

17. Ottoson D, Ekblom A, Hansson P. Vibratory relief for the pain of dental origin. Pain 1981;10:37–45.

18. Melzack R, Stillwell DM, Fox EJ. Trigger points and acupuncture points for pain: correlations and implications. Pain 1977;3:3–23.

19. Francon F. Massage techniques. In: Licht S, ed. Massage, manipulation and traction. New Haven, Conn.: Elizabeth Licht, 1960, pp. 44–50.

20. Wood EC. Beard's massage principles and techniques, 2nd ed. Philadelphia: WB Saunders, 1974.

21. Cyriax J. Textbook of orthopaedic medicine, vol. 1, 4th ed. London: Harper & Row, 1962.

22. Cyriax J. Textbook of orthopaedic medicine, vol. 11, 7th ed. London: Harper & Row, 1965, pp. 11–16.

23. Maigne R. Orthopedic medicine. Springfield, Ill.: Charles C Thomas, 1972, pp. 233–252.

24. Mennell J McM. Joint pain. Boston: Little, Brown, 1964.

25. Mennell J McM. Back pain. Boston: Little, Brown, 1960.

26. Stoddard A. Manual of osteopathic practice. London: Hutchinson, 1969.

27. Maitland GD. Peripheral manipulation, 2nd ed. Boston: Butterworth, 1977.

28. Maitland GD. Vertebral manipulation, 4th ed. Boston: Butterworth, 1977.

29. Harris, R. Traction. In: Licht S, ed. Massage, manipulation and traction. New Haven, Conn.: Elizabeth Licht, 1960, pp. 223–251.

30. Swezey RL. Arthritis: rational therapy and rehabilitation. Philadelphia: WB Saunders, 1978, pp. 139–142.

31. Gupta RC, Ramarao SV. Epidurography in reduction of lumbar-disc prolapse by traction. Arch Phys Med Rehab 1978;59:322–327.

32. McKenzie RA. The lumbar spine mechanical diagnosis and therapy. Uppee Hutt, New Zealand: Wright and Carman, 1981.

33. Macnab I. Backache. Baltimore: Williams and Wilkins, 1977.

34. Farfan AF. Mechanical disorders of the low back. Philadelphia: Lea and Febiger, 1973:206–207.

35. Hood LB, Chrisman D. Intermittent pelvic traction in the treatment of the ruptured intervertebral disc. Phys Ther 1968;48:21–30.

36. Colachis SC, Strohm BR. A study of tractive forces and angle pull on vertebral interspaces in the cervical spine. Arch Phys Med Rehab 1965;46:820–830.

37. Brewerton DA, et al. Pain in the neck and arm: a multicentre trial of the effects of physiotherapy. Brit Med J 1966;1:253.

38. Burton C, Nida G. Gravity lumbar reduction therapy program. Rehabiliation Publication no. 731, Sister Kenney Institute, Minneapolis, Minn., 1976.

39. Nosse LJ. Inverted spinal traction. Arch Phys Med Rehab 1978;59:367–370.

40. Oudenhoven RC. Gravitational lumbar traction. Arch Phys Med Rehab 1978;59:510–512.

41. Cox JM. Chiro-manis treatment manual, 2nd ed. Fort Wayne, Ind.: James C Cox, 1975.
42. Basmajian JV. Muscles alive, 3rd ed. Baltimore: Williams and Wilkins, 1974:294–307.
43. Swezey RL, Swezey ES. The consequences of habitual knuckle cracking. West J Med 1975;122:377–379.
44. Unsworth A, Dowson D, Wright V. Cracking joints. Ann Rheum Dis 1971;30:348.
45. Hollinshead WA. Functional anatomy of the limbs and back, 2nd ed. Philadelphia: WB Saunders, 1963, pp. 199–209.
46. Doran DML, Newell DJ. Manipulation in the treatment of low back pain: A multicentre study. Br Med J 1975;2:161–164.
47. Evans DP, Burke MS, Lloyd KN, Roberts EE, Roberts GM. Lumbar spinal manipulation on trial part I clinical assessment. Rheum and Rehab 1978;17:46–53.
48. Hoehler FK, Tobis JS, Buerger AA. Spinal manipulation for low back pain. JAMA 1981;245:1835–1838.
49. Pratt-Thomas AR, Berger KE. Cerebellar and spinal injuries after chiropractic manipulation. JAMA 1949;133:600–604.
50. Schwarz GA, Geiger JK, Spano AV. Posterior inferior cerebellar artery syndrome of Wallenberg after chiropractic manipulation. Arch Int Med 1956;97:37–42.
51. Green DB, Joynt RJ. Vascular accidents to the brain stem associated with neck manipulation. JAMA 1959;170:520–524.
52. Maitland GD. Lumbar manipulation: does it do harm? A five year follow-up survey. Med J Aust 1961;48:546.
53. Schellhas KP, Latchaw RE, Wendling LR, Gold LHA. Vertebrobasilar injuries following cervical manipulation. JAMA 1980;244:1450–1453.

18

Injection Therapy

Joseph Lee Hollander, M.D., M.A.C.P.

One of the most neglected aids in rehabilitation of the arthritis patient during the past 30 years has been the use of intrasynovial corticosteroid therapy for treatment of joints, tendon sheaths, or bursae. This adjunct is useful when the structure has been persistently painful, swollen, and limited in motion even though the general activity of the arthritis has been at least fairly well controlled by systemic measures. If such recalcitrant problem areas are controlled by judicious local anti-inflammatory drug injections, rehabilitation can begin earlier and progress much faster to that ideal goal of remaking useful citizens from invalids.

In most instances arthritis involves multiple joints and requires appropriate systemic treatment. In certain posttraumatic joint problems the functional impairment is local, and even when many joints have been inflamed it may be only one or two that are persistently stiff and painful after the treatment program is well underway. In such cases the addition of local steroid injections to reinforce the continuing systemic measures will allow earlier ambulation or more active movement without pain or spasm than would be possible without such treatment. Furthermore the palliative effect of such joint injections is obvious within a day and usually will persist for weeks before repetition is needed.

Indications for Intra-articular Corticosteroid Injection

1. Whenever one peripheral joint is persistently painful, swollen, or tender, or only a few are, the local injection of corticosteroid can suppress the inflammation and allow normal function for a period of weeks.
2. Persistently painful joints in osteoarthritis may be made pain-free for long periods, allowing moderate function to preserve muscle strength and mobility with occasional intra-articular steroid injections.
3. Whenever spasm and pain in joints is decreasing range of motion, local

steroid therapy helps prevent deformity and restore muscle strength by permitting more active exercise.

4. Rehabilitation can begin earlier and proceed faster when arthritic pain is minimized by local steroid injection. The fear of inducing pain by motion is eliminated.

5. Local corticosteroid therapy may be utilized even when systemic steroid therapy is contraindicated, such as with diabetes or osteoporosis.

6. Local steroid injection may be helpful in preventing contractures following joint-replacement surgery.

Contraindications to Intra-articular Corticosteroid Therapy

1. Infection is present in or near the joint.
2. Joint destruction is severe or there is marked joint instability.
3. Fracture has occurred in or near the joint or severe local trauma (local steroid can slow the healing process in such cases).
4. Local osteoporosis near the joint is severe.
5. When many joints are actively involved, local steroid injections into one or a few are usually futile.
6. Spinal joints are not usually accessible to the injecting needle.
7. When trial injections (properly placed) have failed to produce definite improvement, further attempts may be futile.

TECHNIQUE FOR INTRA-ARTICULAR STEROID INJECTION

The anti-inflammatory and palliative effect of the cortisone preparation depends on contact with the inflamed or irritated joint surface, so the material *must* be injected *into* not just *near* the synovial space of the joint. Most failures from this technique are caused by inaccurate placement of the needle. An accurate knowledge of the anatomy of each joint to be injected is mandatory to successful results. Special training is needed. Allied health personnel usually have not had sufficient training to perform joint aspirations, and only those physicians who have observed or studied the techniques carefully can achieve the desired effects without causing undue pain with the needling. Primary care physicians can easily be trained to perform this procedure in some joints, such as the knee.

The objective of joint injection is to puncture the synovial sac, aspirate any excess synovial fluid, and inject the cortisone suspension with a minimum of pain and trauma to the joint and adjacent structures. The easiest site for insertion of the needle is usually on the extensor surface of the joint, where the synovium is closest to the skin and remote from major nerves, arteries, or veins. Careful cleansing of the skin around the injection site is important to prevent introduction of infection into the joint. Antiseptic detergent, followed by painting with tincture of iodine, then cleansing with alcohol have proved adequate.

Local anesthesia of the injection site is seldom needed if the insertion is quick and accurate. A local anesthetic agent may be injected into the skin, or a brief spraying with ethyl chloride will give temporary local skin anesthesia. Seldom is larger than a 20-gauge needle needed for joint aspiration, this attached to a syringe of 10- or 20-ml capacity. Both needles and syringes are readily available in individual disposable, presterilized packets.

The steroid suspension is formulated to have a repository effect and so is relatively insoluble in fine particles. Most commonly used, and longest lasting, are triamcinolone hexacetonide (Aristospan, Lederle), prednisolone t-Butyl acetate (Hydeltra T.B.A., M.S.&D), or methylprednisolone acetate (Depomedrol, Upjohn). These are available in concentrations of 20-40 mg per ml. Large joints, such as hip or knee, may require from 20 to 30 mg of the steroid suspension for optimal effect, decreasing down to 3-5 mg for small (finger or toe) joints. It is better not to inject many joints at one sitting, both to avoid undue trauma to the patient and to avoid major systemic absorption of steroid. Injections are seldom recommended oftener than every 6 weeks into any joint, and then only if symptoms and signs have returned markedly.

Techniques for aspirating each peripheral joint cannot be described here in detail but are readily available in several presentations, with illustrations.[1,2]

EFFECTS OF INTRASYNOVIAL CORTICOSTEROID INJECTION

The anti-inflammatory effect of injected corticosteroid suspension may become apparent within a few hours, and even the slower acting preparations such as triamcinolone hexacetonide exert a definite suppressing action on local irritation or inflammation within a day. Maximum effect is usually seen within 72 hours. It has been found advisable to limit activity of the injected joint, particularly a weight-bearing joint, for at least a few days after the local treatment.

The local steroid effect is not simply a relief of pain, which can also be accomplished by potent analgesics, by acupuncture, or by transcutaneous electrical nerve stimulation (TENS). The steroid effect is partial to complete suppression of the local inflammatory process for a period of weeks, thus inhibiting the local tissue destruction by the inflammation. Not only is pain relieved, but swelling is lessened or even eliminated, redness and heat of the part disappear, the stiffness decreases, so the function of the joint improves. This prompt, lasting, and definite effect on a stiff, painful joint thus can speed up rehabilitation greatly. In osteoarthritic joints the reaction to the friction of the roughened joint surfaces is usually obliterated to such a degree that care must be taken to limit activity (vide infra).

REPEATABILITY AND LONG-TERM EFFECTS
FROM INJECTIONS

Injections into an arthritic joint or bursa that is inflamed may be repeated indefinitely for long-term control. Reinjection should not be made oftener than every 6 weeks in osteoarthritic joints or every month in rheumatoid arthritic joints, and then only if symptoms and signs have recurred to a significant degree. The effect from the steroid may persist even for months if the joint is not abused. When symptoms and signs recur quickly after initial improvement, it usually means the patient is overutilizing the joint, the injection was not into the joint space, or the diagnosis needs rechecking. Unstable weight-bearing joints seldom remain asymptomatic for long periods after injection because of the mechanical strains incurred at each step irritating the tissues.

Some of the patients first treated with intra-articular steroid injections in our clinic in 1951 still receive reinjection occasionally on an as needed basis. Several have received more than 100 reinjections into a knee and still experience lasting relief, without deterioration of function of the joint.

FAILURES, ADVERSE REACTIONS, AND LIMITATIONS
OF STEROID INJECTION THERAPY

Failure to achieve improvement in the symptoms in a joint following corticosteroid injection occurs in less than 10 percent of instances, unless the needle has not penetrated the affected joint space. If fluid was aspirated from the joint, proving entrance into the synovial cavity, and the injection of steroid is not followed by decreased inflammation, the diagnosis should be rechecked. Joint inflammation from infection, from gross trauma such as fracture, or from marked instability with mechanical strains at each step is not palliated adequately by steroid injection.

After about 2 percent of injections there may occur a temporary flare, with increased swelling, stiffness, and pain lasting a few hours, then followed by rapid improvement. In this event rest and elevation of the part are advised, and local application of an ice bag for a few minutes at a time until the reaction is ended. Such reactions occur more often after the injected extremity has been actively used within the first day following injection.

Particularly in osteoarthritic joints, the relief after steroid injection may be so marked that the patient will abuse the joint, thinking he is cured of his disability. If the injection simply stops the symptoms allowing the patient to abuse the joint, it is like sweeping dirt under the rug. The roughened joint continues to build up friction on too active use, with the warning symptom of pain obliterated by the steroid. The patient must be cautioned to *moderate* activity: "The injection is to help you do what you *must* do with as little pain as possible, *not* to allow you to do more and more until it hurts again."

If the technique of the injection has not been careful, infection of the injected joint may occur. Although this has been a complication in less than 1 per 10,000 injections the possibility must be kept in mind. Avoidance of infection requires very careful skin cleansing, carefully sterilized needles and syringes, and immediate reaspiration of any joint that has flared up for more than a few hours after injection, with bacterial cultures sent to the laboratory. Prompt treatment of infections when they do occur prevents serious problems that might necessitate surgical intervention.

Joints that have been frequently reinjected, particularly if too often or using excessive steroid doses, may show signs of increasing instability, with laxity of the capsule and supporting ligaments. Whenever this is noted, reinjection should be withheld, activity reduced, and a supporting brace fitted to prevent further laxity. If instability and recurrent pain persist and are severe, surgical replacement of the joint may be needed. Whenever repeated injections fail to give relief, x-rays and an orthopedic consultation are needed.

SUMMARY

Most textbooks on rehabilitation scarcely mention the use of intra-articular corticosteroids. This valuable adjunct in arthritis rehabilitation is often neglected because the physician and therapist have not been made aware of its place in therapy, because they are ignorant of the techniques, or because they are afraid to attempt this specialized form of treatment for fear of introducing infection or producing further breakdown in an arthritic joint.

I have used this form of treatment innumerable times in the 31 years since my colleagues and I developed intrasynovial steroid therapy. It has become a standard form of arthritis treatment all over the world. Although this is *localized* in action, and *temporary* albeit lasting for weeks or even months after each palliative treatment, it can achieve relief repeatedly over years, with judicious reinjections into painful joints, bursae, or tendon sheaths, preventing contractures and deformity. No other treatment for arthritis has given so much relief, to so many, for so long with so few side effects as intrasynovial corticosteroid therapy.

REFERENCES

1.   Hollander JL. Intrasynovial corticosteroid therapy. In: Hollander JL, ed., Arthritis and allied conditions, 8th ed. Philadelphia: Lea and Febiger, 1972, pp. 517–534. Also in 9th ed., McCarty DJ, ed., 1979, pp. 402–414.
2.   McCarty DJ. Special techniques in treating arthritic disorders. In: Hollander JL, ed., Arthritis handbook. West Point, Pa.: Merck, Sharp and Dohme, 1974, pp. 131–140.

19

Biofeedback, Transcutaneous Electrical Nerve Stimulation, Acupuncture, and Hypnosis

Bob G. Johnson, Ed.D.

A variety of procedures have been used over the years to control the pain associated with arthritis. Pain is undoubtedly the greatest single factor leading to the debilitation of people with arthritis. Hence pain control is very important for patients suffering from arthritis. While pharmacotherapy forms the principal modality to compensate for the control of inflammation and pain, other measures also provide help in attaining a state of physiological balance.

BIOFEEDBACK AND THE ARTHRITIS PATIENT

Although the modality of biofeedback has been undergoing research for nearly 80 years in one form or another, it gained clinical prominence only two decades ago. Even more recently it was given its title by Barbara Brown, a physiologist with the Veterans Administration.[1]

Biofeedback is a training procedure utilized for the development of certain kinds of physiological control. In this procedure, subtle bioelectric signals originating in a particular body structure are monitored by sensitive electronic equipment. These signals, once monitored, are amplified and used to power an external stimulus display. The display employed may be in the form of lights or tones or clicks. As the bioelectrical signal varies, so also does the light color or tone frequency or click rate. In this way the patient is supplied with immediate feedback about the behavior of the monitored body function.

Biofeedback refers to any of a wide variety of techniques that use instrumentation to provide a patient with information about changes in his or her own physiologic functions, of which he or she is usually not aware. The information provided is immediate and continuous. When this information is furnished to patients, they are often able to learn to control these previously involuntary functions.

Before voluntary control can be established over some aspect of a patient's physiology, the patient must be aware of the event. Relevant knowledge may include an indication of the level of the event, as is the case with electromyographic feedback or with temperature feedback. Thus the instrument system must be sensitive, accurate, artifact-free, and it must feed back meaningful information. Gradually, through a process of trial and error, the patient evolves strategies for controlling the feedback signals and thereby the physiologic response. The patient learns to associate certain thoughts, as well as proprioceptive and interoceptive sensations with changes in the feedback. A patient may develop some degree of control even before he or she is able to verbalize what is happening. However, the ability to verbalize control strategies enhances transfer of the control from the clinic to real life. Patients are therefore encouraged to describe sensations as well as successful and unsuccessful strategies. Often this incorporates a phrase or series of phrases that will become conditioned to the desired physiological pattern.

One form of behavior is often more desirable than another form, one rate of behavior more profitable than another rate. Therefore patients can rely upon the consequence of behavior to redirect the ways in which they behave to more suitable and healthy patterns. Under certain conditions relaxed muscles are more desirable than tense muscles, a quiet brain healthier than an active brain, and a slowed heart rate better than a rapid one. With biofeedback procedures a patient learns the rate at which a particular body behavior is behaving, as well as how to modify this behavior at will.

Studies have shown that arthritic patients feel more pain when they are under stress.[2] Although a clear-cut connection has not been made, an increase in the production of endocrine hormones that cause inflammation occurs when people are under stress.[3] This may modulate or cause much of an arthritic patient's pain. A patient with arthritis who is exposed to stress will react in an individualized manner influenced by both physical characteristics and developed behavior. Since we all live in a world with considerable stress, it must be recognized that stress cannot be totally eliminated from one's life, nor should it.

Since to eliminate the sources of stress is impractical if not impossible, a more viable alternative is to better manage the existing situation. Arthritis cannot yet be eliminated in most cases, so the remaining choice for patients is to learn to cope more readily with their circumstances. Most people can learn to modify their reactions to stressful situations rather than simply trying to ignore them. Biofeedback procedures are beneficial in that they can help patients obtain information necessary to reach this important goal in a natural manner. In many cases both medication levels and pain levels can be reduced.

Biofeedback procedures employ many standard electronic medical instruments. These are modified to give feedback to the patient via the methods discussed earlier. There are also new instruments designed specifically for biofeedback. Because specialized training in the application of the instruments, as well as the biofeedback procedures, is necessary if it is to benefit the patient, practitioners should produce evidence of certification by the Biofeedback Certification Institute of America,[2] as well as an advanced degree in an appropriate professional specialty. Professionals now applying biofeedback include physicians, psychiatrists, psychologists, rehabilitation counselors, speech therapists, physical therapists, occupational therapists, and nurses. Biofeedback is administered in hospitals, in clinics, and in private offices. Research indicates that the application of electromyographic and temperature biofeedback strategies are most useful in treating patients with arthritis.[4,6]

TRANSCUTANEOUS ELECTRICAL NERVE STIMULATION

Transcutaneous electrical nerve stimulation (TENS) has come to be well recognized as an effective method in the symptomatic treatment of individuals suffering from arthritic pain. Historically it is not a new process. According to Lampe the early Greeks and Romans used electric fish in an attempt to control pain; centuries later, in the late 1700s, man-made devices appeared, replacing natural sources of electricity.[5] In the 1960s, with the publication of the work of Melzak and Wall, the utilization of electrical devices in the control of pain was given new life.[6] For patients suffering arthritis, because pain is usually accompanied by muscle spasms, voluntary protective guarding of painful areas becomes important. The guarding may lead to progressive joint dysfunction with contractures and loss of motion and thereby to more pain. This cyclical tendency leads to circulatory impairment exacerbating the pain.

Transcutaneous electrical nerve stimulation is an innocuous, noninvasive approach to the relief of both acute and chronic pain. Burton states that, "Transcutaneous Electrical Nerve Stimulation (TENS) appears to be a relatively simple and safe means of therapy to manage uncomplicated and well localized pain. TENS is most effective when applied by trained professionals under a physician's supervision. Adequate patient education and clinical trial of the instrumentation are key factors to successful application."[7]

There are a number of theories as to how pain is blocked by electrical neuromodulation. One of the more popular theories is espoused by Melzak as a neurologic "gate" control.[6] More recent evidence suggests that the utilization of TENS units may result in the release of an endogenous morphine equivalent known as endorphin.[5] Regardless of the theoretical base, the pain relief obtained from the use of TENS appears to be real.

The application of TENS units can be an efficacious means of controlling arthritic pain. However, some important considerations should be kept in mind. The use of TENS is effective only if the choices of electrode sites and methods of placement are based upon anatomical and physiological considerations. The choices of electrode sites and the methods of placement are numerous and selection depends upon an awareness of the etiology, location, and character of the pain. Pain can arise from a myriad of superficial and deep tissues and is transmitted by both the central and autonomic nervous systems. The resulting sensation can be perceived locally but may also be referred or radiated to distant areas. Another factor affecting choice of placement is that pain can be referred extrasegmentally from distant trigger points or from such structures as the dura mater.

Furthermore, the choice of equipment, electrode size, single or dual channels, the most effective frequency and duration of treatment must be understood.[8] At least one study has demonstrated the efficiency of TENS units with patients with chronic arthritis.[8,9] The study also shows results favoring specific frequencies to obtain optimal duration of pain relief. Based upon these studies and others the use of TENS units with arthritis patients is well supported.

Therapists using TENS must provide an educational program for their patients in order that unwarranted expectations or counterindications evolving from treatment will not develop.

OTHER APPROACHES TO PAIN CONTROL IN ARTHRITIS

Space does not allow more than a comment regarding additional systems of pain alleviation. Nevertheless, one further approach that has been given considerable attention is acupuncture. Traditional acupuncture includes the utilization of slender, solid needles that are implanted at sites in the skin discerned by the acupuncturist through lengthy periods of study and practice. Acupuncturists subscribe to a theory that states that insertion of the needles leads to an increased flow of "life forces" and the eventual "homeostatic balancing of the person's energy flow."

Some acupuncturists employ needles attached to a device that produces low-voltage electrical flows to increase the effect of the treatment. Many acupuncture points are located over superficial branches of the peripheral nerves that appear to be regions having decreased skin resistance and a high-density input to the central nervous system. These same locations are affective placement points for TENS electrodes as well. As with TENS, it has been suggested that acupuncture stimulates the release of endorphins, which account for the analgesic and anesthetic effects of the treatment. Some controlled studies have suggested at least transient pain relief in patients wth arthritis.

Hypnosis and related altered states have been used in pain reduction for many years. Sigmund Freud probably made the utilization of hypnosis more acceptable to the medical community and lent credibility to the treatment. The Hilgards have studied application of hypnosis to pain control in their laboratory at Stanford University for many years.[10] However, this modality has been accepted in alleviation of arthritic pain only in the past decade. Few studies are yet available as to its efficacy.

SUMMARY

Biofeedback and transcutaneous electrical nerve stimulation have found increasing acceptance in the control of the pain of arthritis within the past two decades. The alleviation of pain from each of these modalities is real, but care must be taken in choosing professionals who are adequately trained and experienced if significant and lasting pain relief is to be obtained by the patient. There has been a tendency for personnel who are relatively unknowledgeable to practice the use of biofeedback and transcutaneous electrical nerve stimulation—with poor results. Other modalities, including acupuncture and hypnosis, have also been demonstrated to obtain acceptable outcomes in pain control.

REFERENCES

1. Brown BB. New mind, new body. New York: Harper & Row, 1974.
2. Schwartz MS. Biofeedback Certification Institute of America. Blueprint knowledge statements. Biofeedback Self Reg 1981;6:253–262.
3. Wickramasekera I. The management of rheumatoid arthritic pain: preliminary observations. In: Truong ST, Bush M, Orr C, eds., Biofeedback, behavior therapy, and hypnosis: potentiating the verbal control of behavior for clinicians. New York: Nelson-Hall, 1976.
4. Brown BB. Stress and the art of biofeedback. New York: Harper & Row, 1977.
5. Lampe GN. Introduction to the use of transcutaneous electrical nerve stimulation devices. Phys Ther 1978;58:1450–1454.
6. Melzak R, Wall P. A new theory. Science 1965;150:971–977.
7. Burton C. Transcutaneous electrical nerve stimulation to relieve pain. Post Grad Med 1976;59:105–108.
8. Mannheimer JS. Electrode placements for transcutaneous electrical nerve stimulation. Phys Ther 1978;58:1455–1461.
9. Mannheimer C, Carlsson CA. The effect of transcutaneous electrical nerve stimulation (TENS) on joint pain in patients with rheumatoid arthritis. Scand J Rheum 1978;7:13–16.
10. Hilgard R, Hilgard JR. Hypnosis in the relief of pain. Los Altos, Calif.: William Kaufman, 1975.

ADDITIONAL READING

Achterberg J, McGraw P, Lawlis FG. Rheumatoid arthritis: a study of relaxation and temperature biofeedback training as an adjunctive therapy. Biofeedback Self Reg 1981; 6:207–223.
Basmajian JV. Muscles alive, 3rd ed. Baltimore: Williams and Wilkins, 1974.
Bresler DE. Free yourself from pain. New York: Simon and Schuster, 1979.
Gaarder K, Montgomery P. Clinical biofeedback: a procedural manual. Baltimore: Williams and Wilkins, 1977.

Green RM. Commentary on electricity. Cambridge, Mass.: Elizabeth Licht, 1953.

Hendler N. Diagnosis and non-surgical management of pain. New York: Raven Press, 1981.

Hilgard ER. Pain as a puzzle for psychology and physiology. Am Psychol 1969;24: 103-113.

Kiviniemi P. Emotions and personality in rheumatoid arthritis: a control study. Helsinki, Finland: University of Helsinki, 1977;6:(suppl. 18).

Loeser JD, Black RG, Christman A. Relief of pain by transcutaneous stimulation. J Neurosurg 1975;42:308-314.

Long BM, Hagfors N. Electrical stimulation in the nervous system: the current status of electrical stimulation of the nervous system on pain relief. Pain 1975;1:109-123.

McGlasham T, Evans F, Orne M. The nature of hypnotic, analgesia, and placebo responses to experimental pain. Psychosomatic Med 1969;31:227-246.

Oka M, Rekonen A, Elomma I. Muscle blood flow in rheumatoid arthritis. Acta Rheum Scand 1971;17:203-208.

Olton DS, Noonberg AR. Biofeedback, clinical applications in behavioral medicine. Englewood Cliffs, N.J.: Prentice-Hall, 1980.

Pelletier KR. Mind as healer, mind as slayer. New York: Dell, 1975.

Shelly CN. Electrical control of the nervous system. Med Program Technol 1974;2:71-80.

Weiner HM. Psychobiology and human disease. New York: Elsevier, 1977.

Williams RC, Jr. Rheumatoid arthritis as a systemic disease, vol. 4, Philadelphia: WB Saunders, 1974.

20

Gait and Ambulation

Carolee Moncur, P.T., M.S., and Marlin N. Shields, R.P.T.

Normal human walking, with its rhythmical movement of body segments, is easily taken for granted in the able-bodied person. To the primary health care physician, the medical care of the arthritis patient is more important than the problems identified by the walking patterns of the patient. Yet these abnormal patterns, prolonged over a long period of time, may cause unnecessary deformities. The physician has a valuable resource in the physical therapist, who, by virtue of training in normal and abnormal gait and ambulation, may assist in the evaluation and care of the arthritis patient. Mechanical problems related to arthritis changes may readily appear during the process of ambulation and give valuable clues to needed treatment.

NORMAL GAIT

Sufficient literature exists that describes various methods for analyzing gait from simplistic methods to more sophisticated methods as utilized in gait analysis laboratories. For the health care practitioner without elaborate resources and the consulting services of a physical therapist, it seems in order to review briefly the components of normal gait.

Normal walking is a sequential progression of standing postures that moves the body forward while retaining balance and security.[1] An effective stride and a stable standing position are the two components necessary for successful walking. The step is therefore divided into two major phases: the *stance* phase (when the limb supports the body weight) and the *swing* phase (when the limb moves forward). Bekey et al. have discussed eight phases of normal gait (figure 20.1). (1) *Initial contact* occurs at heel strike; however, it may also be accomplished with the toe or with the foot flat. (2) *Loading response* has reference to the reaction of the limb segments to being loaded under the circumstance dictated by how the foot

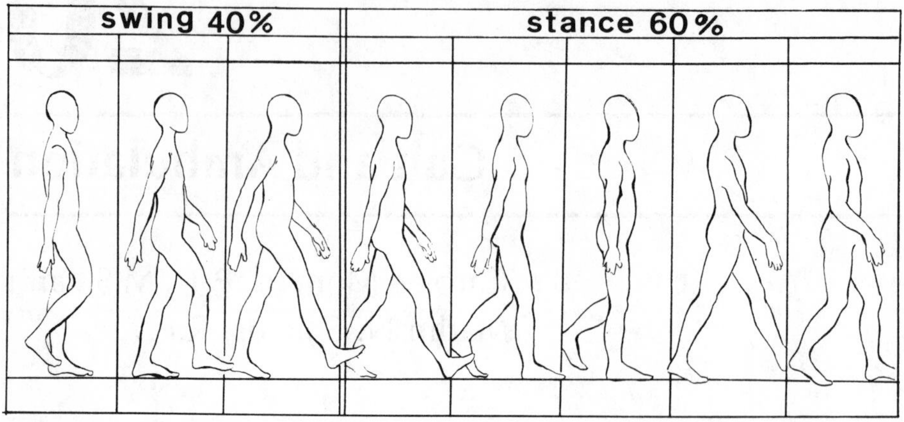

Source: Reprinted by permission of Professional Staff Association, Rancho Los Amigos Hospital, 7413 Golondrinas, Downey, Calif. 90242.
Figure 20.1.   Drawing of the normal gait cycle. (After the representation by the Professional Staff Association of the Rancho Los Amigos Hospital in "Normal and Pathological Gait Syllabus," 1978)

initially contacts a surface. (3) *Midstance* is that period when there is stationary foot support. (4) *Terminal stance* applies to the portion of the single stance period when the body is forward on the supporting foot; normally this occurs at heel off. (5) *Preswing* has reference to the terminal double support period that initiates knee flexion in normal gait. (6) *Initial swing* begins with the occurrence of picking up the foot and advancing the unloaded limb forward. (7) *Midswing* refers to the actions that occur after the swinging limb is forward of the supporting limb; at this time the tibia becomes vertical with respect to the floor. (8) *Terminal swing* is the final period of knee extension prior to initial contact.[1]

Hoppenfeld divides the stance and swing phases into several components. The components of the stance phase are heel strike, foot flat, midstance, and push-off (toe-off). Components of the swing phase are acceleration, midswing, and deceleration. Since the stance-phase limb undergoes the largest amount of stress during walking, the best moment for assessing problems related to gait is during that portion. The person's gait patterns can be observed as the patient enters the examining area.[2]

Characteristics of normal human walking have been described by Inman, Ralston, and Todd.[3] These authors have suggested that during stance phase the width of the base of support should not be more than 2 to 4 inches from toe to heel. During forward motion, the center of gravity of the body (which lies 2 inches in front of the second sacral vertebra) should not oscillate more than 2 inches in a vertical direction. The knee of the swing phase extremity should remain flexed throughout the phase with the exception of heel strike (figure 20.2).

Inman et al. have indicated that the pelvis and trunk will shift laterally

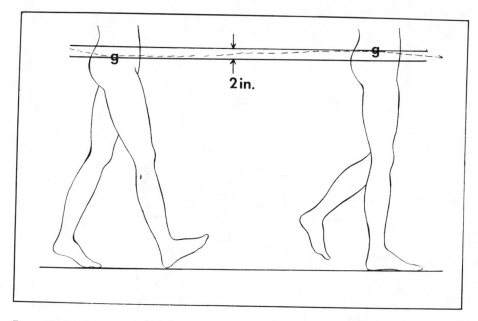

Figure 20.2.   Representation of the vertical oscillation of the center of gravity.

approximately 1 inch toward the stance phase extremity in order to center the weight over that hip. The pelvis rotates forward approximately 40° during swing phase, as the hip joint of the stance phase limb acts as a fulcrum (figure 20.3).

The step length (figure 20.4) is approximately 15 inches in healthy adults and decreases with the aging process. The number of steps per minute (cadence) of the average healthy adult is approximately 90 to 100 steps per minute, utilizing approximately 100 calories per mile.[3,4]

Understanding these basic concepts of the components of normal gait will greatly assist the physician who must assess the gait patterns of patients with abnormal gait.

ABNORMAL GAIT: EVALUATION OF COMMON CLINICAL PROBLEMS

In a person with arthritis any of the events of the gait cycle may be disturbed; however, problems are readily noticeable during the stance phase of walking. Bearing weight on an extremity with painful joints, between any of its segments, will result in the patient unconsciously producing a protective or antalgic gait. In acute injuries, such as a sprained ankle, the patient will assume a similar gait pattern; however, once the injury has healed, the patient will return to the normal

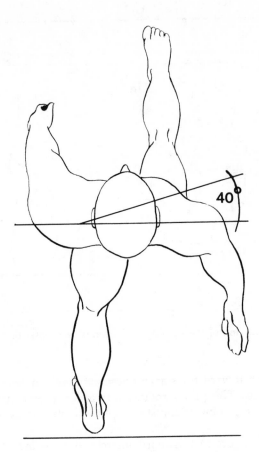

Figure 20.3.   Forward rotation of the pelvis during swing phase.

pattern of walking. The chronicity of arthritis does not facilitate a return to normalcy; therefore the patient with persistent pain may assume a permanent antalgic gait pattern. As a result of attempting to protect painful joints, postural "splinting" may occur, creating the improper use or disuse of the musculature around the joint with resultant muscle weakness and atrophy.

Utilizing the observational gait analysis system of the Pathokinesiology Laboratory at Rancho Los Amigos Hospital,[5] Winchester and Eckerson have identified several pathomechanical problems that might occur in the walking patterns of the patient with arthritis.[6] These will be discussed according to the phase of walking in which they occur, stance or swing.

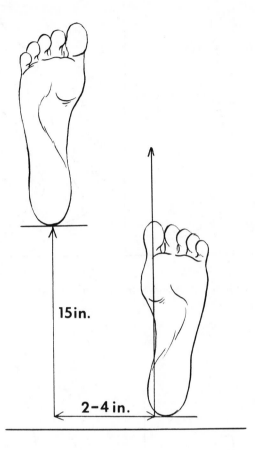

Figure 20.4.   Normal step length.

Stance Phase

Metatarsalgia (painful metatarsal heads) is readily identified during the stance phase of gait (figures 20.5 and 20.6). During midstance the body does not progress over the afflicted foot, whereas at terminal stance the body does not progress ahead of the afflicted foot. The primary and compensatory deviations that occur during midstance are primarily pain and decreased stance time on the involved extremity. During this phase the patient will bear more weight on the heel, decrease the length of the contralateral step, and manifest excessive dorsiflexion of the painful foot. There may be a compensatory increase in subtalar valgus or varus, knee flexion, and hip flexion. At terminal stance, the heel will not rise, thus protecting the forefoot from pain.

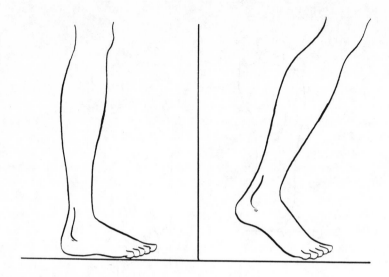

Figure 20.5. Normal foot in mid and terminal stance phases.

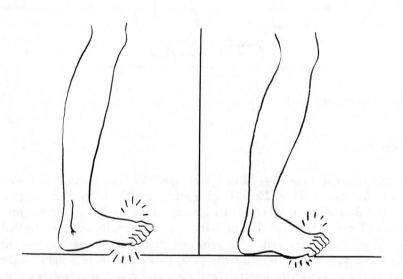

Figure 20.6. Metatarsalgia in mid and terminal stance phases.

Poor *plantar flexor strength* in the patient with arthritis may result because of changes in the ankle joint, subtalar joint, metatarsals, os calcis, and/or disuse of the musculature. During midstance the patient will manifest an improper body alignment in a somewhat flexed position without the body progressing normally over the stationary foot. At terminal stance the body progression ahead of the supporting foot is impaired. The primary deviations demonstrated are excessive dorsiflexion of the foot during midstance and the absence of heel rise during terminal stance. Compensatory deviations manifested during midstance are knee flexion, a forward trunk, and decreased stance time.

Knee flexion contractures will create problems in the gait cycle in both stance and swing phases. During stance phase, however, the heel will not be the initial contact point with the floor. At the loading response there will be reduced or no reaction of the limb to absorbing the impact of weight acceptance. Midstance will reveal an improper body alignment. The primary deviation that will be seen during initial contact is the toe touching the floor first or in a foot flat position. At midstance the primary deviation will be inadequate knee extension with compensatory hip flexion and a forward trunk.

Subtalar valgus will create kinesiologic problems resulting in the posterolateral portion of the heel of the foot not being the first point of contact with the floor during stance phase. During midstance the primary deviation will be the valgus deformity of the foot with a compensatory genu valgus, adduction of the hip and decreased stance time (figures 20.7–20.9).

A *hip flexion contracture of 40°*, for example, will cause a malalignment of the body posture during midstance and terminal stance phase. The primary deviation will be inadequate hip extension in the stationary limb. Compensatory deviations will be manifested as a forward bending of the trunk, tilting of the symphysis downward, and excessive knee flexion with dorsiflexion of the foot.

The *hip abductors* may decrease in strength in the arthritis patient. For example, if a patient has a "fair" grade abductor group of muscles, during both mid- and terminal stance phase the body will not be in proper alignment. The primary deviation that will be observed will be contralateral pelvic drop with compensatory lateral trunk flexion and forward trunk flexion due to the increased length in the unaffected limb. In order to correct the muscle weakness, the abductors of the hip should be increased in strength to a "good" grade.[6,7]

Swing Phase

Poor *plantar flexion strength* will not create abnormal kinesiologic manifestations in the swing phase limb.

Knee flexion contractures will not allow the swinging limb to extend fully at the knee (terminal swing). The primary deviations that will be observed will be inadequate extension of the knee and a decreased step length. Consequently the compensatory mechanisms that will occur will be excessive pelvic and trunk rotation with flexion of the contralateral stance phase limb.

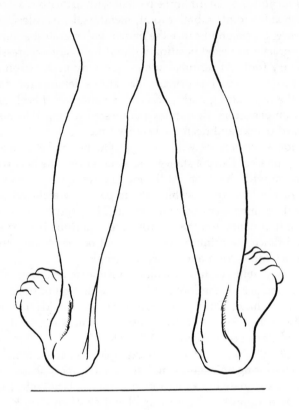

Figure 20.7.   Subtalar and genu valgus.

During swing phase the patient with *metatarsalgia* (painful metatarsal head) will be able to meet all of the demands of the phase. There will be no manifestations of primary or compensatory deviations. The same is true for *subtalar valgus deformity* and *hip abductor weakness.*

With a hip flexion contracture of 40°, for example, the normal demand of lifting the limb and advancing it forward during the initial swing phase will not be met. The primary deviation noted is excessive hip flexion. Compensatory deviations with a hip flexion contracture will be backward trunk motion and limited active hip flexion, and the symphysis pubis will tip forward.[6,8-12]

TREATMENT OF A COMMON CLINICAL PROBLEM

Although it is outside the scope of this chapter to suggest treatment for all of the previously discussed gait-related problems, one common problem that affects the walking pattern of arthritis patients warrants discussion. *Metatarsalgia* is

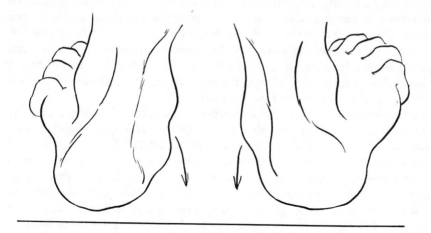

Figure 20.8. Subtalar valgus.

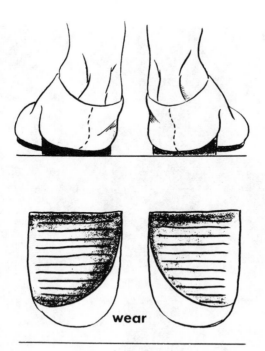

Figure 20.9. Posterior and heel views of shoes of patient with subtalar valgus.

recognized as a painful condition that not only affects the forefoot but also affects the utilization of the musculature and therefore motion of the ankle, knee, and hip joints. The patient subconsciously creates an antalgic gait pattern by attempting to avoid pain during the gait cycle. The patient avoids plantar flexion and complete knee and hip extension, thus facilitating the potential for loss of muscle function and joint range of motion in the joints of the lower extremity, and the potential for permanent loss of function exists.

Early metatarsalgia may be unobtrusive; however, the symptoms may become quite obvious during terminal stance (toe-off) and upon palpation with pressure over the metatarsal heads (figures 20.10, 20.11). Early diagnosis will allow changes to be made that may improve the gait patterns, prevent deformities, and protect painful joints. A custom-fitted soft orthotic with a metatarsal pad placed just behind the metatarsal heads will redistribute pressure during the foot flat portion of the stance phase of gait. A soft, closed-cell material, such as Spenco, placed directly under the metatarsal heads will absorb the shock and friction of the terminal stance phase (prior to toe-off) of walking (figure 20.12). At this time the foot orthosis is now able to redistribute any weight effectively away from the metatarsal heads.

Extra-depth shoes with a removable liner will allow for the custom orthotic

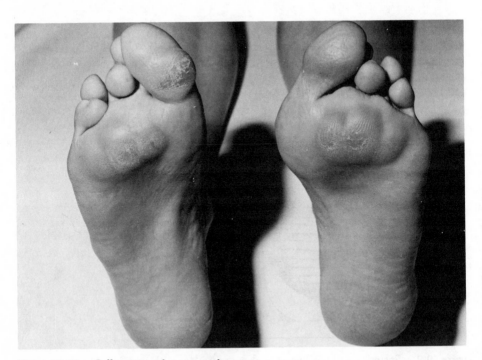

Figure 20.10. Callousities of metatarsalgia.

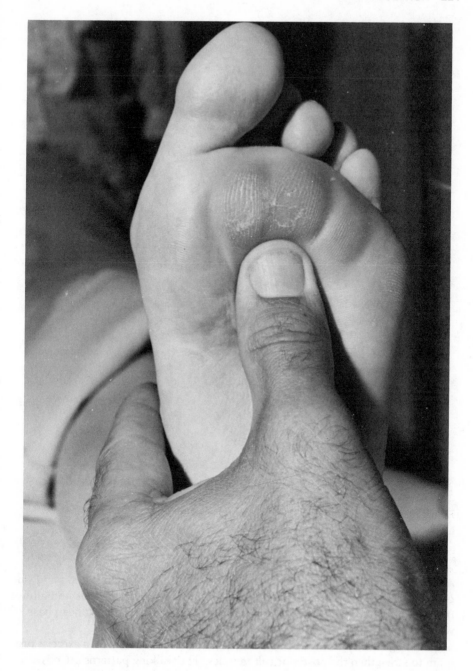

Figure 20.11.   Palpation of the metatarsal heads.

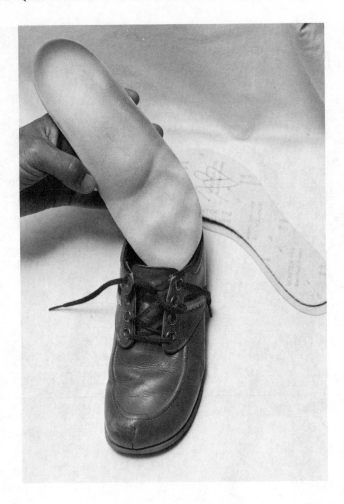

Figure 20.12.   A custom-fitted soft orthosis for metatarsalgia.

and the patient's foot to be accommodated without pressure on the top and side of the foot from the shoe. This reduces pain in the metatarsal heads and allows the patient to return to a more normal gait pattern during the stance phase of walking (figure 20.13).

Along with appropriate footwear the patient is instructed in an exercise program to strengthen the posterior calf muscles. The walking patterns are observed by the therapist and correction of habits are suggested to the patient. Objective data utilizing the foot switch stride analyzer (figure 20.14) are collected before and after the placement of the orthosis in the shoe in order to assess cadence, velocity, time spent in stance, swing and double-support phases, and the foot

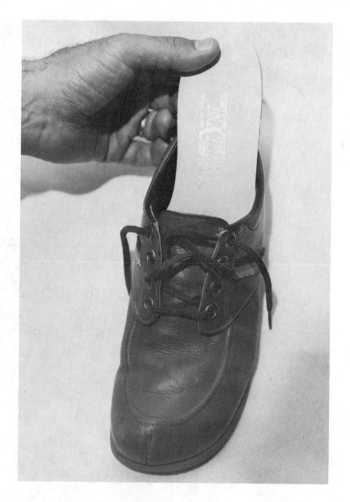

Figure 20.13. Extra depth shoes.

patterns of the patient. These data are compared to normal subjects' data of the same measures. Periodic follow-up is accomplished to monitor the status of the patient and his or her compliance patterns and progress.

PRINCIPLES FOR USE OF ASSISTIVE DEVICES DURING GAIT AND AMBULATION

When gait and ambulation training is required for the person with arthritis, certain general principles apply to this activity. The major goal will be to correct any

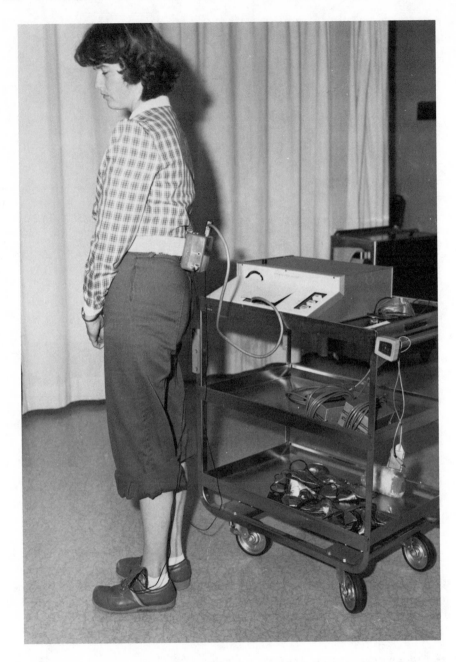

Figure 20.14. Footswitch stride analyzer.

deviations occurring in the gait cycle. This may be done by unloading the painful joint(s) that might be creating the antalgic gait pattern and by instructing the patient to assume different habits of walking. An important principle to remember is that ambulation in the person with arthritis may not be strictly a lower extremity function. To avoid tunnel vision, the health care practitioner must not forget that unloading a painful joint in the lower extremity may require the use of an assistive device that will load the joints of the upper extremity. Prolonged use of such a device may create pain and deformity in the upper extremity joints and subsequently minimize the functional ability of the patient to ambulate. The principles of joint protection, rest, and pain management apply during ambulation. Another important principle to recall when using assistive devices for joint protection during ambulation relates to the size of the joint. The largest and strongest joints of both the upper and lower extremities tolerate weight-bearing much more readily than do the small joints of the hand, wrist and, feet. It is important when making decisions about the assistive device to be used, that one consider the patient's life-style, employment, energy level, ability to rest, and tolerance to gadgets. If the patient is given a device that requires a high level of energy consumption to walk, compliance will be low. In summary, assistive devices should be designed for the individual and the environment in which the individual will be living and working.

In general the assistive device to be used will be determined by the physician's decision regarding the patient's weight-bearing status. Kathrins[13] has suggested that the weight-bearing classifications are predetermined by the physician as outlined in table 20.1.

Assistive devices not only facilitate ambulation but also general mobility such as getting in and out of bed, from lying to sitting, sitting to standing, and the reverse.[14] Wheelchairs are suited to the person with arthritis on both a temporary

Table 20.1.   Weight-bearing Classifications

Weight-bearing Status	Description	Assistive Devices
Non-weight-bearing bed to chair	Affected extremity's foot must touch ground	No ambulation
Non-weight-bearing	Affected extremity's foot must never touch ground	Two-handed device
Partial weight-bearing	50 percent of body weight onto affected extremity	Two-handed device
Full weight-bearing guarded	Total body weight on affected extremity	Two-handed device
Full weight-bearing	Total body weight on affected extremity	One- or two-handed device

Source: Reference 13. Reprinted with permission.

or permanent basis. When deformity is so extensive that ambulation is an unrealistic goal, then a wheelchair that is fitted to the width and height of the patient is necessary. Removable arm and leg rests can be placed on the chair. The physical therapist, collaborating with the patient, physician, and supplier, can prefit the chair to the satisfaction of the patient.

Ambulatory aids such as canes, crutches, or walkers are utilized to unload painful joints of the lower extremity. Which to use is determined by the joint(s) involved, the weight-bearing classification, and the status of the upper extremities. Forearm or platform crutches may be the most beneficial for the person with arthritis because they load the joints of the shoulder and elbow and decrease the loads on the hand and wrist. Canes must be fitted according to the stability of the patient in terms of balance as well as considering the involved joints. A cane with a straight or T handle is preferred to the C-shaped handle as the former tends to disperse the weight born on the upper extremity to the larger joints. The patient should be cautioned to avoid ulnar deviation of the hand whenever possible while using the cane.

When deciding upon the type of walker to be used, one should consider the weight-bearing status of the patient including pain, the time it takes for a patient to walk a certain distance, the energy costs involved, and the safety factors necessary for the patient. Although it might appear that walkers with four legs and crutch tips on each leg may be the choice for the person with arthritis, the energy and gait pattern required to move this type of walker may not provide the greatest benefit for the patient. Walkers with front wheels or gliders may be a better choice to reduce the energy costs and improve the gait pattern while being equally safe for the patient. If there is a concern about the patient bearing weight on the hands, the walker can be adapted with platforms to change the weight-bearing loads of the upper extremities to the elbows and shoulders.

SUMMARY

Several kinesiologic problems that are common in the patient with arthritis and appear during walking have been presented. Evaluation of the walking patterns is a valuable tool for assessing the status of the lower extremity. Should an assistive device be necessary for gait, ambulation, or general mobility, a thorough understanding of the disease process, joint protection, rest, pain management, and the patient's life-style must be sought. The evaluative and treatment skills of a physical therapist in gait analysis and ambulation, in concert with the diagnostic skills of the primary care provider, will reveal a more complete picture of the patient's physical status and allow for improved treatment programs.

REFERENCES

1. Bekey GA, Chang CW, Perry J, Hofer MM. Pattern recognition of multiple EMG signals applied to the description of human gait. Pro Inst Electrical and Electronics Engineers, May 1977;65, no. 5.
2. Hoppenfeld S. Examination of gait. In: Physical examination of the spine and extremities. New York: Appleton-Century-Crofts, 1976.
3. Inman VT, Ralston HJ, Todd F. Human walking. Baltimore: Williams and Wilkins, 1981.
4. Inman VT. Functional aspects of the abductor muscles of the hip. J Bone Joint Surg 1947;29:607.
5. Pathokinesiology Service and Physical Therapy Department. Normal and pathological gait syllabus. Professional Staff Association of Rancho Los Amigos Hospital, Downey, Calif., 1978.
6. Winchester P, and Eckerson L. Pathomechanics of gait in the patient with arthritis. Unpublished paper presented at the Western Regional Arthritis Health Profession Association Conference, Newport Beach, Calif., 1982.
7. Steindler A. Kinesiology of the human body. Springfield, Ill.: CC Thomas 1955.
8. Colson JM, Bergland G. An effective orthotic design for controlling the unstable subtalar joint. Orthotics Prosthetics 1979;33:39–49.
9. Eyring EJ, Murray WP. The effect of joint position on the pressure of intra-articular effusion. J Bone Joint Surg 1964;46A:1235–1241.
10. Murray MP, Gore DR, Clarkson BH. Walking patterns of patients with unilateral hip pain due to osteoarthritis and avascular necrosis. J Bone Joint Surg 1971;53A:259–274.
11. Sutherland DH, Cooper L, Daniel D. The role of the ankle plantar flexors in normal walking. J Bone Joint Surg 1980;62A:354–363.
12. Vahvanen V. Rheumatoid arthritis of the pantalar joints. Acta Orthop Scand 1969; Suppl 107.
13. Kathrins B. Orthopedics. In: Logigian MK, ed. Adult rehabilitation: a team approach for therapists. Boston: Little, Brown, 1982, p. 73.
14. Silverman EH. Rheumatic diseases: evaluation and treatment. In: Logigian MK, ed., Adult rehabilitation: a team approach for therapists. Boston: Little, Brown, 1982, p. 134.

21

The Role of Surgery in Rehabilitation of the Arthritis Patient

Lawrence M. Haas, M.D.

Rehabilitation of the arthritis patient presents a difficult yet rewarding challenge to the health care team. The role of the surgeon has changed considerably in the past decade. It is now widely accepted that the combined skills of primary care physicians, rheumatologists, surgeons, podiatrists, nursing personnel, physical therapists, occupational therapists, counselors and psychologists, social workers, and vocational counselors are needed to achieve the optimum rehabilitation of a person afflicted with arthritis.[1] In former years the surgeon was called upon as a last resort when other methods of treatment failed. Today early surgery may be an important factor in rehabilitation. Total joint replacement may rehabilitate an arthritis patient much more rapidly than years of gait training, exercises, and therapy. However, surgery may not always be the best method of rehabilitation. This chapter will discuss when to consult the surgeon, when to perform surgery, and what rehabilitation is necessary before and after surgery.

SURGICAL SPECIALISTS

The orthopedic surgeon is most often the surgical specialist caring for the arthritis patient. Other surgeons are often consulted, however. Difficult spinal problems can require the skills of a neurosurgeon or orthopedic surgeon specializing in spine surgery. Certain temporomandibular problems are treated by oral surgeons or maxillofacial surgeons. The specialty of hand surgery is very important to the arthritis patient. Orthopedic surgeons, plastic surgeons, and some general surgeons subspecialize in surgery of the hand and are valuable members of the arthritis team. The podiatrist can also make significant contributions to foot surgery. Orthopedic surgeons have the best background to evaluate totally the extremity problems of arthritis patients. They also can perform surgery when indicated and will defer to various subspecialists when the occasion dictates.

SURGICAL CONSIDERATIONS

Surgery cannot cure arthritis. It must be considered one of the available methods of treatment. Surgery can alleviate pain, correct deformities, and restore function. The timing of surgery in the patient with arthritis is critical. If surgery is delayed until all function is lost and the patient's condition has severely deteriorated, then the chance of optimal rehabilitation is poor. The wise surgeon does not proceed with surgery until the patient has had a trial of other methods of treatment. One cannot accurately predict the incidence or duration of remission. Seldom can surgery be considered preventive or be given full credit for improvement in the disease status. It is possible to define indications for surgery in arthritis patients, however. When surgery is performed, the results of surgery can be considered temporary if the disease continues unchecked.

Adequate surgical treatment of patients can best be performed when they are seen relatively early in their disease.[2] Surgery is performed as indications become evident. To ask for a surgical consultation does not mean that surgery is requested. The surgical specialist is asked to evaluate the patient's history of problems, perform a physical examination oriented toward the surgical problem, and make recommendations for current or future treatment. The surgeon is more than happy to see the patient for "consultation only." Many factors influence the decision to operate. One of the most important factors is the attitude of the patient. Cooperation of the patient is essential. Many patients with arthritis have waxing and waning episodes of depression, and surgery probably should be delayed during symptomatic phases. Persons with long-standing arthritis with marked disability may become apathetic and depressed. However, sometimes small gains attained at surgery can restore enthusiasm and improve the outlook on life.

It is not recommended that one persuade a patient to undergo surgery. It is beneficial to have patients speak with others who have had similar operations. An operation is indicated if it is within reasonable probability that reduction of pain and improvement of function can be expected for at least 1 year following surgery.

The timing of surgery is critical.[3] The operation should not be delayed until the patient's condition is end stage. It is not important to wait until the disease is completely quiescent and the sedimentation rate has fallen. However, surgery should be delayed during an acute generalized exacerbation. It is a misconception, however, that surgery usually causes exacerbation of arthritis.

If surgery is delayed too long the patient may become accustomed to being totally disabled and be too dispirited to be willing to make the necessary efforts to improve. The person with arthritis often develops progressive disability over a period of many years. Both the patient and his or her personal physician may fail to assess accurately the exact degree of deterioration since the functional loss occurs slowly over a long period of time. It is of great value to consult with rehabilitation specialists, who can give an accurate and objective assessment of the degree of disability and the rate of progression.

THE TEAM APPROACH

Surgery cannot be used alone in the treatment of arthritis. It can be successful only when combined with other treatment modalities. Physical and occupational therapy are valuable in the preoperative and postoperative care of arthritis patients. The therapist can give valuable information to the surgeon. Accurate preoperative measurement of deformity, range of motion, grip strength, muscle function, and patient attitudes and goals are essential. Occasionally the surgical treatment plan is altered based on the preoperative data obtained. Postoperatively the same team is the key to success. The most technically perfect surgery will fail if adequate rehabilitation is not done postoperatively. Muscle strengthening, range-of-motion exercises, and instructions in activities for daily living are given. Social workers can begin personal and vocational planning. The therapist can encourage the patient. Often handicapped persons become so dependent that after surgery they lapse into their preoperative lethargy unless persistent encouragement is given by the health team.

Surgery itself can be a powerful rehabilitation tool. For example, consider a rheumatoid arthritis patient who has such severe knee and hip disease that he or she has to walk constantly with the external support of crutches. Occasionally a total knee and total hip replacement can allow the patient to use the upper extremities in a much more normal fashion. Even without hand surgery, the hand function has been improved by decreasing the need for crutches and allowing upper extremity function. Correct surgical treatment cannot be administered unless the signs of early deterioration of function are recognized. *There is very little indication for a "wait-and-see" attitude.* Six months or less is usually an adequate time to assess whether medical therapy, occupational therapy, physical therapy, splinting, or bracing have sufficiently relieved symptoms and improved function to recommend against surgery. In the early stages of arthritis and in juvenile arthritis nonsurgical therapy is usually indicated. Splinting is of great value. Muscle strengthening is very important. Later in the disease these methods may not succeed. Prophylactic surgery can be of great value for instance in preventing tendon ruptures of the hand.[3]

PATIENT AND PROCEDURE SELECTION

The highly motivated and cooperative patient who has not responded to the nonoperative therapy should be considered for evaluation by the appropriate surgical specialist. The primary care physician often asks "When should you operate?" As soon as it is established that there is a significant symptomatic and functional problem that is not responding to nonoperative measures, surgery should be considered. The patient should be motivated and have reasonable cardiovascular function and general good health. Advanced age is not a contraindication, since there are satisfied patients with excellent results beyond age 80. Youth *is* a relative contraindication to total joint replacement, since the components may not last long enough to be of prolonged value. However, a younger patient who is severely incapacitated by multiple joint involvement may wear the total joint out very slowly because far less "mileage" will be put on that joint than normal because of the person's other disabilities.

Another frequently asked question is "What joints should you operate on?" Careful evaluation and consultation with the health care team will often reveal which areas would be most benefited by reconstructive surgery. Multiple surgeries may be contraindicated. After two, three, or more operations, some patients appear to run out of gas. Even though further surgery might benefit them, they often state that they have had enough hospitalizations, have spent enough personal and insurance funds, and are often willing to accept what residual disabilities they have. It is therefore very important for the surgeon and other team members to assess which areas are most important to operate on first. An operative plan should be laid out for the patient. The procedures should be performed in the order of maximum benefit to the patient. For personal, health, family, or financial reasons, the patient may decide not to proceed any further. He or she will still have achieved considerable benefit from the surgical experience.

TYPES OF PROCEDURES

There are many operations that can help in rehabilitating the arthritis patient.[4]

Synovectomy. Synovectomy originally was felt to be of great prophylactic benefit in preventing further joint destruction in patients with rheumatoid arthritis. In recent years the role of synovectomy has become less well defined. A patient who has one or two swollen, painful joints, particularly the knee or metacarpophalangeal joints of the hands might be a candidate for early synovectomy, particularly if there is no evidence of joint destruction. If the patient's arthritis subsequently goes into remission, there may be long-term benefit from this surgical procedure. If exacerbations occur, however, synovitis can recur in these operated joints. There is no guarantee that a synovectomy will produce lasting relief. It is a way of buying time in one or two severely affected joints while waiting for long-term medical therapy such as gold to become effective.

Arthrodesis. Fusion of joints, or arthrodesis, is accomplished by removing involved joint surfaces and fixing the two bones together by one of several methods. Although joint function is lost, the joint is fused in a position of optimum function. The greatest benefit of the arthrodesis is the relief of pain. It is reserved for patients in whom other more functional procedures cannot be accomplished.

Total Joint Replacement.   The single major advance in the relief of pain and restoration of function of damaged major joints, particularly the hip and knee, has been total joint replacement. Total knee and hip arthroplasties in selected patients are now accepted as standard procedure. Silastic arthroplasties of the hands and wrists have also become standard. Less well defined are procedures to the ankle, shoulder, and elbow and other joints.

Total joint arthroplasty implies replacing both surfaces of a joint. This usually is accomplished by replacing one side of the joint with a metal component and the other side with a polyethylene component. These two surfaces can glide with little friction and do not require lubrication other than that supplied by body fluids. Wear characteristics are favorable, and there is little reaction or rejection by the host tissues. The components are usually fixed to the bone using methyl methacrylate bone cement. Newer methods are developing that may soon eliminate the need for bone cement. Infections and loosening of components are complications that can develop in the immediate postoperative period or as long as years later. When loosening alone develops, total joint revision can be accomplished to salvage function. When major infections occur, the artificial joint components usually have to be removed, resulting in shortening of the limb, loss of motion, and occasionally dictating arthrodesis of the joint.

Soft-Tissue Procedures.   Often of great benefit are tenosynovectomy, tendon repair, release of nerve entrapments, and other soft-tissue procedures. In the hand these procedures can be combined with silastic arthroplasty.

The following are specific anatomic areas where surgical treatment can facilitate the rehabilitation of the arthritis patient.

SPECIFIC JOINT SURGERY

Temporomandibular Joint.   Patients with arthritis, particularly those with ankylosing spondylitis and rheumatoid arthritis, can develop pain and limitation of motion of the temporomandibular joint.[5,6] When this involvement becomes severe, patients have difficulty eating and nutrition becomes a significant problem. Treatment in the acute phase consists of analgesic and certain anti-inflammatory drugs. When symptoms of subluxation occur, an occlusal splint can be constructed. If this therapy, along with medical therapy, is not successful, a single injection of long-acting steroids into the temporomandibular joint is indicated. This requires specialized knowledge of the anatomy of this area. In chronic phases where pain persists and jaw opening becomes more restricted, surgical treatment may be indicated. Surgery is performed by oral and maxillofacial surgeons and consists of menisectomy with arthroplasty, resurfacing the condylar head with an interposition alloplastic inlay graft such as Proplast Teflon sheeting. Surgery has been successful in elimination of pain and masticatory dysfunction.

Cervical Spine. Painful neck and arm symptoms are very common in arthritis patients.[7] They often respond to nonoperative therapy. Patients who do not respond to bracing, physical therapy, and medication and who develop neurologic findings of a myelopathy deserve careful investigation by the surgical specialist, usually a neurosurgeon. Patients with osteoarthritis often develop cervical disc disease and may benefit by cervical discectomy, foraminotomy, or anterior and posterior surgical fusions. Patients with advanced rheumatoid arthritis can develop the same problems, but in addition can develop severe C-1, C-2 subluxation. This complication has resulted in sudden death in these patients when the condition is so advanced that it causes marked subluxation with compression of the cervical cord and invagination of the odontoid process into the foramen magnum. These patients, when symptomatic, and when they do not respond to bracing, require posterior cervical wiring and fusion. However, while the patient is waiting for surgery, his or her head must be "sandbagged" or placed in a four-poster brace. Soft cervical collars will not give sufficient support.

Thoracic Spine. On rare occasions a patient with severe ankylosing spondylitis can benefit from osteotomy of the spine. This procedure should be performed only by an orthopedic surgeon who specializes in spinal surgery. There is a postoperative risk of paraplegia.

Shoulder. The surgeon is often consulted by a patient with early shoulder bursitis associated with arthritis. Injection, ultrasound, and range-of-motion exercises can be administered. If the patient develops a pericapsular fibrosis (frozen shoulder), a careful manipulation of the shoulder, under general anesthesia, can restore satisfactory function. The joint must be intact and relatively normal in order to consider manipulation. In a mild shoulder-impingement syndrome with catching or locking, removing the cause of the impingement, usually the underside of the acromion and outer clavicle, restores range of motion. Chronic bicipital tendonitis can be relieved by rerouting or tenodesing the long head of the biceps tendon. Loss of active range of motion due to rotator cuff insufficiency may require repair of the rotator cuff tear. Calcific tendonitis can be relieved by surgery if injections have failed. When arthritis of the glenohumeral joint (shoulder joint) has developed, total shoulder arthroplasty can be of benefit.[8] The results of total shoulder arthroplasty are not as predictable as those of total hip and total knee replacements. In a cooperative patient with a functioning rotator cuff, results of total shoulder replacement approach 90 percent success.[8]

Elbow. Conservative medical therapy is indicated for the great majority of elbow problems. Occasionally injections are of benefit. In severe involvement, as in a patient with rheumatoid arthritis with marked limitation of motion and pain, surgery should be considered. Pain with pronation and supination and elbow synovitis can be relieved by resection of the radial head and elbow synovectomy.

Elbow arthroplasty might be indicated when severe pain and limitation of motion is present. In younger patients an interposition arthroplasty using either a fascial graft, skin graft, or muscle pedicle, can produce a mobile, although not normal elbow, with significant pain relief. In older patients total elbow arthroplasty has produced satisfactory early results (figures 21.1 and 21.2). The long-term results are uncertain, since there has not been as extensive follow-up as there has been with total hip replacement. Many upper extremity surgical procedures can be performed safely without general anesthesia, even as an outpatient.[10]

Wrist and Hand. Rheumatoid arthritis particularly attacks the joints of the hand and wrist.[11] Synovitis affects the hand and wrist at two sites: the extensor tendons and the joints. The synovial tissue can cause necrosis of tendons under tight compartments. The swelling also deforms joint capsules and promotes tendon dislocations. On the extensor surface of the wrist, the synovium beneath the extensor retinaculum can cause tendon ruptures and dislocations. One of the few prophylactic operations a surgeon can perform in an arthritis patient is to remove the tenosynovium from the dorsum of the wrist and transfer the extensor tendons above the extensor retinaculum. This procedure can prevent or delay rupture of extensor tendons. Extensor tendon ruptures that have already occurred can be repaired at the same time. The distal ulna can be resected simultaneously to promote an improved function of the radial ulnar joint. Severe pain and deformity in the radiocarpal wrist joint is treated by arthrodesis or arthroplasty (figure 21.3).

Silastic and cemented total wrist arthroplasty have been performed with success. In patients with intact tendons on the flexor and extensor side, arthroplasty is preferred over arthrodesis since subsequent motion, although not normal, will improve overall hand function. In laborers or the very young, arthrodesis is probably still better.

The wrist flexor synovium can also hypertrophy and produce a carpal tunnel syndrome by compressing the median nerve. Flexor synovectomy and release of the carpal tunnel are indicated. The ulnar and radial nerves can occasionally be involved in arthritis.

The joints in the hand that can respond most satisfactorily to surgical rehabilitation are the metacarpophalangeal joints. Synovectomy may be indicated in the younger patient that has isolated involvement without evidence of joint destruction. In most patients there is multiple tissue involvement including intrinsic contracture, tendon dislocations, flexor and extensor tenosynovitis, joint destruction, and ulnar drift. In a relatively young patient with little joint involvement, soft-tissue procedures such as tendon transfers, intrinsic releases, and extensor tendon centralizations are indicated. In the majority of patients with advanced disease and joint involvement, soft-tissue reconstruction is combined with silastic metacarpophalangeal joint arthroplasties (figures 21.4 and 21.5). The smaller joints of the hand also can be improved in their function. The proximal and distal interphalangeal joints in patients with arthritis may require reconstructive surgery. These complex deformities include swan-neck deformities, bouton-

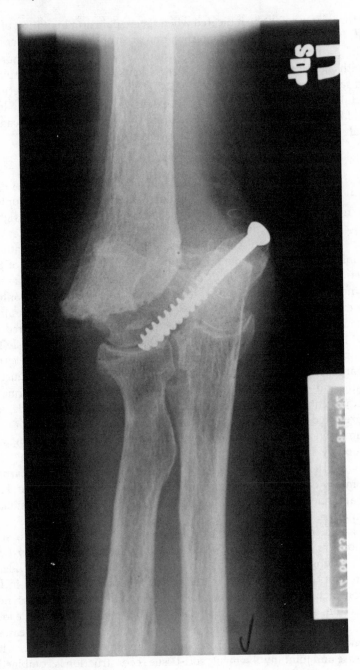

Figure 21.1.   A failed attempt at open reduction in a 61-year-old woman with rheumatoid arthritis and ununited fracture of the right distal humerus.

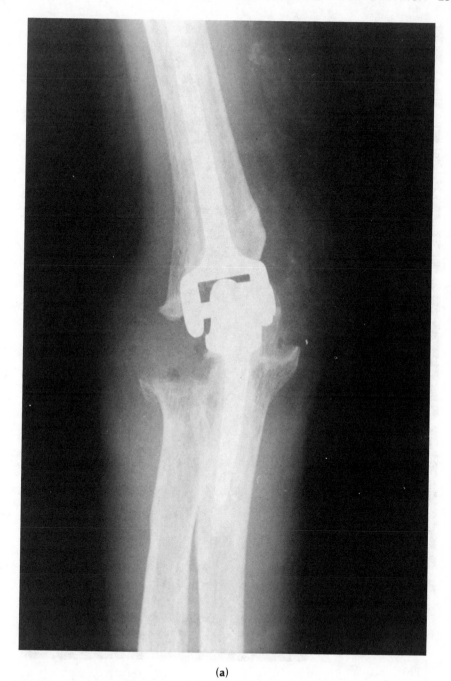

(a)

Figure 21.2.   Postoperative replacement of the elbow joint shown in figure 21.1 with a Pritchard total elbow, (a) AP x-ray; (b) lateral x-rays.

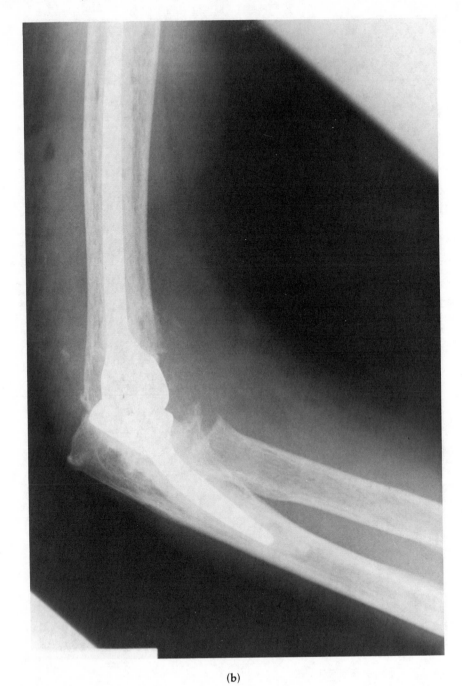

(b)

Figure 21.2. *(continued).*

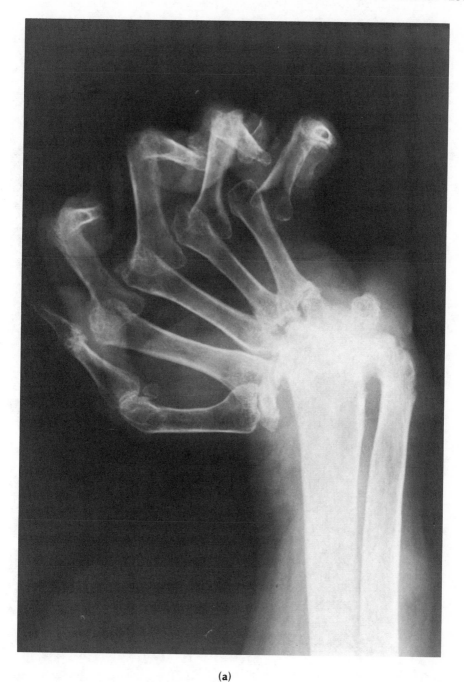

(a)

Figure 21.3.   Right hand and wrist of a 57-year-old man with rheumatoid arthritis. (a) Severe deformity preoperatively. (b) Postoperative appearance after arthodesis of the right wrist using an intermedullary rod through the long finger metacarpal and radius.

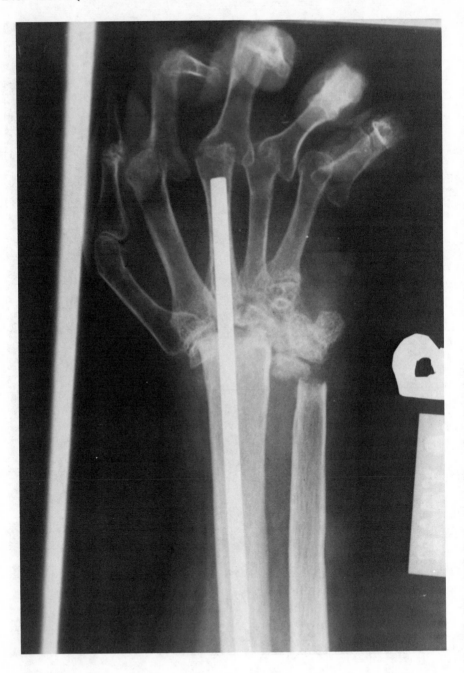

(b)

Figure 21.3. *(continued)*.

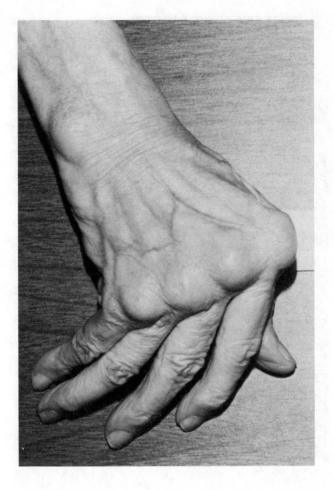

(a)

Figure 21.4. Hand of a 77-year-old woman with advanced rheumatoid arthritis.
(a) Deformity preoperatively. (b) Postoperative appearance after silastic arthroplasties of
the thumb, index, long, ring, and little fingers.

niere deformities, mallet fingers, tendon ruptures, dislocations, and painful
joints.

As stated previously, a major function of the upper extremity in the
severely involved arthritis patient is to assist in gait by using crutches, walkers, or
canes. With the advent of total hip and knee replacement, more attention can be
given to the intricate and precise function of the hand, since it is then always
needed to assist in walking. The use of the hand therapist is critical in improving
the functional results following reconstructive surgery. He or she is a physical or

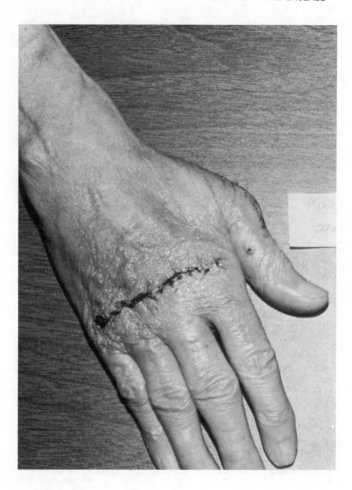

(b)

Figure 21.4.   *(continued).*

occupational therapist with specialized training in hand rehabilitation and splint fabrication. The hand therapist is of great value in the preoperative assessment of the hand and to assist in planning the functional goals for both the patient and the surgeon. Postoperatively the hand therapist assist the patient in early motion and rehabilitation of muscles, joints, and tendons. The therapist also can assist patients in redirecting their activities of daily living to include the improved capacity to function with their hands.

Ankle and Foot.   The orthopedic surgeon can, with the podiatrist and physical therapist, evaluate ankle and foot problems. Gain analysis should be performed.

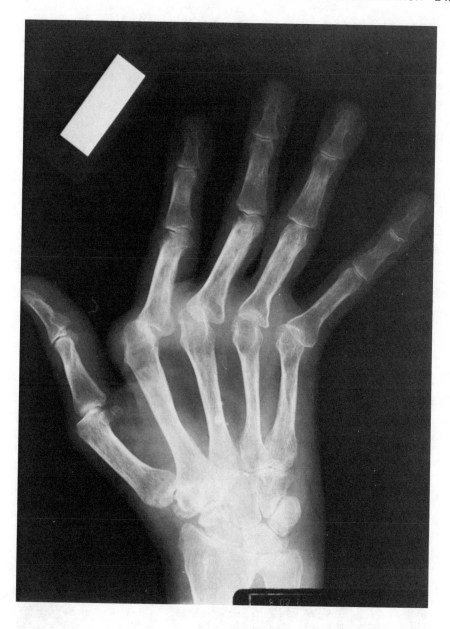

(a)

Figure 21.5.   The x-ray appearance of the hand of a 55-year-old woman with progressive deformities associated with rheumatoid arthritis. (a) Preoperative deformity. (b) The postoperative x-ray after arthrodesis of the metacarpophalangeal joint and silastic arthroplasties of the remaining metacarpophalangeal joints.

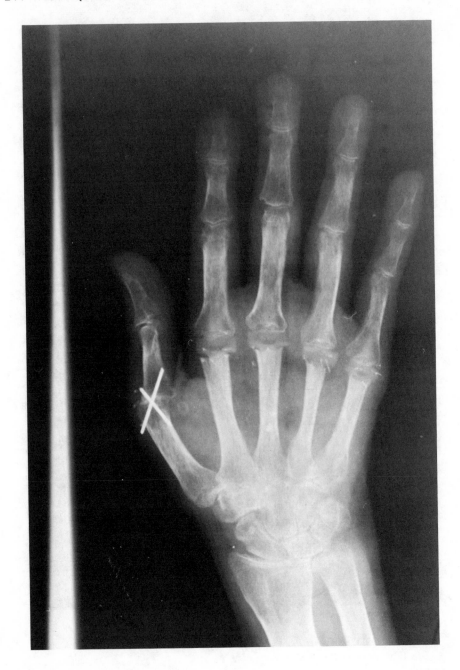

(b)

Figure 21.5. *(continued).*

Orthotics, braces, and supports may be of great benefit. When nonoperative treatment is unsuccessful, surgery is considered. Severe bunion deformities can be corrected either by soft-tissue procedures alone or combined with bone surgery or silastic joint replacement or both. Painful metatarsalgia, if not responsive to supports, can be relieved, particularly in advanced rheumatoid arthritis, with metatarsal head resection. These patients may require prolonged postoperative supports to prevent recurrence. Hammer toes and calluses, when unresponsive to nonsurgical treatment, can be corrected very easily with surgery. Total ankle replacement has not had an adequate follow-up to dictate its constant use. When ankle arthritis is severe, the operation that has the highest degree of success is arthrodesis.

Knee. In early knee involvement with arthritis, arthroscopy can provide an anatomic diagnosis.[12] Operative arthroscopy can be used to remove torn menisci, loose bodies, and occasionally to perform synovectomy. When knee damage is limited to either the medial or lateral compartment, and there is angular deformity an osteotomy is occasionally indicated. In the older patient with severe arthritis, rehabilitation can be facilitated with the use of total knee replacement.[13] (See figures 21.6.) A metal alloy femoral component and polyethylene tibial component is cemented in place. Often a patellar resurfacing is performed. Knee deformity can be corrected and range of motion restored. This operation has met a high degree of success in the hands of the skilled orthopedic surgeon. Pre- and postoperative physical therapy enhances the final result. Both muscle strengthening and range-of-motion exercises are important. In the well-selected patient a total knee replacement can be expected to provide many years of satisfactory function. However, rare complications of infection and/or loosening of components may develop. The complication requires removal or revision of the component as well as appropriate medical treatment.

Hip. The most significant orthopedic operation developed for the arthritis patient is the total hip replacement[14] (see figure 21.7). John Charnley conceived this procedure in the 1960s. This operation was the model for all subsequent total joint procedures. It utilizes an alloy metal femoral component, a high-density polyethylene acetabular cup, and is fixed to the patient's bone with methyl methacrylate cement. As part of the procedure, synovectomy can relieve pain, capsulectomy and muscle release can correct contractures, and the choice of neck length can reduce inequality of leg length. Preoperative and postoperative physical therapy and instruction improves muscle function, increases range of motion, facilitates patient cooperation, and improves the results of surgery. This procedure has the highest degree of success of any total joint replacement and is an excellent aid in rehabilitation of the arthritis patient.

    In younger patients who are too active to be candidates for total hip replacement, other procedures are considered. Double cup or resurfacing preserves the femoral neck bone, but it has mixed reviews as far as long-term results

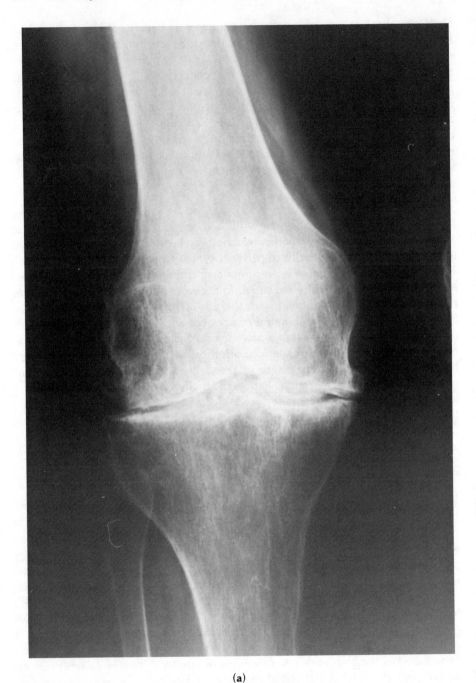

(a)

Figure 21.6. X-ray of knee of a 68-year-old woman with severe knee pain associated with rheumatoid arthritis. (a) PA x-ray. (b) Lateral x-ray. (c) AP x-ray of total knee arthroplasty (TKA) in this patient. (d) Lateral x-ray of TKA.

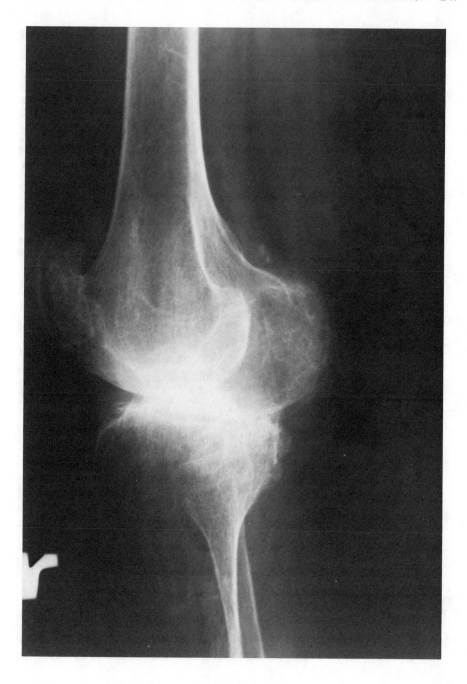

(b)

Figure 21.6. *(continued).*

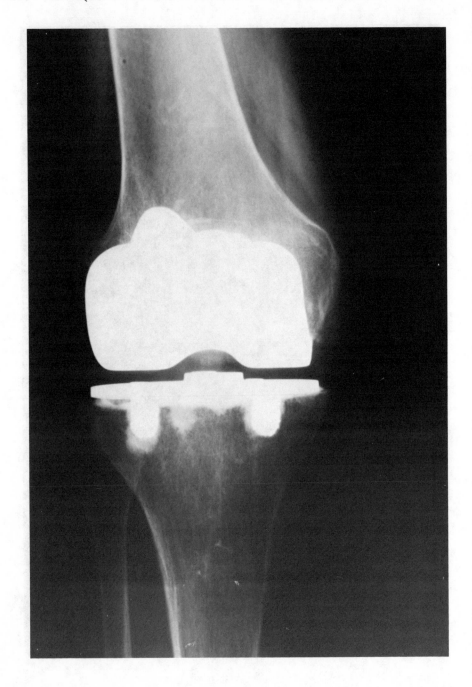

(c)

Figure 21.6.   *(continued).*

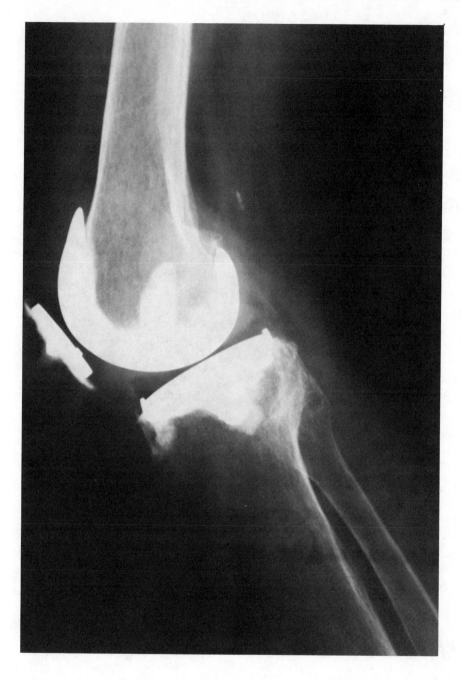

(d)

Figure 21.6.   *(continued).*

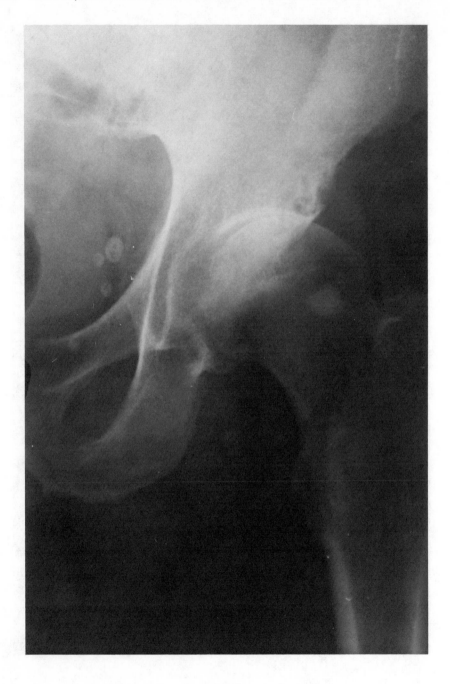

(a)

Figure 21.7. (a) Preoperative radiograph of a rheumatoid arthritis patient with a painful hip demonstrating loss of the joint space. (b) Postoperative x-ray of the patient; a total hip replacement has been performed.

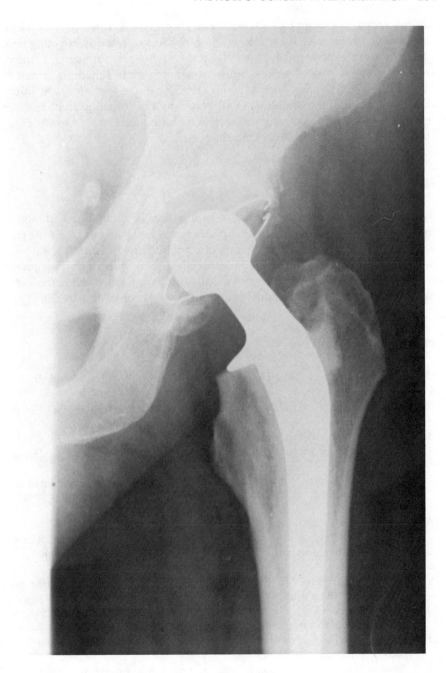

(b)

Figure 21.7. *(continued).*

are concerned. In certain patients who meet strict criteria, osteotomy of the proximal femur occasionally is considered. In rare cases of arthritis in young people, hip arthrodesis is performed. However, total hip replacement is by far the most frequent surgical procedure and leads to a much more functional result than fusion. Loosening of components requires revision of the operation, and infection dictates removal of the component with resultant leg shortening and limitation of motion. On occasion vigorous and early long-term antibiotic treatment of septic total hip replacements has salvaged the joint.

SUMMARY

The role of the surgeon in arthritis rehabilitation is multiple. He should be a member of the multidisciplinary health care team. He should evaluate the patient early and assist in formulating therapeutic goals. Surgery is not a treatment of last resort, but one to restore function and relieve pain. When a trial of nonoperative therapy has failed, the surgeon's skills can be integrated with those of the health care team to facilitate the optimum rehabilitation of the arthritis patient.

REFERENCES

1. Hunder GG, Bunch TW. The treatment of rheumatoid arthritis. Bull Rheum Dis 1982;32:1-8.
2. Preston RL. The surgical management of rheumatoid arthritis. Philadelphia: WB Saunders, 1968.
3. Flatt A. The care of the rheumatoid hand. St. Louis: CV Mosby, 1968.
4. Crenshaw AH, Edmonson AS. Campbell's operative orthopedics. St. Louis: CV Mosby, 1980.
5. Farrar WB, McCarty WL. A clinical outline of temporomandibular joint diagnosis and treatment, 7th ed. Montgomery, Ala.: Normandie Publications, 1982, pp. 23-27.
6. Kirsch, T, DDS. 1983, Personal communication. Tucson, Ariz.
7. Goldfarb RP. Surgical aspects of arthritis of the neck. Ariz Med 1978;35(1):26-29.
8. Cofield RH. Symposium: total shoulder replacement. Contemp Orthop 1982;5(6) 99-127.
9. Rosenfeld SR, Anzel SH. Evaluation of the Pritchard total elbow arthroplasty. Orthopedics 1982;5(6):713-719.
10. Haas LM, Landeed FH. Improved intravenous regional anesthesia for surgery of the hand, wrist and forearm: the second wrap technique. J Hand Surg 1978;3(2)194-195.
11. Swanson AB. Flexible implant resection arthroplasty in the hand and extremities. St. Louis: CV Mosby, 1973.
12. Arthroscopic surgery of the knee: seminar 3 transcript. Arthroscopic Surgery of the Knee Seminars, 1981, 3-218. Available from Robert Metcalf, M.D., 339 E. 3900 South, Salt Lake City, Utah 84107.
13. Katz JA. 1983, Personal communication. Tucson, Ariz.
14. Roberts MD. 1983. Personal communication. Tucson, Ariz.

22

Joint Protection and Energy Conservation

Dena M. Shapiro-Slonaker, O.T.R., M.S.Ed.

Learn the theory, not the methods. If one understands the theory, they can devise their own methods.

Dr. James Dean Mays, 1971

In the history of the philosophy and application of joint protection Joy Cordery's work is recognized as the first of its kind.[1] Her monograph has served to popularize a set of principles pertaining to the preservation of joint structures. She substantiated her set of rules with biomechanical theory and an understanding of the results of inflammation.

Originally the goal of joint protection was to prevent deformity.[2] Achievement of this goal has remained insufficiently documented, due to the variability of the disease and perhaps the long-term compliance necessary.[3] There appears to be a consensus among practitioners that the objective for joint protection should be redefined as pain relief, reduction of internal and external stress to the joint, and decreasing inflammation within the patient's life-style. Success in obtaining these objectives should be clinically evident.

Efforts to develop the theory upon which these principles are based necessitated exploring the areas of biomechanics, pathology of disease and inflammation, anatomy, and patient and staff education.

Definition of Terms

There is much discussion regarding the meaning of *joint protection.* Some prefer to think in terms of preservation of structural components in a biomechanical frame of reference, with a cause-and-effect relationship—slowing progression of joint deterioration. Others direct their concern to the enhancement of joint utilization in a functional sense—by avoiding pain and increasing function.

Protection varies for different diseases. Increasing joint activity may be helpful in some diseases and harmful in others. Moreover, since each joint operates interdependently with those adjoining it, what may be protective to one may redirect the forces to another in a stressful manner. Protection therefore can be thought of as the center of a hub with many spokes, all interacting together in an effort to produce movement, function, and the ability to work in an atraumatic manner with the least effort.

The term *energy conservation* does not suggest saving the energy available but, rather, spending it wisely. An analogy that has proved helpful is the bucket: everyone gets one bucket of energy a day to spill off any way the individual likes. It can be replenished with rest but has a limited supply. Use of energy must take into account the systemic features of disease, general state of deconditioning, and the total needs of the patient in regard to psychosocial, recreational, and vocational demands.

USE VERSUS ABUSE OF JOINTS

People with arthritis are faced with difficult self-management problems. They have a multitude of decisions to make daily regarding how, how much, and when to use the joints. It is the responsibility of the health care providers to teach the patients the principles of joint protection. Learning the concepts and principles on which these decisions are made enables patients to use and not abuse their joints.

Rest

There are two kinds of rest: *systemic* and *local*. Bed rest is a controversial issue. Prolonged bed rest is avoided for fear of the patient developing contractures and severe muscle atrophy. However, complete bed rest is suggested during an acute, generalized exacerbation with severe systemic reactions. As the patient improves, the regimen is changed to partial bed rest until the normal daily activity is resumed.[4-6] Because of the systemic nature of rheumatoid arthritis, relatively little activity can cause fatigue. The bucket runs dry easily. Most health professionals recommend that the patient continue to rest a minimum of a half hour daily and get 8 to 10 hours of sleep at night.

Resting in bed does not imply adequate joint rest, especially when movement in bed can cause stress to inflamed joints.[4] When a specific joint is inflamed, splinting provides support to the individual joint structures, reduces stress to the capsule, and allows the muscles to relax around the joint with a resultant decrease in inflammation.[3,7-10]

When a patient's disease is in remission, it must be stressed that rest is different from *inactivity*. Because of chronic pain, early morning stiffness, easy fatigability, and depression, the patient may withdraw from social, vocational, and recreational pursuits. As the patient becomes less active, a process of deconditioning begins, which, if allowed to progress, may result in bony demineralization, muscle atrophy, loss of joint range of motion, and deterioration of personality.

Exercise versus Activity

A common misconception on the part of patients is that if they are doing their housework or job, they are getting enough exercise. There are specific goals for exercise though, with specific benefits not necessarily obtained during routine activity. General activity cannot control for frequency, duration, and intensity of a specifically prescribed exercise regimen.[1] Neglecting the prescribed exercise program therefore is abusive to the joint. (See chapter 14.)

Doing versus Doing Correctly.   Once it is established that patients should keep active, it becomes essential that the manner in which they perform their activities be guided so as not to produce excessive strain to unstable or painful joints. Cordery suggests that an attempt should be made to distribute and use forces in proportion to the strength and vulnerability of the parts of the joints involved in performance of the activity.[1] The patient must learn to be cognizant of which activities cause pain or strain and adapt behavior accordingly. Specific principles of joint protection when employed resolve the symptoms of externally produced pain and positively reinforce the patient's decision to use the principles consistently.

When to Apply Principles

It is generally accepted that joint-protection principles should be used during an active exacerbation of disease. This is done to avoid overstretching soft tissues, increasing intra-articular pressure and causing pain. When the joint is in remission, do the principles still need to be followed? There is controversy over this issue presently, but use of joint protection principles is consistently mentioned in the medical literature as necessary to increase or improve function.[1-3,5,6,11,12]

In pending deformity—when joint structures are lax and muscular support of the joint is diminished—external pressures and forces can push the joint beyond its limits of stability. When the articulating surfaces of the joint are worn, excessive, continuous pressure at that location can be damaging. This concern lends to application of principles that tend to avoid a persistently damaging influence.

Pain Relief

Pain can be caused by several situations. Acute inflammation is clearly related to pain. Exceeding the capabilities of the joint to resist the forces applied can result in pain. When a joint, limited in mobility, is stretched too far at the end of the range of motion, pain is elicited. Acute strain to myotendonous or ligamentous structures is frequently a cause of pain in the normal population. It would stand to reason that avoidance of these circumstances would be beneficial.

An occupational therapist who has rheumatoid arthritis and has diligently applied joint-protection principles said, "Using joint protection is a coping mechanism to limit functional loss. It gives the patients some element of control over what happens to them."[13]

AIDS TO PROTECT THE JOINT DURING FUNCTION

Assistive Devices

The most significant of considerations regarding the use of assistive devices is whether or not a device is really necessary. The patient should use every joint to its maximum rather than substitute for motion with long-handled equipment. Strength should be used in a degree consistent with the disease process. Assistive devices are used to reduce pain and preserve joint integrity by minimizing extraneous stress. Additionally they should be utilized to increase the patient's independence in a task that otherwise could not be performed because of physical limitation.[3]

Specific purposes of equipment include the following in the frame of reference of joint protection. They are outlined here and discussed in more detail in chapters 20 and 23.

1. Support weakened joints. Removing the forces of weight-bearing from inflamed or unstable lower extremity joints can be accomplished with ambulatory devices. The design of crutches, canes, or walkers should minimize stresses to the small joints of the hand and to the wrist.
2. Provide leverage to increase force with decreased exertion.
3. Help joints maintain the most stable anatomical (neutral) alignment. Much literature is available that carefully evaluates positions, duration, and arrangements most helpful to maintaining anatomical alignment.[1-3,11,22]
4. Extend reach when joints are limited in passive range of motion or status after surgery when specific motion must be avoided.
5. Avoid unnecessary use or strain. Holding a hand of cards or a book requires maintaining one position for an extended period of time. This position demands sustained contraction of the intrinsic muscles, which may remain tight. Intrinsic tightness may proceed to swan-neck deformity. By using card holders or reading racks to preclude sustained intrinsic contracture, the effect may be lessened and intrinsic muscle length retained.

Insurance may cover the cost of assistive devices, but since the patient's and family's financial resources are frequently severely limited, expense is a vital concern. Many aids that would make the difference between independence and dependence are passed up because they simply cannot be afforded. All efforts should be made to explore the creative resources within the family to fabricate these items at much less expense.[14]

Patients hesitant to accept these items, viewing them as crutches, should be encouraged to see them as tools instead. For example, an assistive device may be used by the patient in the clutches of the "gel" phenomenon during morning stiffness. Once patients feel they have some choice they are more receptive to protecting those joints that should not continue to take stress while performing activities in the usual manner.

Self-help catalogues, articles, and books are abundant. Excellent bibliographies can be obtained from books by Melvin,[3] Klinger,[15] Lowman,[16] the Canadian Arthritis and Rheumatism Society,[17] and the Arthritis Foundation.[18,19]

Splinting

Though splinting was discussed earlier in the context of resting the joint, other objectives of splinting pertinent to this chapter include supporting the weak joint during function, relief of pain, and resisting deforming forces. Emphasis is placed on preventing the dynamic forces from overcoming the pathologic joint. Correcting deformities has not been substantially documented except in the surgical literature. Splinting is discussed in detail in chapter 16.

GENERAL PRINCIPLES OF JOINT PROTECTION

The patient's life-style is critical to the determination of treatment goals. The patient's role in the family, community, job (in or out of home), with spouse or partner, and during recreational pursuits must be carefully analyzed to establish realistic rules, simple rules, and most important, understood rules. The Arthritis Information Clearinghouse lists many of the patient education materials available, with examples of the principles too numerous to mention here.[19] Cordery[1] and Melvin's[3] work are suggested as primary references.

ENERGY CONSERVATION

Theory of Energy Conservation

Energy conservation can be associated with many of the same concerns explained in protecting joints. Excessive strain or pain uses extra energy to cope. Associated medical conditions such as cardiac, pulmonary, and diabetic disorders must be taken into account in the population of patients with rheumatic diseases. Systemic disease, chronicity of disease, and accompanying demands of coping use more energy. Depression is a common source of fatigue.

Energy conservation literature is abundant in the area of cardiac rehabilitation.[20] The effort required to ambulate is addressed in literature relating to the lower extremity amputee. In the patient with arthritis, there is an increased energy demand to ambulate at a slower pace because of the extra muscle contraction needed to stabilize weakened joints.[21] The strength required to perform activities efficiently is usually reduced secondary to motor inhibition by pain, poor general nutrition, health, and psychological status.[12] Shontz's theory of restricted energy due to intense threat of illness is described[20] and clinically observed. Therefore more energy is expended and the necessity for learning how to conserve it becomes essential.

For the Patient: General Principles of Energy Conservation[1,3,20]

1. Plan ahead.
   a. Write out a diary of activities for a week or two. Circling active periods in red, rest activities in blue, provides a handy way to see at a glance the distribution of activity per day and week.
   b. Perform an analysis of the activities to be done and space out over time the more demanding aspects of each activity. Write a new schedule of activity based on the analysis performed.
   c. Gather all supplies and equipment before starting an activity.
2. Organize and arrange space.
   a. Work areas should be arranged so that everything needed will be on hand next to the area where you perform the task.
      i. Stove area. Pans and lids could be stored on sliding drawers or pull-out racks; keep spices, stirring utensils, oven mitts, and strainers near the stove.
      ii. Sink. Keep knives, utensils for vegetables and salad preparation, colander, cleaning supplies, and wastebasket here; use a pull-out board and a high chair so that you can sit to work.
      iii. Counter top. Bowls, spices, sugar, flour, hand mixer, spatulas, measuring cups, and spoons should be kept here.
      iv. Laundry area. Have table for sorting and folding clothes, chair to set basket on (or use basket on wheels) for loading and unloading clothes from the machines; keep detergents, hangers, etc., here.
      v. Workshop and garage. Arrange yard, wood, electrical, and plumbing supplies together. Use carts or large containers on wheels to hold items.
   b. Storage
      i. Think about every cupboard you have; put what you use most in front, at a good height.
      ii. Put lighter objects higher up.

      iii.   Keep refillable small containers in easy reach and keep economy-size jars, bottles, or boxes out of the way.

      iv.   Use commercial organizers. Rubbermaid and Grayline produce many organizers found in hardware, department, and grocery stores. These include turntables, pull-out drawers, and racks to hold dishes, pot lids, cups, and saucers; storage for ironing and sweeping equipment; boxes for foils and plastic wraps, etc.

      v.   Hang items up within reach to avoid clutter and having to dig through drawers to locate them. Cup hooks, peg boards, and magnetic hooks are available in hardware and home improvement stores.

3.   Eliminate steps involved or the activity itself.[20]

    a.   Use easy-care garments.

    b.   Make bed completely on one side before moving to the other side.

    c.   Soak dishes before washing and use easy-care surface pots and pans (Silverstone or Teflon).

    d.   Reuse washed dishes instead of replacing them in the cupboard after every washing.

    e.   Use the same dish for freezing, cooking, and serving.

    f.   Use canned or frozen prepared foods.

    g.   Establish individual family member's responsibility for picking up after themselves and performing assigned tasks.

4.   Sit to work.

5.   Keep proper equipment in excellent repair.[15,20]

    a.   Use self-cleaning oven, frost-free freezer, automatic dishwasher if finances permit.

    b.   Test equipment for ease of operation before purchase.

6.   Take intermittent rest periods.

    a.   Rest before fatigued.

    b.   Arrange to stop and rest during walks in community or even down hallways or grocery aisles.

SUMMARY

Health professionals often assume personal responsibility for the patient's progression of disease and attempt to intercede to prevent it from getting worse. They suggest how, when, where, and what activities are to be performed, but seldom tell why. While this may seem an overstatement, let it be said that it remains the patient's responsibility to attempt to learn how to live to the fullest within the limitations of the disease.

It is the professional's duty to learn the theories and teach pertinent explanations to the patient. Patient participation and cooperation are essential for a good treatment outcome, but success is unlikely if patients do not understand the disease, how it may change their life-style, and what may be done to help. There is documented evidence that careful planning and timing of patient education is beneficial in achieving behavioral changes.[21] If adequately instructed in theory, the patient can transfer the principles from one activity to another with more ease, resulting in an overall improvement of physical, vocational, recreational, and ultimately emotional function.

REFERENCES

1. Cordery JC. Conservation of physical resources as applied to the activities of patients with arthritis and the connective tissue diseases. In: Study course III, 3rd International Congress, World Federation of Occupational Therapy, Dubuque, Iowa: WC Brown 1962, pp. 22–38.

2. Cordery JC. Joint protection: a responsibility of the occupational therapist. Am J Occup 1965;19:285.

3. Melvin JL. Rheumatic disease: occupational therapy and rehabilitation, 2nd ed. Philadelphia: FA Davis, 1982.

4. Fried DM. Rest vs activity. In: Licht, S, ed., Arthritis and physical medicine. Baltimore: Waverly Press, 1969, ch. 12, p. 271.

5. Ruddy S. The management of rheumatoid arthritis. In: Kelley WN, Harris ED, Jr., Ruddy S, Sledge CB, eds., Textbook of rheumatology. Philadelphia: WB Saunders, 1981, ch. 63, p. 1004.

6. Lightfoot RW. Treatment of rheumatoid arthritis. In: McCarty DJ, ed., Arthritis and allied conditions, 9th ed. Philadelphia: Lea and Febiger, 1979, ch. 35, p. 514.

7. Partridge REH, Duthie JJR. Controlled trial of the effect of complete immobilization of the joints in rheumatoid arthritis. Ann Rheum Dis 1963;22:91.

8. Gault SS, Spyker JM. Beneficial effect of immobilization of joints in rheumatoid arthritis and related arthritides: a splint study using sequential analysis. Arthritis Rheum 1969;12:34.

9. Ehrlich GE, ed. Total management of the arthritic patient. Philadelphia: JB Lippincott, 1973.

10. Smith RD, Polley HT. Rest therapy for rheumatoid arthritis. Mayo Clinic Proc 1978;53:141–145.

11. Lowman EW. Employability of rheumatoid arthritics. Arch Environ Health 1962; 5:502–504.

12. Swezey RL. Arthritis: rational therapy and rehabilitation. Philadelphia: WB Saunders, 1978.

13. Personal communication, Theresa Brady, O.T.R., Minneapolis, 1982.

14. Grainger SE. Making aids for disabled living. London: BT Batsford, 1981.

15. Klinger JL. Mealtime manual for people with disabilities and the aging. Camden, N.J.: Campbell Soup Co., 1978.

16. Lowman EW, Klinger JL. Aids to independent living. New York: McGraw-Hill, 1969.

17. Aids and adaptations. Compiled by Occupational Therapy Department, Canadian Arthritis and Rheumatism Society, British Columbia Division, Vancouver, Canada.

18. Self-help manual, 2nd ed. Arthritis Health Profession Association, Arthritis Foundation, Atlanta, 1980.

19. Arthritis Information Clearinghouse, P.O. Box 9782, Arlington, Va. 22209.

20. Trombly CA, Scott AD. Occupational therapy for physical dysfunction. Baltimore: Williams and Wilkins, 1977, p. 326.

21. Gerber LH. Principles and their application in the rehabilitation of patients with rheumatoid disease. In: Kelley WN, Harris ED, Jr., Ruddy S, Sledge CB, eds., Textbook of rheumatology. Philadelphia: WB Saunders, 1981, ch. 112, pp. 1849–1863.

22. Garee B, ed., Ideas for making your home accessible. Bloomington, Ill.: Accent Special Publications, Cheever Publishing, 1979.

23

Assistive Devices, Aids to Daily Living

Helen Schweidler, O.T.R.

Assistive devices and adaptive equipment are terms used interchangeably to describe a wide range of tools and appliances used by individuals with physical limitations to simplify activities of daily living. The items may vary from simple, inexpensively constructed, homemade gadgets to complex equipment custom designed by a rehabilitation engineer. The items may be specifically designed for individuals with disabilities or distributed by medical suppliers. Tools and appliances available in hardware department stores may also serve as assistive devices. Assistive devices serve four basic functions:

1. *To compensate for lost function.* Individuals who could not otherwise perform a task may become independent by using a device. For example, a man whose pinch strength is not sufficient to hold the tab on a zipper may use either a zipper pull or a loop or cord through the tab to manage the fly of his trousers. An individual who lacks lower extremity strength to rise from a standard-height toilet may be able to rise to standing from an elevated toilet seat.

2. *To alleviate internal and external joint stress.* Assistive devices are important in joint protection. They are used to reduce the force transmitted across joints by muscle-tendon units and to reduce outside pressures. For example, an enlarged handle on a cooking utensil allows the hand to be used with metacarpophalangeal joints in less flexion and ulnar deviation. A knife designed with a vertical handle is held in line with the palmar crease rather than with pinch of thumb against index finger, so that pressure toward ulnar deviation is reduced.

3. *To decrease energy demands.* Fatigue is an important factor in an individual's ability to function independently. Assistive devices may be used to conserve energy. A wheeled cart makes it possible to carry many items at one time so that steps are saved. The cart also eliminates the need to carry heavy items.

4. *To increase safety.* Many devices aid in preventing injury. A cane may help to promote balance. A bag or basket attached to a walker may make carry-

ing objects from place to place safer. Bathing and dressing aids with long handles are used to protect the back and hips.

The selection of assistive devices requires assessment of skills and problems in activities of daily living. There are no standard equipment lists appropriate to all individuals. Considerations that should influence the choice of a device include the individual's acceptance of an assistive device, the individual's physical abilities, the cost and availability of items, and safety.

Acceptance of Assistive Devices

Frequently people who are severely limited in function enthusiastically accept devices that provide them with some independence. Other individuals who manage tasks more independently, but at a cost of joint stress, fatigue, or safety risk, may be less accepting.

Individual attitudes may discourage the use of aids. It must be clear that the patient does wish to be able to perform the selected task more independently or with improved efficiency and safety. Equipment provided for tasks the patient views as unimportant or too difficult to master are not likely to be used.

Fear of disability or deformity, along with negative self-image and other emotional concerns, may interfere with acceptance of assistive devices. The patient may be unwilling to be seen doing something differently. The emotional defense process of denial may prevent such a person from seeing the need for equipment. Financial concerns also may prevent purchase, because some items of equipment are expensive.

Low tolerance of frustration and fear of failure may cause the person to reject equipment. Use of many items requires skill and practice. This is particularly true for those who have multiple joint involvement. Additional physical or cognitive problems such as diminished vision or poor learning ability may make it necessary for an individual to have instruction and supervision to be successful in using a particular device.

Acceptance of assistive devices is improved when the individual has some knowledge of joint protection and energy conservation principles. Instruction and supervised practice in the methods for using a device may be necessary. It is important for assistive devices to be as attractive, or at least as unobtrusive, as possible. This not only aids in acceptance, but also supports a more positive self-image for the user.

Physical Abilities

When a person is physically able to complete a task without excessive joint stress, fatigue, or risk of injury, it is always preferable to continue without an assistive device. In some instances a task can be made manageable by changing the method rather than by using or adapting a tool. Persons with limited active range of motion and strength in the shoulder can comb their hair using a long-handled comb. If they have adequate passive range of motion, they can also comb their hair by supporting the weight of the elbow either with the opposite hand or with some supporting surface (a table).

Devices should not be used when it is possible to maintain independent function. The demands of daily activities help maintain strength and range of motion. It is important to remember that an individual's physical abilities may vary greatly from morning to evening or from day to day. Use of assistive devices may be indicated during periods when daily living tasks are more difficult, yet is unnecessary at other times.

If the person's physical ability to use a particular device is marginal, safety should be considered even more strongly. Garden tools with long handles reduce stooping and bending, but raised planter boxes or a work stool may be a safer solution for the person with ambulation problems.

When an assistive device is needed, the body mechanism involved in using it should be carefully noted. Stressful forces should not be shifted from one damaged joint to another. A wooden scissors-type reaching device can be stressful to hands and wrists. (See figure 23.1). The weight, distance, and direction of forces should be changed to the individual's advantage by either changing the style of

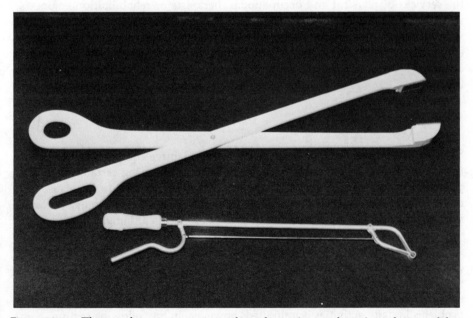

Figure 23.1. The wooden scissors-type reaching device (upper device) can be stressful to the hands and wrists. An aluminum passive reacher (lower device) eliminates the need for prolonged, forceful grasp.

reaching device or changing the method of using it. The lightweight aluminum passive reacher (which requires grasp to open the tongs, but not to close them) eliminates the need for prolonged, forceful grasp. Because this reacher holds the object without grasp at the handle, the person may place the hands closer to the mass of the object and therefore reduce the length of the lever from the load. This also enables positioning wrists and hands with better alignment. Thus some of the weight can be supported on the forearm if necessary.

Cost and Availability

Unfortunately insurance coverage for assistive devices is generally not available. The cost of some items can be prohibitive. Some community agencies and volunteer groups provide equipment or even fund purchase.

Individuals should be encouraged to investigate several resources before making a purchase. Comparison shopping may allow considerable saving or even more important, reveal a number of alternatives that will solve specific problems in activities of daily living. For example, when a raised chair seat height is needed, alternatives include chairs with electric lifts, "catapult" cushions with spring lifts, cushions of varied sizes and materials, platforms, or blocks placed under a chair. The therapist can often assist in steering a patient to several potential resources for an item.

Concern for cost and availability applies not only to equipment, but also to the services of physical and occupational therapists or rehabilitation engineers, which may be needed. It is in many instances wasteful to purchase equipment without professional guidance about design, selection, and use of the item. Nearly all assistive devices are nonprescription items. However, third-party payers who do reimburse for equipment require the physician's approval or prescription for items.

Safety

Safety is another of the four basic functions of adaptive equipment. It is important to think also of the risks that may be involved in using certain items. It is possible for accidents to occur as a result of faulty construction or misuse of a device. Sharp edges (especially on dressing and bathing aids) risk injury to fragile skin. A wheeled cart used improperly as an ambulation aid might hazard a fall.

Attention to joint protection must be emphasized. Excessive stress due to some devices may increase inflammation or further injure or possibly rupture diseased ligaments or tendons.

In the discussion of the purposes and selection of assistive devices, some examples of aids are given. The number and variety of possible solutions to problems in daily activities is unlimited, however. In the following section, common functional problems in daily activities are identified. Devices that are frequently used are listed with a brief comment and resources for more information.

COMMON FUNCTIONAL PROBLEMS

Bathing. Limitations in ambulation and transfer skills may make getting in and out of the tub or shower fatiguing, unsafe, or impossible. Loss of upper extremity strength and range interferes in managing faucets, washcloths, soap, shampoo, and so on. Limited range in proximal upper and lower extremity joints creates problems in reaching body parts, and fatigue could prevent the person from completing a bath independently. (See table 23.1)

Toileting. Limitations in knee and hip flexion and extension and in transfer skills create difficulty getting on and off a toilet. Decreased range in proximal upper and lower extremity joints or loss of hand skills may interfere with managing toilet paper as well as cause problems in dressing and undressing for toileting. (See table 23.2)

Grooming. Decreased proximal upper extremity range impedes hair care, applying makeup, shaving, and dental hygiene. Loss of hand dexterity also interferes with these tasks as well as nail grooming. Temporomandibular joint disease may complicate dental care. (See table 23.3)

Table 23.1. Bathing Aids

Devices	*Comments*
Safety aids[4, 8, 11] 　Safety mats 　Grab bars	Aid transfer. Increase safety. Vertical pole or bars that attach to tub assist weak grasp since forearm may be substituted.
Tub/shower seats[1, 4, 8]	Aid transfer. Increase safety. Wide variety of styles and heights available.
Taps or faucets[1, 4, 6, 8] 　Lever faucet handles 　Tap-turning devices	Aid limited upper extremity strength and range. Reduce joint stress.
Hand-held shower heads[8]	Aid limited range. Save energy. May be mounted at side of tub for easier access.
Bathing supplies[8] 　Shower caddies 　Tub trays 　Soap dispensers	Aid limited strength and range. Wide variety available.
Washing and drying[1, 6, 8] 　Long-handled sponges 　Wash mitts 　Adapted washcloths 　Terry robes	Aid limited range in proximal joints. Long-handled sponges impractical if wrists/hands involved. Mitts aid limited grasp. Terry cloth robe saves energy required for drying after bath.

Table 23.2. Toileting

Devices	Comments
Elevated toilet seats[1, 4, 6, 8] Commodes	Wide variety of temporary and permanent adaptations possible.
Grab bars[1, 4, 8]	Aid transfer and increase safety.
Dressing[1, 2, 5, 8, 9] Adapted clothing Dressing aids	See dressing section and table 23.4.
Toilet paper holdings[8]	Device holds paper and extends reach for cleaning after elimination. See figure 23.2.

Table 23.3. Grooming

Devices	Comments
Enlarged or extended handles on toothbrush, comb, razor[1, 6, 8, 10-12]	Lightweight materials to build up handles include cylindrical foam, adhesive foam, small wooden doweling, and aluminum tubing. Plastic coating or applications of low-temperature plastic splinting materials foster better grip.
Dental hygiene aids[8] Electric toothbrushes Water jet appliances Floss and toothpick holders Toothpaste tube key	Careful selection of these devices is advised as some are heavy, have clumsy grip, or require too much pinch.
Nail care devices: electric nail files, buffers[1, 8]	Compensate for weakness and loss of fine pinch. Clippers may be mounted on a wooden block or extensions may be placed on the handles.
Adaptations for cosmetic containers[1, 7, 8, 12]	Attachment for aerosol spray can provides lever to press spray button. Cosmetics may be selected for accessible containers (push-up lipsticks, deodorants with larger tops).

Dressing. Limited range in proximal upper and lower extremity joints may make it difficult to get clothing over the feet or over the head. Poor grasp strength and loss of fine prehension skills create problems in manipulating fasteners. Upper extremity weakness interferes with putting on coats or jackets. (See table 23.4).

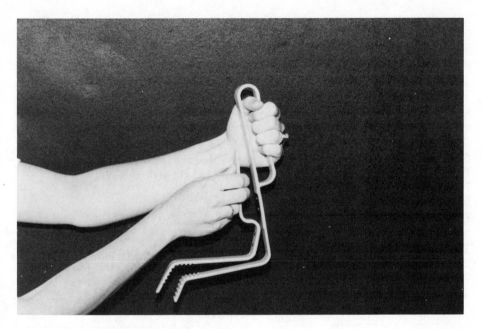

Figure 23.2.   Toilet paper holder.

Eating. Limited proximal upper extremity range may impair the person's ability to get food to the mouth and lack of supination or fine prehension, the ability to manipulate utensils. Weakness may make it difficult to cut food or lift a glass or cup. (See table 23.5)

Meal Preparation. The person with arthritis may need special aids to compensate for impaired mobility, limited range in reaching and bending, or lack of strength and endurance. Because many kitchen tasks are resistive or repetitive, it is especially important to consider joint protection and energy conservation. (See table 23.6)

Housekeeping. Aids and adaptations may be necessary due to problems in mobility, proximal upper and lower extremity range of motion and strength, or hand problems. As noted in meal preparation, it is important to consider aids that will promote early joint protection and energy conservation. (See table 23.7).

Transportation and Shopping. The ability to drive and ride in a car, to manage social and recreational outings and shopping may be limited by problems in mobility and transfer, upper extremity strength and range, and endurance. (See table 23.8)

Table 23.4.   Dressing

Devices[1, 6, 8]	Comments
Dressing stick (figure 23.3) Reaching devices	Reachers are appropriate for individuals who have no arthritic hand and wrist involvement. The lightweight passive reacher may solve upper extremity problems.
Shoe/sock aids Stocking donner Long-handled shoe horn Boot jack Elastic shoe laces Adapted shoe closures	A wide variety of commercial and homemade styles. Shoes can be adapted with Velcro, zippers, and clip-style closures.
Button hook Zipper pull Zipper loop or ring (figure 23.4) Zipper tab	Difficult closures may also be replaced with simpler fasteners or Velcro strips. Clothing may be selected with elasticized waists, front closures, and for wraparound style.
Adapted clothing[1-3, 5, 8, 9]	Patterns or specially made garments may be purchased.

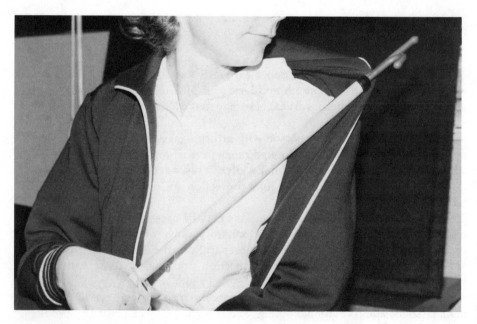

Figure 23.3.   Dressing stick.

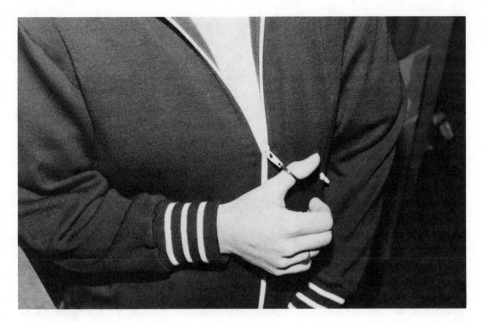

Figure 23.4.   Ring in zipper.

Table 23.5.   Eating

Devices	Comments
Adapted utensils Enlarged or extended handles Utensil cuffs Swivel forks and spoons[1, 6-8]	Attractive utensils are commercially available with enlarged handles. Handles or cuffs of standard utensils may be enlarged with foam or plastic to eliminate tight grasp of utensil. Swivel handles compensate for loss of supination.
Aids for drinking Long straws Lightweight and spillproof cups Thermal mugs[1, 6-8]	Thermal mugs with wide handles allow both hands to be used with MP joints in less stressful position.
Trays Table height adjustments[1, 6, 7]	Severely disabled or hospitalized patients may need meals served at more accessible table height.

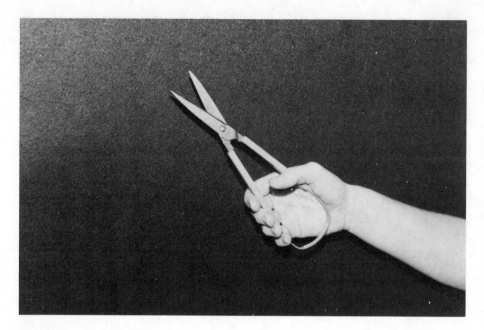

Figure 23.5.   Spring-style scissors.

Table 23.6.   Meal Preparation

Devices	*Comments*
Lightweight utensils, cookware, and dishes[7, 8]	Less strength and energy are required; reduce joint stress. Ceramic plates may range in weight from 24 oz to 11 oz each.
Devices to open containers: jar openers, can openers[1, 6-8]	Compensate for weak grasp and/or loss of fine prehension. Electric appliances must be selected so that controls are easy to operate.
Aids for cutting and chopping[1, 6-8]	These compensate for weak grasp and loss of fine hand skills and reduce joint stress. Knives and scissors should be maintained with sharp cutting edges to reduce the force required in cutting. Spring-style scissors are less stressful to joints (figure 23.5). Cutting board may be adapted with rustproof nails to hold food.
Labor-saving appliances[7, 8]	Generally lessen joint stress, because less strength and energy are required. Examples include microwave ovens, electric skillets, blenders, and food processors. Appliances should be selected so that controls are easy to operate and parts that must be lifted are lightweight.

Table 23.6.   Meal Preparation *(continued)*

Devices	Comments
Adaptations for storage: pegboard, vertical storage, pull-out shelves[7, 8]	Conserve energy. May compensate for loss of range and strength. Work areas should be arranged so that tools and equipment are stored at the place where they are first used. Adaptations may be permanent and built-in, or temporary commercially available items.

Table 23.7.   Housekeeping

Devices[7,8]	Comments
Kitchen or utility carts	Conserve energy, reduce joint stress, compensate for limited strength. Wheeled carts eliminate lifting and carrying with many items carried in one trip.
Lightweight sweepers Self-propelled vacuums Shortened handles on broom and dustpan for wheelchair use	Conserve energy. Reduce joint stress. Lightweight sweepers may be used to reduce frequency of heavier vacuuming.
Laundry aids Platforms to raise washer/dryer height Lowered clothes racks and lines Adjustable height ironing board Lightweight "travel" iron	Compensate for strength and range limitations. Automatic washers and dryers should be selected for accessibility, and easy-to-operate controls; clothes for easy care, little ironing.

Table 23.8.   Transportation and Shopping

Devices	Comments
Car door openers (figure 23.6)[6, 8]	Reduce stress on thumb. Devices are commercially available or may be simply constructed.
Key holders (figure 23.7)[1, 6, 8]	Compensate for weak lateral pinch by providing leverage.
Seat cushions[8]	Aid transfer. Covered in slick materials, these facilitate sliding and pivoting. Catapult cushions may be placed sideways on car seat to aid standing.
Wide-angle rear-view mirrors[8]	Compensate for limited neck range.
Devices for loading and unloading wheelchair	Wide variety available. May be needed by individual or the person who assists him.

Table 23.8. Transportation and Shopping *(continued)*

Devices	*Comments*
Seat canes[8]	Conserve energy and provide means to rest periodically during long walk or long period of standing.
Wheeled shopping carts[7, 8]	Conserve energy and compensate for loss of strength. Attention should be given to height of the handle to allow erect posture.
Shoulder bags[8] Back packs	Reduce joint stress of prolonged grasp by allowing larger joints to carry items. Also frees hands for ambulation aids.
Ambulation aids	Canes, crutches, walkers, and wheelchairs need to fit the individual and instruction in their proper use must be given. It may be appropriate to use a wheelchair for safety or energy conservation during outings even though the individual can ambulate. Powered chairs such as the "Amigo" are useful for long distances and uneven terrain.

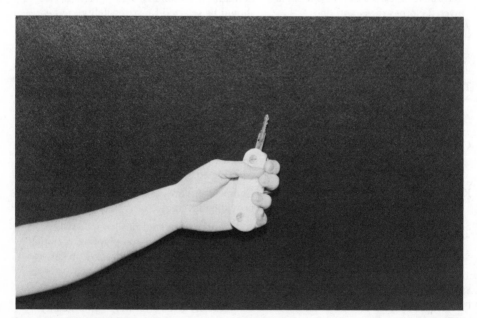

Figure 23.6. Key holder.

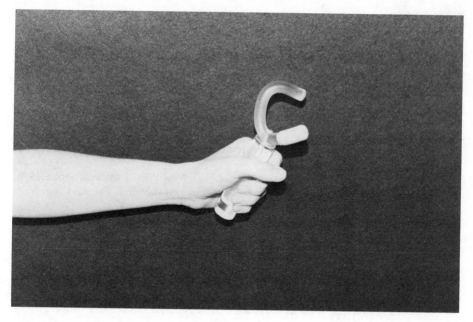

Figure 23.7.   Car door opener.

SUMMARY

Assistive devices and adaptive equipment serve to compensate for lost function, to reduce joint stress, to save energy, and to increase safety. If a person is physically able to complete a task without excessive joint stress, fatigue, or risk of injury, it is always preferable to continue without an assistive device. However, it is important to consider that an individual's physical abilities may vary greatly from morning to evening or from day to day.

If aids are needed, the individual's success in using them is increased by instruction and supervised practice as well as knowledge of joint protection and energy-conservation principles.

The selection of adaptive equipment must be done carefully with particularly close attention paid to safety and joint stress. Ideally, services of a rehabilitation engineer and physical and occupational therapists are provided to assist the person in identifying, analyzing, and solving problems in activities of daily living.

Nearly all assistive devices are nonprescription items. However, third-party payers may require a physician's approval or order.

REFERENCES

1. Aids and adaptations, compiled by the Occupational Therapy Department, Canadian Arthritis and Rheumatism Society (CARS), British Columbia Division, Vancouver, Canada. (Available from CARS, 45 Charles St. E., Toronto, Ontario, Canada.)
2. Beasley MC, Burns D, Weiss J. Adapt your own: a clothing brochure for people with special needs. Birmingham: University of Alabama, Division of Continuing Education, 1977.
3. Bowar MT. Clothing for the handicapped. Minneapolis, Minn. Sister Kenny Institute, 1978.
4. Cary JR. How to create interiors for the disabled. New York: Pantheon Books, 1978.
5. Clothing fastenings for the handicapped and disabled. London: Central Council for the Disabled (39 Victoria St., London, S.W. I, England), 1968.
6. How to make it cheap, vols. 1–3. Middletown, Ohio: Independence Factory (P.O. Box 597, Middletown, Ohio 45042).
7. Klinger JL. Mealtime manual for people with disabilities and the aging. New York: Institute of Rehabilitation Medicine, New York University Medical Center, 1978.
8. Klinger JL. Self-help manual for patients with arthritis. Atlanta: Arthritis Foundation, 1980.
9. Kramer J. Gardening without stress and strain. New York: Charles Scribner's Sons, 1973.
10. Lorig K, Fries JF. The arthritis helpbook: what you can do for your arthritis. Reading, Mass.: Addison-Wesley, 1980.
11. Melvin J. Rheumatic disease: occupational therapy and rehabilitation. Philadelphia: FA Davis, 1977.
12. Watkins RA, Robinson D. Joint protection techniques for patients with rheumatoid arthritis. Chicago: Rehabilitation Institute of Chicago, 1974.

24

Architectural and Environmental Barriers

William L. Woods, Jr., B.S.M.E.

This chapter attempts to educate the reader about ways, not already touched on, that will increase independence in everyday living of people with arthritis. Removing architectural and environmental barriers is an area well suited to the application of a team approach. Information gained in the chapters on physical evaluation, needs assessment, exercise programs, hydrotherapy, gait and ambulation, joint protection and energy conservation, assistive devices, and psychosocial aspects all is relevant to the removal of architectural and other environmental barriers. It is myopic to believe that considering only one or two details of an environment, however important, like architectural or even psychological barriers, is fulfilling the health professional's responsibility in helping an individual achieve his maximum potential for independence.

Rehabilitation professionals need to evaluate the patient's total life in order to enhance and complement each other's skills and particular areas of expertise. One goal should be to improve a person's quality of life by suggesting and initiating modifications in mechanical or architectural barriers. Whatever the modality of change, two primary results should occur: independence and safety.

Secondary benefits result from a person gaining independence. These are enhanced feelings of self-worth or self-esteem, increased independence, saved energy and time, a wider choice of activities or options, increased freedom for the individual *and* other members of the family, and improvement of the financial situation if the handicapped individual or another family member can return to work.

The achievement of these objectives is often the role of an occupational or physical therapist. In order to maximize the success of any life-style modification, the team should first understand the person's handicaps, which may be multiple, then evaluate and design any final environmental adaptation.

After the individual's medical situation, long-term prognosis, and unique physiological and functional abilities are defined, a list can then be developed that specifies activities that are beneficial and appropriate (some may be destructive) to the patient. The next step is the prescription and administration of the list or preventive maintenance program to maintain or improve the individual's physical situation. It is essential for the patient to subscribe to this program. Without motivation on the part of the patient, all previous and future attempts at environmental or medical intervention by the team are almost assured failure. Major limitations for independent living are often lack of motivation of the patient or the lack of financial resources.

It is important to remember that the person with "the problem" has the ultimate control over the change process and may stop the project by doing nothing. The role of the psychologist or counselor can be fundamental to ensuring the success of environmental modifications in patients' lives by helping them cope, accept limited conditions, and dare to do more.

Listening by the rehabilitation team is essential. Since no one is closer to the problems than the patient himself, he may have a good start on how to solve his own problems because of his personal interest and involvement in the outcome.

At this conceptual planning stage, the traditional medical or rehabilitation team should involve another team member who can turn concepts and plans into practical, safe hardware and structures. Because of the multiple skills this person may possess, the role may be designated "technologist." The technologist is knowledgeable about what is being made or can be made from bolts, mortar, or transistors, as well as about the physics of body mechanics. The same person may serve as any or all of the following:

Therapist (occupational or physical)

Engineer (rehabilitation, biomedical, mechanical, electrical)

Architect/designer (building, landscape, interior, industrial)

Contractor (mason, carpenter, plumber, electrician, handyperson)

Technician (machinist, mechanic, welder, electronic specialist)

Orthotist/prosthetist

Computer specialist

There are two types of technologists: generalists, who have more academic training and a wider, general knowledge of many fields (therapists, engineers, architects), and specialists, who have expertise mainly in one particular area (orthotists, machinists, cabinetmakers). Skills and knowledge can overlap, however, and awareness of multiple options for the patient, creativity, and flexibility are valuable characteristics for the technologist (and anyone else) to possess.

The technologist can be enlisted in the team as either a coprofessional or a service-delivery contractor. He must be sensitive to the fact that the person with a physical problem is the boss and what the patient wants to accomplish is all that will be achieved. Furthermore, he should be aware of the rolls of the other team members and be willing to help them achieve their tasks (physical evaluation, exercise program, motivation). He should know what other team members have done and actually cannot proceed until these objectives are accomplished.

One of the technologist's primary concerns should be safety for the client and for others around him. Aids that can be potentially destructive should not be devised or considered. Here again a decision by the team, including the patient, would be most helpful in deciding the appropriateness of some aids (the patient may not have the cognitive or perceptual skills to drive a car or electric wheelchair even though his physical deficits can be remedied through technological intervention).

The technologist must also be careful not to let his imagination and technology run away with the project. Sophisticated technology is only seldom needed. Many people can become prematurely physically limited by being *too* reliant on seductive aids that result in the loss of strength and range of motion. A simple rule in technological intervention is that the more simplistic and natural a solution, the better will be its long-term ramifications. A practical result of such a rule is that it keeps costs down, increases reliability, and prevents or decreases maintenance problems in the future.

The technologist must also show patience. The best long-term solution may require the disabled individual to learn new physical skills and techniques (transfers) or to break old habits. Repeated adjustments of equipment and motivation of the patient are often required ultimately to reach a successful conclusion to the environmental modification.

Technology is developing at such a rapid rate today that there are few physical problems that cannot be improved by the appropriate application. In each design the technologist should strive to maximize safety, independent function as well as functional range of motion in the patient, and esthetic quality and to minimize cost and energy consumption.

Architectural design improvements position storage (clothes, dishes, tools) areas and work stations (sinks, desks, tables) in optimal locations, or equipment may be modified and controlled from distances. Aids that increase the effective length of the arm, such as custom-designed reachers to pick things up off the floor, extended hair combers, and toothbrush holders, also fall under this category.

Functional strength can be improved by using simple, passive, mechanical devices such as the lever or inclined plane to help with opening jars and doors or getting up a hill through the use of complicated, externally powered devices such as electric wheelchairs or electrohydraulic power lifts for loading into vans.

Other areas in which the technologist can be of significant value to the handicapped individual are

General security, safety, and physiological care (door security, fire)

Communication (TV, telephone, emergency messages devices)

Transportation (walking aids, wheelchairs, vehicles)

Employment (educational aids, worksite modification)

Daily living activities (personal hygiene, dressing, eating, cooking, laundry)

Recreation (game modifications, TV, stereo)

It is impossible to provide the multitude of specific environmental modification solutions briefly. This problem is compounded by the need to customize many solutions to the special requirements of each individual. However, there are a myriad of basic areas in modifying each person's home environment.[1,2] These follow, along with general recommendations in design specifications for people with arthritis. Recommendations have been developed through testing of several hundred handicapped individuals at the NIH-sponsored Southwest Arthritis Center and by other studies conducted by the author.[3]

Exterior Concerns

A. Transportation and independent mobility
    1. Aids required
        a. Walking aids
        b. Electric wheelchair
        c. Modified automobile or van
    2. Vehicular needs
        a. Control systems
            i.   Steering
            ii. Braking
        b. Equipment storage
            i.   Wheelchair (location, style)
            ii. Walking aids
        c. Restraint systems
            i.   Humans
            ii.   Equipment
            iii. Occupied wheelchair

B. Removal of transportation barriers
    1. Parking area
        a. Surface. Concrete, no more irregular than stiff brushed finish (asphalt not good in hot climates)
        b. Width. Sufficient to accommodate full-size van and side-loading wheelchair lift (12 feet +)
        c. Length. Sufficient to accommodate van with tailgate lift system (25 feet)
        d. Slope. Away from house or flat over total parking area (maximum 1 inch in 4 feet)
        e. Lighting. Sufficient to see keys and locks.

      f.   Covered. For rain or summer sun protection (excessive heat in car interior is hazardous to spinal cord and sensory impaired)

2. Sidewalks/ramps
   a. Surface
      i. No irregularities greater than 1/8 inch vertical or 1 inch horizontal
      ii. Some texture (not polished smooth), no more irregular than stiff brushed concrete
   b. Width. No less than 3 feet
   c. Edging
      i. Should be present on sidewalk regions where there is greater than a 1-inch vertical difference between the sidewalk surface and the surrounding terrain
      ii. The height of the edging should not be less than 3 inches and of sufficient strength not to break with wheelchair abuse (3-inch-thick rebar), round off intersection corners
   d. Slope
      i. As flat as possible
      ii. As straight a run as possible
      iii. Do not exceed a rise of 1 inch in 12 inches of run (5°)
   e. Switchbacks
      i. 4 feet by 4 feet minimum U turn area
      ii. Zero slope
   f. Railings
      i. Helpful to many on ramp or level, consider
      ii. Railing height between 32 and 36 inches for adults, 18 and 24 inches for children
   g. Lighting
      i. Sufficient to seek keys, locks, and any hazards
      ii. Sufficient for others to see you
   h. Roof
      i. Primarily to provide cover in rain
      ii. Sun stroke, temperature extremes, and wet clothing can be especially dangerous for quadriplegics and other disabled individuals
   i. Paths. Sufficient routes to allow use of backyard or garden as a recreation area

3. Entrance/exit doors
   a. Emergency exits. Two or more accessible routes for fire, etc.
   b. Door width. 36 inches minimum
   c. Door knob. Lever style or panic bar
   d. Lock. Pushbutton or electronic key with interior mechanical override
   e. Porch. 5 feet by 5 feet level area minimum
   f. Door swing. *"In"* preferred (otherwise minimizes porch maneuvering area)

    g. Lighting. Sufficient to see keys, locks

    h. Porch. Rain and sun protection while opening and unlocking the door

    i. Security. Intercom or close circuit TV on door, used in conjunction with solenoid door latch and automatic door opener (manual override)

    j. Door closer system. Lightest system possible or equipment with overriding latch system to remove door closer force

Interior Concerns

A.   Entrance hall

   1. Width. Minimum 36 inches, 48+ inches preferred

   2. Length. 7+ feet (door swing in and chair allowance)

   3. Surface

      i. Smooth tile surface preferred

      ii. No irregularity greater than 1/8 inch vertical allowable

      iii. No horizontal irregularity greater than 1/2 inch

      iv. Carpets generally unacceptable; best carpet is indoor-outdoor style (no throw rugs)

   4. Slope. As close to zero as possible

B.   Interior halls

   1. Width. 36+ inches

   2. Surface. Smooth tile, parquette preferred, indoor-outdoor carpet acceptable

   3. Slope. Zero preferred, no stairs

   4. Lighting. Sufficient to spot floor irregularity or obstacles

   5. Railing. When needed, 32 to 36 inches height above floor

C.   Interior doors/room entrances

   1. Width. 32 inches minimum

   2. Knobs. Lever style

   3. Threshold. 1/2 inch maximum; zero preferred

   4. Closures. Minimum spring, none (preferred), or automatic

   5. Surfaces

      a. No stairs

      b. Tile or parquette, indoor-outdoor carpet (second choice)

D.   Interior light switch, controls, power outlets—32 to 36 inches above floor throughout house

E.   Bathroom
1.   Equipment
   a.   Shower. Most common need
      i.   Threshold, roll in (walk-in) preferred, maximum height 3 inches
      ii.   Surface
            (a) Rough tile (Falcon-trak paint)
            (b) 3-M Nomad carpet (removable)
      iii. Grab bars
            (a) Vertical at entrance
            (b) Horizontal on at least two adjacent walls (32 to 34, inches, 1 1/2 inch diameter
      iv.   Shower control. Single lever control 32 inches from floor
      v.   Shower head.* Multiple or hand held with multiple wall attachments
      vi.   Temperature control.* Scald guard regulator.
      vii. Seat. Fold-up, wall-mounted bench or permanent corner seat
      viii. Wall storage for paraphenalia*
      ix.   Sloped crown at entrance for water retention, slope = 1 inch in 48 inches to drain
   b.   Tub. Individual taste or needs may require starred items above
      i.   Surface. 3-M Nomad carpet (removable)
      ii.   Grab bars. Place vertical bars on both ends of tub
            (a) Place 36 + -inch wide bar on long wall
            (b) Consider mounting 36-inch bar at an angle on long wall
      iii. Seat. Consider bench or stool in tub
   c.   Toilet
      i.   Preferred height for wheelchair transfer 22 inches, higher seats at custom height good for weakness in legs
      ii.   Grab bars (1 1/4 to 1 1/2 inches diameter above toilet tank (rear) and at each side wall.
      iii. Consider power lift
   d.   Sink
      i.   Wheelchair height, 30 inches clear under sink
      ii.   Opening under counter for drive-in chair
      iii. Mount faucet in middle (front to back) or at front edge (limited range of motion)
   e.   Mirror
      i.   Bottom edge at 30 inches for wheelchair user
      ii.   Top edge at 72 inches for standing disabled
   f.   Infrared lamps. Provide warmth while drying; mounted in ceiling
   g.   Light switch. Palm-size toggle preferred, mount at 34 inches above floor (pushbutton, mercury switch good)

  h. Door
    i. Pocket door best to maximize space
    ii. Consider automatic open/close
 2. Space
  a. 5′ × 5′ turnaround space for wheelchair a minimum
  b. 5′ × 5′ clear in front of toilet for left or right hand and head-on transfers
  c. 5′ × 4′ - minimum roll-in shower space

F. Bedroom
 1. Closet
  a. Roll-in/walk-in best
  b. Doors
    i. Pocket door (which slides into the wall) or swing-out door to maximize interior space
    ii. Bifold or accordion good
    iii. Consider automatic or large easy grip handles for closure
  c. Shelves on doors and walls at 24 to 48 inches height (shoes, sweater storage)
  d. Clothing rails. 5 feet and 30 inch heights, allows long dresses and two-level shorter item storage
  e. Consider making all features vertically adjustable in 1 inch increments
 2. Bedside organization table
  a. Pull-out lap boards (for writing or eating)
  b. Pull-out phone or storage tray
  c. Book shelves
  d. Power controls for house lighting and appliances
  e. Lighting for reading
 3. Bed
  a. Consider "Habitat" style, heated water bed for prevention of pressure sores
  b. Height. Appropriate for wheelchair transfer or raised for weak legs
  c. Consider power lift (hoist)
 4. Consider wall-hung work or study area
  a. Cantilever desk and shelves
  b. Vertically adjustable
 5. Space. 5′ by 5′ minimum turnaround for wheelchair
 6. Lighting/outlets/controls
  a. Pushbutton or palm toggle
  b. 30 to 36 inches above floor
 7. Floor surface
  a. No stairs
  b. No slope

      c. Smooth tile or parquette preferred; consider indoor-outdoor carpet (second choice)

      d. No throw rugs

G.   Dining room/kitchen

   1. Dining table

      a. Adequate height (30 inches clear), width (30 inches clear) for wheelchair

      b. Consider bar counter in kitchen for everyday

         i.   Multilevel

         ii. Vertically adjustable sections

      c. Stool is good for many disabled

         i.   Back support

         ii. Arm rests

         iii. Foot rests

         iv. Stable base

      d. Dishes/utensils

         i.   Plate with raised rim preferred (unbreakable)

         ii. Utensils with large-diameter wooden handle preferred

   2. Storage/sink

      a. Cantilever hung and vertically adjustable cabinets, counter 24 inches wide

      b. Removable modules under cabinet allows for wheelchair vertically and horizontally (30 inches by 30 inches minimum)

      c. Brim on counter edge to reduce spills into lap

      d. Faucet. Single-control lever style mounted on side of sink rather than back edge

      e. Sink

         i.   Double compartment

         ii. Stainless steel (to prevent chipping)

         iii. Shallow (trailer) model (5 inches deep) or Kohler "Epicurian" style sink

         iv. Garbage disposal

      f. Lazy susan, roll-out drawers in cabinets for hard-to-reach areas

      g. Ball-bearing rollers on all drawers

      h. Touch latch on all doors and cabinets (no handles)

      i. Space. Consider U cabinet or counter layout with 5 × 5 foot center

   3. Equipment

      a. Built-in dishwasher very helpful

      b. Range

         i.   Front control

         ii. Programmable lock (a safety feature where there are small children)

         iii. Consider inductive heat style (no hot spot or burner on counter)

     c. Oven
       i. Built-in at convenient height
       ii. Consider toaster oven on counter
       iii. Microwave. Cook on paper (lightweight/no wash)
          Short time/Defrost preprepared meal
          Container stays cool (relatively)
     d. Utility cart-seating table, one trip, carrying hot food
     e. Stool. Consider sitting to work to save energy
       i. Backrest
       ii. Arms
       iii. Foot rest
       iv. Stable base
     f. Refrigerator
       i. Side-by-side style
       ii. Magnetic latch or door pedal open
       iii. Consider ice cube and water dispenser on door
     g. Lighting, outlet, switches
       i. At 30- to 36-inch height
       ii. Pushbutton or palm toggle style

H. Laundry area
  1. Counter/shelf
     a. Storage, folding clothes (24 inches wide at 32 inch height)
     b. Wheelchair clearance (30 inches high by 30 inches wide)
     c. Cantilever adjustable-height mount
  2. Automatic washer
     a. Front controls
     b. Front loading
     c. Consider changing height by placing on box
  3. Dryer very helpful
     a. Front control
     b. Front loading
     c. Consider raising on box to more comfortable height
  4. Clothesline
     a. Adjustable height
     b. Sidewalk to line and under line
     c. Consider retractable line on the porch
  5. Ironing
     a. Permanent press fabrics (use dryer, no iron)
     b. Travel iron (lightweight)
     c. Fold-down or pull-out (from counter top) ironing board
  6. Space. 5' by 5' in front of equipment for turnaround

I. Living room/recreation room
  1. No steps

2. Surface. Smooth tile, parquette preferred; indoor-outdoor carpet (second choice)
3. Good recliner. When appropriate (custom fit, registered therapist)
   a. Appropriate height
   b. Proper length seat
   c. Lumbar support
   d. Flat back support in shoulder region
   e. Adjustable position; seat, back, legs
   f. Adjustable foot rest
   g. Consider power lift
4. Work/study area. Designed to suit needs
   a. Height
   b. Width
   c. Writing surface
   d. Environmental controls
   e. Book holder/page turner
   f. Lighting
   g. Storage/organization
   h. Proper seating
   i. Modified hobby equipment (woodwork, sewing)
5. Remote and automatic controls for electrical systems
   a. TV/radio
   b. Stereo. Consider tape deck
   c. Lighting
   d. Home computer
   e. Air conditioning system
6. Consider ability to go places independently
   a. Modified van/car
   b. Electric wheelchair
7. Modified games/hobbies

SUMMARY

The removal of architectural and environmental barriers and the promotion of independence of the person with severe arthritis often requires the assistance of many health professionals. Among the many benefits to accrue from barrier removal are increased self-esteem, increased "freedom," saved energy and time, and improvement of family finances. Achievement of such a program, however, cannot succeed without the full cooperation and much motivation on the part of the patient.

The role of the technologist (a biomedical engineer most often) is to assist the health professional and patient team in securing a safe, effective architectural or environmental modification. Creativity, flexibility, patience, and an extensive knowledge of hardware involved in environmental modifications are the essential characteristics of a good technologist. Multiple exterior and interior environmental problems of the arthritis patient can be solved.

REFERENCES

1. Bruck B. Access: the guide to a better life for disabled Americans. New York: Random House, 1978.
2. Hale G, ed. The source book for the disabled. New York: Paddington Press, 1979
3. Woods W. Disability and building codes: a quantitative study. Southwest Arthritis Center, Tucson, Ariz. 1981.

25

Arthritis Patient Education

Kate Lorig, R.N., Dr.P.H.

Everyone agrees that patient education is an important part of arthritis care. Various studies have estimated that between 19.3 percent and 35.4 percent of physicians' time is spent in patient education.[1-5] Arthritis health professionals (AHP) also spend a large part of their time with patient education activities. Despite the importance of this subject, however, patient education is seldom part of either AHP or physician education.

To provide a framework for understanding patient education, it is important to define terms. Patient education includes all planned educational activities aimed at assisting patients in achieving voluntary health-behavior changes.[6] It should be noted that the aim of patient education is more than just providing the patient with knowledge about his or her disease. Many health professionals believe that, given the correct information, patients will change their behavior. However, many studies indicate that there is little correlation between changes in health knowledge and changes in health behavior.[7,8] On a more intuitive level, if knowledge was all that was needed to change health behaviors, we would be a nation of sleek nonsmokers. Thus if patient education is more than the supplying of knowledge, it is necessary to examine how it can be successfully applied to the field of rheumatology.

To begin with, patient education should be based on the beliefs, needs, and concerns of the patient. The importance of patients' beliefs in determining future health action has been explored by the health belief model that postulates that behavior is based on a patient's belief and that he or she has the disease and that the treatment will be efficacious.[9] With arthritis, patients usually believe that they have the disease but often, because of the simplicity of the treatment (for example, aspirin) or because of the influence of the media or friends, do not believe in the efficacy of the treatment.

Miller and Fishbein each suggest that salient beliefs are instrumental in determining a patient's actions.[10,11] They state that if behavior is to be changed, these beliefs must be considered. Green suggests that health behavior is determined by predisposing, enabling, and reinforcing factors.[6] For example, most people with arthritis do not seek medical care until they experience pain, disfigurement, or deformity. These could be considered predisposing events. Enabling factors include being able physically to get to medical care and being able to pay for the care. Reinforcing factors include the support of family and friends in maintaining the suggested treatment regime. Hochbaum expanded the concept of reinforcing factors by exploring the barriers that prevent patients from complying with medical suggestions.[12,13]

Using these theoretical models on a frame, arthritis as well as other patient education should be based on the patient's beliefs. When the Stanford Arthritis Center asked 100 middle class patients about their greatest concerns, the most frequent response was pain, followed by disability and deformity.[14] However, most arthritis patient education is based on avoiding disability and deformity; pain is a secondary concern. When 50 Latino patients were questioned about what causes arthritis, the majority gave answers that dealt with rapid changes from hot to cold, for example, working hard all day and then taking a cold shower, or ironing and then washing one's hands. Thus patient education for these patients must consider the importance of heat and cold, such as, suggesting a hot shower or bath before exercising.

The easiest way to determine patient needs, beliefs, and concerns is to ask. An interview is usually part of any good medical encounter. However, often the importance of patient responses is not considered when giving patient education. The reason for the discounting of patient responses is that health professionals often think they know what is best for the patient. Patient education often reflects the expertise and beliefs of the health professionals without considering the knowledge and beliefs of the patient. Physical therapists teach exercises, occupational therapists joint protection, and nurses medication schedules.

The following is a discussion of suggested content and methodology to be used in arthritis education. Much of this discussion is based on experience gained from the more than 2,000 patients who attended Arthritis Self-Management (ASM) courses given by the Stanford Arthritis Center. The overall assumptions underlying this discussion are:

1. Patients are intelligent human beings who can make appropriate decisions about their own health care.
2. There is no specific set of fixed treatments that have always proven efficacious, and thus, within the limits of conventional practice, each patient should help decide what is best for him.
3. Treatment, if at all possible, should not contradict the belief system of the patient.
4. Pain is the major concern of most patients, and thus all interventions should be discussed in terms of pain relief.

Exercise.   In keeping with the assumption that patients can make their own decisions, patients can be taught how to design an exercise program including both stretching and isometric exercises. Many need not be given specific exercises but rather should be given guidelines for every major joint.[15] They should also be given guidelines for when to expand and when to cut back on their program. These guidelines are based on the amount of pain experienced 2 hours after completing exercise.[16] Thus if there is no pain 2 hours after exercising for 4 days, the program can be expanded. If exercise-induced pain does continue for 2 hours or more, the program should be cut back. The advantage of teaching principles rather than specific exercises is that patients have the tools to change their exercise program as needed. Exercise should be targeted on specific joints chosen by the patient. This decision is based on two factors. First, any program that is too complex tends not to be followed for any length of time.[17,18] Behavior changes should fit into life patterns as easily as possible. Research conducted at the Stanford Arthritis Center provided evidence that the arthritis pain is more reflective of the most painful joint than it is of mean overall joint pain. Thus if the pain can be relieved in the most painful joints, the patient will probably experience an improvement in overall well-being.

Joint Protection.   Joint protection and use of aids, like exercise, can be taught in terms of what the patient would like to do. Three or four principles can be taught such as use of larger joints whenever possible. The patient can then be asked, "What would you like to do that you now find difficult?" Based on the response, the patient is asked to figure out how the principles might be applied to the problem. When education is done in a group or family setting, all members of the group can participate in the problem-solving sessions. Emphasis is placed on assisting the patient to continue leading as normal a life as possible. When aids are necessary, try to suggest and encourage low-cost adaptations utilizing things from everyday life. Again, the philosophy in this approach is to treat the arthritis patient as a basically well person with a problem instead of as a sick patient. This encourages the well rather than the sick role.[19]

Relaxation.   Formal relaxation techniques have not traditionally been a part of arthritis patient education. The role of relaxation in pain management has been documented, however.[20,21] It seems reasonable to assume that relaxation has a place in arthritis pain management. No one relaxation technique has proven to be more successful than any other. Patients can choose between Benson, Schultz, Jacobson, or other techniques.[22,23] Meditation and prayer are equally acceptable. The point is not to force any philosophy but to have the patient set aside some time each day to relax both the body and the mind in ways acceptable to him. This is not too different than the more traditional advice to have the patient take frequent rests. The difference is that relaxation techniques allow the patient to relax the mind as well as body.

Nontraditional Diets and Other Treatments.   A major topic of concern to rheumatologists is patients' use of nontraditional diets and other treatments. The reasons for this concern are many. In some cases, nontraditional treatments are harmful or at least very expensive without being helpful. In addition many physicians are concerned that patients will utilize nontraditional therapies in place of recommended medical treatments. Unfortunately most patient education has been shown to be ineffective, especially if alternatives are not given.[24,25] In some cases education against nontraditional treatment may actually cause patients to doubt the reliability of traditional treatment. For example, if a patient believes that drinking wine makes arthritis worse but is told this is not true or is belittled for this belief, he is not likely to believe anything else suggested by the physician.

One possible solution to this dilemma is to teach patients how to evaluate treatments, both traditional and nontraditional, and to then make an informed decision. Patients should ask the following questions about any treatment: (1) Is the source of information reliable? (2) Were there clinical trials or just anecdotes? (3) If anecdotes, were the people like me? (4) Is there another possible explanation for the cure or success of the treatment? (5) Are there side effects or dangers? (6) Can I afford this treatment? Thinking through the answers to these questions, patients can decide whether or not to try a treatment. To help patients in this process, physicians and other health professionals need to know about current trends in nontraditional treatments and be ready to give patients factual information. For example, the patient who asks about wine might be told that there is no evidence that wine has any effect on arthritis but that if he thinks wine negatively affects arthritis, it might be best not to drink wine. Such a neutral statement gives factual information without contradicting the patient's belief system. Research has indicated that attitudes are best changed by giving information on both sides of controversial issues.[26]

If a patient asks about a potentially dangerous treatment such as some given in foreign clinics, the physician might say that the drugs usually given are a combination of steroids and tranquilizers that give short-term relief but have serious long-term side effects. If a patient insists on seeking such treatment, it is important to keep the door to communication open by telling the patient you would like to hear about his or her experiences and to give the patient information about where the drugs can be analyzed.

The line between nontraditional and accepted treatment is thinner than many of us like to believe. For example, patient education is considered by many an unproven therapy; similarly, although treatment with gold is well-accepted, there is little information on how it affects arthritis as it does.

As important as the content of patient education are the various processes or methods by which patient education is presented. In recent years there has been a great deal of study in the field of behavioral medicine, the results of which can be applied in clinical practice.

Questioning.   How questions are asked and when they are asked is important. For example, work by Roter has shown that patients who are encouraged to ask questions early in the medical encounter are more likely to keep future appointments than those who do not ask questions.[27] To get patients to ask questions and express concerns, it is best to use open-ended as opposed to yes/no questions. For example, ask, "What questions do you have?", not "Do you have any questions?"

Demonstration/Return Demonstration.   Physicians should demonstrate what the patient should do and have the patient *return* the demonstration before leaving the office. Handing a patient a list of exercises is not enough; the patient should actually *do* the exercise or practice the joint protection techniques while in the physician's office. The importance of the return demonstration was illustrated in a study where it was shown that the single most important factor in predicting the practice of breast self-examination was having the woman examine her own breast in the doctor's office or self-examination class.[28] One of the most difficult problems in arthritis care is achieving medication compliance. One way of helping this problem is to have hospitalized patients take their own medications, while still hospitalized.

Contracting/Use of Diaries.   Having patients give a verbal or written commitment to specific actions is a powerful tool for behavioral change. Ureda has shown that patients who sign contracts concerning losing weight and have these contracts cosigned by relatives or friends lose more weight than those people who do not sign contracts.[29] Verbal contracts can be easily elicited by asking a patient at the end of an encounter to list or state those things which he or she is going to do. To reinforce the importance of the contract, it is important to ask about these activities early in the next encounter. Contracted activities should be entered in the medical record.

Sometimes keeping a diary helps to reinforce a contract. A patient can note what exercises he or she is doing, and keep track of daily medication and pain levels. Diaries are especially helpful in the short term as in establishing a new program but should generally not be kept for more than a few weeks.

Giving Information.   Patients need specific information. For example, "Isometric exercises should be held for 6 seconds and repeated two to four times a day"; "Take this medication with food, 2 tablets 3 times a day."

Although we want to teach patients general principles, these need to be taught in specific terms. Less specific directions often lead to trouble. For example, some patients have been known to have joint flares because they practiced isometric exercises 30 or 40 times a day. In their enthusiasm to carry out their doctor's or therapist's suggestion that they exercise a few times every day, patients sometimes overdo. Often patients are told to take medication with meals, the assumption being patients eat three times a day. However, meals per day can range from one to seven. Lack of compliance is often due to communication errors.

Group/Normative Pressure.   Probably the strongest reinforcing factor is the support of family and friends. Evidence of the importance of social support in achieving behavior change has been demonstrated by several studies.[30,31] This support can be elicited in several ways. The influence of opinion leaders and peers is important.[32] Modeling's effectiveness has been demonstrated.[33] A well-known demonstration is provided by Alcoholics Anonymous. The importance of support groups in arthritis patient education has also been demonstrated.[34,35] The implications for medical practice are that physicians should involve patients' family members or friends whenever possible. Another way of providing reinforcement is by forming patient education classes, support groups, or patient

Table 25.1. Arthritis Patient Education Studies

Study	Subjects	Design	Independent Variables	Outcomes
Vignos, Parker, Thompson[37]	20 RA patients	Pretest/posttest comparison of two interventions.	1. Group education and literature versus 2. Literature only	Knowledge increased in both groups, but more for group 1 than group 2.
Holsten, Morris, Moeschberger[38]	57 RA patients hospitalized for arthritis	6 month pretest/posttest comparison of two groups.	1. Patients hospitalized on an arthritis ward. 2. Arthritis patients hospitalized on a general ward	Knowledge—no differences. Compliance—higher for group 1.
Schmitt, McBrair[39]	30 RA patients; 25 insurance company employees	Posttest comparison of three groups.	1. RA patients seen by rheumatologist while receiving group education 2. RA patients seen by rheumatologist 3. Patients-insurance company employees	Knowledge increase for patients attending group sessions when compared to other two groups.
Moll et al.[40]	50 gout patients	Comparison of two groups.	1. Group receiving literature with illustrations 2. Group receiving literature without illustrations	Knowledge—no differences between groups.
Strass, Mikkelsen[41]	OA patients	Pretest/posttest one group	A slide tape presentation	Knowledge increase 8 weeks after seeing presentation.
Kaye, Hammond[42]	48 RA patients	Pretest/posttest for knowledge. Posttest only for other factors.	One-time audiovisual program and consultation with a health educator	Knowledge increase reported. enhanced family communication, behavior changes, and more meticulous medication use.

Study	Sample	Design	Intervention	Results
Ferguson, Bole[43]	40 RA patients	Survey interviews	Family support belief in benefit of treatment	Noncompliance is related to lack of belief in benefit of treatment.
Knudson, Spregel, and Furst[44]	12 RA patients	Pretest/posttest descriptive data.	1. 6-session group patient education course 2. Nonrandomized controls	Group 1 had improved knowledge and behaviors and decreased self-care activities.
Udelman and Udelman[34]	Hospitalized arthritis patients	Posttest	Group therapy sessions	Increased understanding of illness, improved coping techniques, healthier family communications.
Schwartz[35]	RA patients	Posttest	Group therapy sessions	Improved communication, improved clinic attendance and compliance. Fewer flares during group.
Gross, Brandt[36]	Ankylosing spondylitis patients	Pretest/posttest comparison groups	1. Support group education 2. Control group	Group 1 showed increased knowledge and exercise and expressed improvement in coping ability and family communication.
Lorig, Kraines, Holman[45]	309 arthritis patients	Pretest/posttest randomized controlled crossover time series	12-hour patient education course	Increased knowledge, exercise, relaxation, decreased pain, number of physician visits. No change patient satisfaction with physicians, locus of control, disability.

clubs. While such groups provide information about arthritis, it may be that their most important function is providing social support.

At any age arthritis tends to be an isolating illness. Therefore one of the most important forms of therapy is the encouragement of social contact. Because a physician often serves as both an opinion leader and a role model, he or she can be very instrumental in encouraging social activities.

Evaluation. Patient education is often criticized because of the lack of rigorous evaluation. However, a number of studies have demonstrated the effectiveness of arthritis patient education, as shown in table 25.1.

While we still have much to learn, we are fortunate in having an increasing number of validated, self-administered instruments that are helpful in evaluating health status as it applies to arthritis.[46,47] Although it is not possible for all physicians and arthritis health professionals to conduct clinical research, it is now possible to conduct some pre- and posttesting of patient education efforts.

SUMMARY

Arthritis patient education involves much more than the giving of information. To be successful, such education should take into account the belief system of the patients and incorporate presupposing, enabling, and reinforcing factors. This can be done by being aware of the process of patient education and its importance in producing health behavior change.

REFERENCES

1. Bartlett EE. The contribution of consumer health education to primary care practice: a review. Med Care 1980;18(8):862-871.
2. Bergman A, et al. Time-motion study of practicing pediatricians. Pediatrics 1966; 38(2), part 1:254-263
3. Donaldson MC, London CD. Time study of doctors and nurses at two Swedish health care centers. Med Care 1971;9:457-467.
4. Hessel SJ, Haggerty RJ. General pediatrics: a study of practice in the mid 1960's. J Ped 1968;73:271-279.
5. Parrish HM, et al. Time study of general practitioner's office hours. Arch Environ Health 1967;(14):892-898.
6. Green LW, Kreuler M, Partridge KB, Deeds SG. Health education planning: a diagnostic approach. Palo Alto, Calif.: Mayfield, 1979.
7. Marston MV. Compliance with medical regimens: a review of the literature. Nurs Res 1970;170(19):312-323.
8. Young M, Buckley P, Wechsler H, Demone H, Jr. A demonstration of automated instruction for diabetic self-care. Am J Public Health 1969;59:110-122.
9. Rosenstock I. The health belief model and preventive health behavior. Health Ed Monographs 1974;2(4):254-386.

10. Miller G. The magical number seven, plus or minus two: some limits on our capacity for processing information. Psychol Rev 1956;63(2):81–97.

11. Fishbein M, Ajzen I. Belief, attitude, intention and behavior. Reading, Mass.: Addison-Wesley, 1976.

12. Hochbaum GM. Patient counseling vs. patient teaching. Topics Clin Nurs 1980; 2(2):1–7.

13. Hochbaum GM. Strategies and their rationale for changing people's eating habits. J Nutrition Ed 1981;13(15):S59–65.

14. Lorig K. Arthritis self-management: a joint venture. Unpublished Ph.D. dissertation. Berkeley, University of California, School of Public Health, 1980.

15. Lorig K, Fries J. The arthritis helpbook. Reading, Mass.: Addison-Wesley, 1980.

16. Swezey R. Arthritis: rational therapy and rehabilitation. Philadelphia: W.B. Saunders, 1978.

17. Ley P. Psychological studies of doctor-patient communications. In: Rachman S, ed., Contributions to medical psychology. Oxford: Pergamon Press, 1977, pp. 9–42.

18. Becker MH, Malmon LA. Strategies for enhancing patient compliance. J Commun Health 1980;6(2):113–135.

19. Parsons T. Definitions of health and illness in light of American values and social structure. In: Juco, E Gartley, ed., Patients, physicians and illness. New York: The Free Press, 1958.

20. Varni JW. Behavioral medicine in hemophilia arthritic pain management: two case studies. Arch Phys Med Rehab 1981;62:183–187.

21. Varni JW. Behavioral medicine in pain and analgesia management for the hemophilic child with VIII inhibitor. Pain, in press. 1981;11:121–126.

22. Benson H. The relaxation response. New York: Avon Books, 1975.

23. White J, Fadiman J, eds. Relax. New York: Confusion Press, 1976.

24. Kirscht JP, Haefner DP. Effects of repeated threatening health communications. Int J Health Ed 1973;16:268–277.

25. Leventhal H. Fear appeals and persuasion: the differentiation of a motivational construct. Am J Public Health 1971;61:1208–1224.

26. Hovland C, Janis I, Keley H. Communication and persuasion. New Haven, Conn.: Yale University Press, 1953.

27. Roter DL. Patient participation in patient-provider interaction: the effects of patient question asking on the quality of interaction, satisfaction and compliance. Health Ed Monographs 1977;5:281–315.

28. Lieberman Research Inc. A study of the effectiveness of alternative breast cancer PE programs. Prepared for The American Cancer Society, 1977. Available from Lieberman Research, Inc., 919 Third Avenue, New York, N.Y. 10022.

29. Ureda JR. The effect of contract witnessing on motivation and weight loss in a weight control program. Health Ed Quart 1980;7(3):185–196.

30. Nuckolls KB, Cassel J, Kaplan BH. Psychosocial assets, life crisis, and the prognosis of pregnancy. Am J Epidem 1972;95:431–441.

31. Berkman LF, Syme SL. Social networks, host resistance and mortality: a nine year follow-up study of Alameda County residents. Am J Epidem 1979;109:186–204.

32. Rogers E, Shoemaker F. Communication of innovations. New York: The Free Press, 1971.

33. Bandura A, Blanchard E, Ritter B. Relative efficiency of desensitization and modeling therapeutic approaches for inducing behavioral, affective and attitude changes. J Personality Social Psychol 1969;13:173–179.

34. Udelman H, Udelman D. Group therapy with rheumatoid arthritis patients. Am J Psychotherapy 1978;32:288–299.
35. Schwartz L, Marcus R. Multidisciplinary group therapy for rheumatoid arthritis. Psychosomatics 1978; 19:289–293.
36. Gross M, Brandt KD. Educational support groups for patients with ankylosing spondylitis: a preliminary report. Patient Counseling Health Ed 1981;3:6–12.
37. Vignos P, Parker W, Thompson H. Evaluation of a clinic education program for patients with rheumatoid arthritis. J Rheum 1976;3:155–165.
38. Holsten DJ, Morris AD, Moeschberger M. Effects of an organized educational program on patient understanding of rheumatoid arthritis and compliance with medical treatment. Presented at the 12th Scientific Meeting of the Allied Health Professions Section of the Arthritis Foundation, Miami Beach, Fla., December 1976.
39. Schmitt A, McBrair W. Assessing the quality of education provided to rheumatoid arthritis patients in a suburban-rural setting. Presented at the 14th Scientific Meeting of the Allied Health Professions Section of the Arthritis Foundation, Denver, Colo., June 1979.
40. Moll JMH, Wright V, Jeffrey MR, Goode D, Humberstone PM. The cartoon in doctor-patient communication. Ann Rheum Dis 1977;36:225–231.
41. Stross J, Mikkelsen WM. Educating patients with osteoarthritis. J Rheum 1977;4:313–316.
42. Kaye R, Hammond A. Rheumatoid arthritis. JAMA 1978;239:2966–2967.
43. Ferguson K, Bole GG. Family support, health beliefs, therapeutic compliance in patients with rheumatoid arthritis. Patient Counseling Health Ed 1979;1:101–105.
44. Knudson KG, Spiegel TM, Furst DE. Outpatient education program for rheumatoid arthritis patients. Patient Counseling Health Ed 1981;3:77–82.
45. Lorig K, Kraines RG, Holman HR. A randomized prospective controlled study of the effects of health education for people with arthritis. Arth Rheum (Suppl.). 1981;24:590. (Abstract.)
46. Fries JF, Spitz P, Kraines RG, Holman HR. Measurement of patient outcome in arthritis. Arth Rheum 1980;23:137–145.
47. Meenan RF, German PM, Mason JH. Measuring health status in arthritis: the arthritis impact measurement scales. Arth Rheum 1980;23:146–452.

26

Understanding and Enhancing Patient Cooperation with Arthritis Treatments

Alan M. Jette, P.T., Ph.D.

The quality of health care depends in the final analysis on the interaction of the patient and provider. There is abundant evidence that in current practice this interaction all too often is disappointing to both parties. Systematic surveys confirm widespread dissatisfaction among patients with health professionals and among health professions with their patients' lack of cooperation.[1,3]

Many different factors have been found to contribute to the generally low level of patient cooperation with professional recommendations. Haynes classifies them into six areas: demographic features of patients, features of the disease, features of the therapeutic regimen(s), characteristics of the therapeutic source, features of the patient-practitioner interaction; and sociobehavioral features of patients.[4] Attention here is focused on the role of health-care providers in increasing patient cooperation with therapeutic recommendations. In particular, this chapter will concentrate on how the nature of the patient-provider relationship affects patients' cooperation with health care recommendations, suggest ways in which health professionals might improve the current state of affairs, and highlight outstanding research issues in this important area.

The term "patient compliance" is intentionally avoided. This unfortunate term evokes the image of a passive, subservient, and unfeeling patient who "complies" with the wishes of the omniscient and omnipotent practitioner. The phrase "patient cooperation" is used instead, as recommended by Friedman and Di-Matteo.[5] This term reflects the more constructive view that health care involves the give-and-take characteristic of all social interaction.

STATEMENT OF THE PROBLEM

The advice of persons acknowledged to be health experts is frequently ignored.[6] There are many implications of a patient's failure to follow a health professional's recommendation. The most obvious consequence is that the patient does not receive the full benefit of the expertise of his or her health care provider. The specific effects, or course, will vary with the nature of the recommendation. For example: Failure to take a prescribed dosage of a remission-inducing rheumatologic drug may lead to an exacerbation of the disease. If a physician assumes his or her patient is indeed taking the prescribed amount (but the patient is not), and then the physician increases the dosage, the patient may begin to take the higher dose. This may lead to an overdose. Undetected patient noncooperation may also lead to the misevaluation of the efficacy of a particular treatment regimen. A treatment that is in fact effective may be judged ineffective because of patient noncooperation. In fact some investigators would go so far as to propose that clinical trials not be published unless they include an adequate assessment of compliance.[7]

Reported rates of compliance vary greatly according to the type of behavior studied and the particular circumstances under which care is offered. One early review of thirty-three carefully done studies that included a wide variety of medical problems found a median of 43 percent of patients who did not cooperate with health advice.[8] An estimated one-third of all patients fail to follow fully the treatments prescribed to them.[9]

One study of forty-six patients with rheumatoid arthritis affecting the hand revealed that only one-third of the patients cooperated with the recommendation to wear a hand splint.[10] Another investigation of sixty-six patients with rheumatoid arthritis found that 3 percent of the subjects did not use a prescribed hand splint at all, 32 percent wore it less than half of the time, and 65 percent cooperated at least 50 percent of the time.[11] Ferguson and Bole reported that 75 percent of patients at the University of Michigan Arthritis Center were not cooperating with the recommended use of a splint; 60 percent did not cooperate with prescribed exercise regimens, in contrast to 22 percent who reported not taking aspirin at least some of the time.[12] A 1967 drug study of arthritis out-patients reported that only 50 percent had taken their medication exactly as prescribed.[13] This finding is similar to the findings of a study in 1976 where 55 percent of the rheumatoid arthritis patients studied were found to be following an exercise regimen prescribed for the disease.[14] Another study of 123 rheumatoid arthritis patients found that 67 percent neither took their medications fully nor came to the clinic as often as advised.[15]

These preliminary disease-specific estimates of the magnitude of this problem should be interpreted cautiously. All six studies just mentioned involved small, unrepresentative samples of rheumatoid arthritis patients drawn from teaching hospitals. Nevertheless these data do suggest that patient noncooperation with arthritis treatment recommendations is a serious problem that has important ramifications for the management of the rheumatic diseases.

Based on our current level of scientific knowledge, what can health practitioners do about patient noncooperation?

INCREASING PATIENT COOPERATION

The health expert's role in improving cooperation from patients is poorly defined. Studies have found that physicians tend to overestimate the degree to which their patients are cooperating and are unable to judge which of the patients are cooperating with therapeutic recommendations and which are not.[16] In order to increase patient cooperation, health professionals must first understand what factors influence degree of cooperation. Patient noncooperation can be categorized as involuntary and voluntary. The different factors leading to each type of noncooperation must be understood before the professional can respond appropriately.

Involuntary Noncooperation

Patients must know and understand what recommendations have been made to them if they are to cooperate with those recommendations. This certainly seems basic enough; yet it has been widely demonstrated that the language and concepts that we in the health field use with our patients are not widely understood.[17] Not only are many of our technical words not understood by patients, but many commonly used bits of advice do not convey the meanings as intended. Instructions on prescriptions, for example, are frequently ambiguous.[18] In one study of patients from a medical service who were asked to interpret instructions on drug labels, only 36 percent correctly stated what "every 6 hours" is supposed to mean. Interpretations of what is meant by "evening" and by "with meals" varied considerably.[19] Health professionals have a clear responsibility to communicate their recommendations accurately and clearly to patients.

Two investigations shed considerable light on the problem of inadequate communication between the health expert and his or her client and its influence on patient cooperation. Svarstad and her colleagues studied patients and physicians in a neighborhood health center.[20] They tape-recorded and carefully analyzed patient-physician encounters. In doing so, they discovered many instructional failures: medications were prescribed but not discussed with the patients; few indications were given on how long the patient should continue taking the medication; and written instructions were, at best, incomplete. For those patients with misinformation regarding their regimen, only 17 percent cooperated with the physician's instructions. In contrast, 60 percent of those patients with accurate information cooperated. Note, however, that even with accurate information, 40 percent still did not cooperate.

Hulka and colleagues further explored this issue with a sample of patients of general practitioners.[21] The patients in this study had either congestive heart failure or diabetes mellitus. The investigators examined the assumption that degree of cooperation is a patient-related phenomenon; that noncompliance behavior represents the patient's volitional choice. Patients were interviewed in their home by a nurse interviewer after an office visit to the general practitioner. Patients produced for the nurse all medications that they were taking. Patients reported how often they took each medication, the dosage taken each time, the reason they took it, and whether they were taking it as prescribed by the physician. These data were supplemented with pharmacy records and when necessary by the physician.

Discrepancies in drug-related behavior were classified into four categories: (1) Omission rate. The proportion of drugs that a patient was not taking of those prescribed by the physician. (2) Commission rate. The proportion of drugs that a patient was taking that the physician had not prescribed. (3) Scheduling misconception rate. The proportion of prescribed drugs taken by the patient for which the patient did not know the correct schedule. (Scheduling was defined as the frequency of consumption per 24 hours and the number of units to be taken each time. (4) Scheduling noncompliance. The proportion of prescribed drugs taken by the patient for which the patient knew the correct schedule but did not take as prescribed.

Patients were omitting an average of 18–19 percent of the drugs prescribed, taking 19–20 percent more drugs than their physicians realized, and making scheduling errors on about 17 percent of the drugs. The average total error rate for all physician-patient pairs was 58 percent. Scheduling noncompliance was only 3 percent.

The results from both studies illustrate that much of what we label as unco-operative patient behavior is involuntary and may be attributed to incongruity between what the patient thinks she or he is supposed to do and what the provider thinks the patient is doing. Findings such as these suggest that exclusively focusing on volitional patient uncooperativeness as the target for improving medication-taking behavior may have less potential than reviewing the aspects of the patient-provider encounter that may contribute to involuntary noncooperation. The generalizability of these results has not yet been studied in a rheumatologic population.

A number of implications for practice can be extrapolated from existing research on involuntary noncooperation. A carefully thought-out approach to educating patients, for example, may substantially reduce the levels of involuntary patient noncooperation.[22] Patient education will be more effective if it follows the following principles: Education should be *individualized*. Learning is a process accomplished by individuals at different rates by individual means; thus patient education should be tailored to each patient. Learning is facilitated by rapid and complete *feedback* on the extent to which what is required is being learned. Learning occurs more rapidly and effectively if patients *understand* clearly what they are expected to learn. Learning is enhanced when the learner is *motivated*. Learning is more efficient and effective when patients perceive that what they are expected to learn is *relevant* to them.

Health professionals need to develop communication skills to be able to follow these principles effectively. At the least we must try to ensure that patients hear and understand what is being recommended. Specifically:

1. Instructions to the patient should be written, legibly.
2. Jargon should be avoided in written and verbal instruction. Many patients simply do not understand medical or technical terms but will frequently not admit it.

3. Carefully instruct the patient in the regimens being recommended and provide opportunities for feedback from the patients.
4. Coordinate your efforts with other professionals; seek their help to ensure that regimens are understood and that patients have the necessary skills to complete the recommendation.
5. The family and other members of a patient's informal support network should be tapped as potential resources to assist the patient.

Voluntary Noncooperation

Patient perceptions of relevance of the information or task and patient motivation both influence voluntary cooperation with health recommendations. Can the patient-provider interaction be structured to motivate the patient to undertake the recommendations and to change patient attitudes that may influence whether or not they follow therapeutic recommendations? One approach that has had some success is an attitudinal examination.[23]

Attitudinal Examination

In an experiment with physicians who were treating patients with essential hypertension at a general medicine clinic, a tutorial program involving the physician was used to try to increase patient cooperation.[24] Participating physicians met with the researcher and discussed how to identify the uncooperative patient. Physicians were instructed in strategies of patient education. The relationship of patients' attitudes regarding the seriousness of the disorder, their perceptions of personal susceptibility to complications, perception of the efficacy of their therapy, and potential barriers to carrying out the recommendations were stressed. Physicians were trained to examine such perceptions and attitudes of patients along these four areas and to gear their educational intervention to what they found in this attitudinal examination. For example, if a patient did not believe a treatment would be effective, the physician would emphasize this aspect in the therapeutic encounter. After exposure to a 1-hour teaching session, tutored physicians allocated an increased percentage of clinic visit time to patient education than did control physicians. This led to an increase in patient knowledge, more appropriate patient beliefs regarding hypertension and its therapy, and increased the cooperation with the regimen leading to subsequent decreases in blood pressure.

Attitudinal examinations deserve further study and if found to be effective in reducing voluntary noncooperation, could be incorporated into the standard history-taking process of patient visits.

Characteristics of the Recommendations

Chronic illness regimens, especially those of long duration, elicit the lowest levels of cooperation. One study, for instance, found a 30 percent incidence rate of dosage errors in diabetic patients with an illness of 1–5 years duration but an 80 percent dosage error rate in patients who had had the disease for over 20 years.[16] While health professionals cannot do much about the chronicity of arthritis, degree of cooperation is also affected by the complexity of the treatment regimen.

Cooperation rates drop off sharply as the complexity of the treatment regimen increases. Hulka found that for patients with diabetes or congestive heart failure, errors were less than 15 percent when only one drug was prescribed, increased to 25 percent when two or three drugs were to be taken, and exceeded 35 percent when five or more drugs were involved.[21] In other words the more drugs a physician prescribes, the more the patient omits; the more drugs the patient takes, the greater the number about which the physician is uninformed. In general the more the patient is told to do, the greater the likelihood of failure.[25]

This is obviously a problem for the arthritic patient who is frequently on multiple regimens: medications, exercises, use of assistive devices, splints, and more. Whenever possible complex treatment regimens must be simplified. This requires that the health expert know exactly what the patient is doing and tailor the regimen to be as simple as possible. The physician can do the following:

Reduce the number of medications whenever possible.

Simplify the dosage and frequency schedules.

Have patients take all of their drugs at the same time when possible.

Provide drugs that can be taken less frequently, such as a nonsteroidal drug with once daily dosing rather than four times per day if available.

Provide patients with drug calendar schedules to help them remember to take their drugs.

Have instructions clearly written out in advance.

These changes may all assist the patient to implement therapeutic recommendations.

Socioemotional Aspects

Patient satisfaction with the quality of specific visits to health providers affects cooperation. In two studies involving mothers of children with acute illness, when patient expectations were met, they were much more likely to follow the recommendations and return for follow-up visits.[26,27]

Patients want to feel accepted, appreciated, and respected. Indications of respect for patients do not arise solely in the actual interaction between provider and patient. Excessive waiting time, for example, which is probably interpreted by patients as disrespectful, has also been associated in a study of rheumatoid arthritis patients with poor patient cooperation and high treatment-dropout rates.[15]

However, it is by no means clear exactly what behaviors on the part of providers lead to good rapport. In the study by Geersten et al. involving arthritis patients, those who described the physician as personable cooperated better than those who described him or her as businesslike.[15] In contrast, a study with diabetic patients found that patients cooperated better when they described their preferred physician as authoritarian.[28] Davis found that interaction described as friendly and relaxed was not related to cooperation, but the presence of antagonism, tension, and confrontation did predict noncooperation.[29] For his sample of adult patients, deviations from expected patterns of relationships were associated with noncooperation regardless of the specific pattern. These findings suggest that compliance is a function of a delicate balance of direction and evaluation presented in a manner that is acceptable to the patient. The diversity of these findings, however, highlights the need for much more empirical study of the socioemotional aspects of health care.

Situational Factors

Health professionals are urged to explore systematically the unique circumstances of each patient, not only with regard to the presenting problem for which consultation is being sought, but also to identify situational factors that may affect the patient's ability and inclination to receive and carry out the recommendations. Therapeutic recommendations are not made in a social vacuum, but are filtered through the social roles people play. Davis, for example, in his study of farmers with heart disease, found that those whose work orientation was high were more likely not to cooperate with the physician's advice to curtail work activity.[30] Others have found that patients are less likely to stay in treatment when following therapeutic recommendations which would involve a high degree of interference with their daily activities—a common element of recommendations for treating arthritis.[31]

SUMMARY

This review of the literature on patient cooperation with arthritis treatment recommendations is categorized into two sections: involuntary and voluntary noncooperation. Extrapolating primarily from investigations of patients with other chronic diseases, five strategies for reducing involuntary patient noncooperation and four recommendations for improving voluntary patient cooperation are discussed. These are illustrated in table 26.1. Although much remains to be learned about factors that influence patient cooperation with arthritis treatment recommendations, the application of existing knowledge can improve current levels. Determined efforts by health professionals are necessary if the excessive waste resulting from patient noncooperation is to be reduced.

Table 26.1 Strategies for Increasing Patient Cooperation

Involuntary Noncooperation	*Voluntary Noncooperation*
Individualize and write out instructions	Perform an attitudinal assessment
Avoid jargon	Reduce treatment complexity
Elicit feedback	Reduce waiting time and be sensitive to the
Use other professionals	patient's psychological needs
Involve the patient's family	Explore each patient's situational
	constraints

REFERENCES

1. Sackett DL, Haynes RB, eds. Compliance with therapeutic regimens. Baltimore: Johns Hopkins University Press, 1976.
2. Koos, E. "Metropolis"—what city people think of their medical services. Am Public Health 1955;45:1551-1557.
3. Doyle BJ, Ware JE. Physician conduct and other factors that affect consumer satisfaction with medical care. J M Ed 1977;52:793-801.
4. Haynes RB. A critical review of the "determinants" of patient compliance with therapeutic regimens. In: Sackett DL, Haynes RB, eds., Compliance with therapeutic regimens. Baltimore: Johns Hopkins University Press, 1976, pp. 26-39.
5. Friedman HS, DiMatteo MR. Health care as an interpersonal process. J Social Issues 1979;35:1-11.
6. Sackett DL. The magnitude of compliance and non-compliance. In: Sackett DL, Haynes RB, eds., Compliance with therapeutic regimens. Baltimore: Johns Hopkins University Press, 1976, pp. 9-25.
7. Soutter BR, Kennedy MC. Patient compliance assessment in drug trials: usage and methods. Australia, New Zealand Med J 1974;4:360-364.
8. Marston M. Compliance with medical regimens. Nursing Res 1970;19:312-323.
9. Stone, GC. Patient compliance and the role of the expert. J Social Issues 1979;35(1): 34-59.
10. Moon MH, Moon BAH, Black WAM. Compliancy in splint-wearing behavior of patients with rheumatoid arthritis. New Zealand Med J 1976;6:360-365.
11. Oakes TW, Ward JR, Gray RM, Klauber MR, Moody PM. Family expectations and arthritis patient compliance to a hand resting splint regimen. J Chron Dis 1970;23: 757-764.
12. Ferguson K, Bole GG. Family support, health beliefs, and therapeutic compliance in patients with rheumatoid arthritis. Patient Counseling Health Ed 1979;1:101-105.
13. Mason RM, Barnardo DE, Fox WR, Weatherall M. Assessment of drugs in outpatients with rheumatoid arthritis. Ann Rheum Dis 1967;26:373-388.
14. Carpenter JO, Davis LJ. Medical recommendations—followed or ignored? Factors influencing compliance in arthritis. Arch Phys Med Rehab 1976;57:241-246.
15. Geersten HR, Gray RM, Ward JR. Patient non-compliance within the context of seeking medical care for arthritis. J Chron Dis 1973;26:689-698.
16. Charney E. Patient-doctor communication. Ped Clin N Am 1972;19:263-279.

17. Pratt L, Seligman A, Reader G. Physicians' views on the level of medical information among patients. Am J Public Health 1957;47:1277–1283.
18. Kirscht JP, Rosenstock IM. Patients' problems in following recommendations of health experts. In: Stone GC, Cohen F, Adler NE, eds., Health Psychology. San Francisco: Jossey-Bass P, 1979, pp. 189–216.
19. Mazzullo J. Methods of improving patient compliance. In: Lasagne L, ed., Patient compliance, New York: Futura, 1976.
20. Svarstad BL. Physician-patient communication and patient conformity with medical advice. In: Mechanic D, ed., The growth of bureaucratic medicine. New York: Wiley, 1976, pp. 220–238.
21. Hulka BS, Kupper LL, Cassel JC, Efrid RL, Burdette JA. Medication use and misuse: physician-patient discrepancies. J Chron Dis 1975;28:7–21.
22. Newfeld VR. Patient education: a critique. In: Sackett DL, Haynes RB, eds., Compliance with Therapeutic Regimens. Baltimore: Johns Hopkins University Press, 1976, pp. 83–92.
23. Haefner D, Kirscht JP. Motivational and behavioral effects of modifying health beliefs. Public Health Rep 1970;85:478–484.
24. Inui TS, Williamson JW. Improved outcomes in hypertension after patient tutorials. Ann Int Med 1976;84:646–651.
25. Blackwell B. Drug therapy, patient compliance. New Eng J Med 1973;289:249–252.
26. Becker MH, Drachman RH, Kirscht JP. Motivations as predictors of health behavior. Health Services Rep 1972;87:852–862.
27. Francis V, Korsch BM, Morris MJ. Gaps in doctor-patient communication. New Eng J Med 1969;280:535–540.
28. Williams TF, Martin D, Hogan M, Watkins J, Ellis E. The clinical picture of diabetic control, studied in four settings. Am J Public Health 1967;57:441–451.
29. Davis MS. Variations in patients' compliance with doctors' orders: practice and doctor-patient interaction. Psychiatry Med 1971;2:31–53.
30. Davis MS. Variations in patients' compliance with doctors' advice: an empirical analysis of patterns of communication. Am J Public Health 1968;58:274–288.
31. Tagliacozzo D, Ima K, Lashof JC. Influencing the chronically ill: the role of prescriptions in premature separations of outpatient care. Med Care 1973;11:21–29.

27

Psychosocial Aspects of Rheumatic Disease

Marilyn Gross Potts, M.S.W.

A patient with a chronic rheumatic disease typically faces numerous psychosocial stresses in addition to the normal everyday stresses. Some, obviously, are imposed by the major changes in life-style that result from the disease and its effects, particularly on the musculoskeletal system. Others arise from the reaction of the patient to a wide variety of losses, the most important being functional ability, independence, and self-esteem. The ability of patients to deal with these psychosocial factors greatly affects their ability to benefit from medical care.[1] In addition, in the view of some researchers, psychological factors may play a role in the etiology of rheumatoid arthritis.

THE MYTH OF THE "RHEUMATOID PERSONALITY"

Several reports written during the 1950s and 1960s suggest that patients with rheumatoid arthritis share a specific premorbid personality characterized by rigidity, self-punitive behavior, passivity, and difficulty dealing with hostility and aggression. In the aggregate these reports present conflicting data. Some findings suggest that suppressed hostility and heightened aggressive tendencies are characteristic of the rheumatoid personality; others indicate that passivity is typical.[2] In addition the methodology employed in these studies has been questioned.[3] Data in support of the rheumatoid personality are based primarily on studies that are retrospective rather than prospective and that do not include adequate comparison groups.

Furthermore, studies utilizing standardized tests may fail to control for items that relate to physical symptoms, resulting in spuriously elevated scores for patients with rheumatoid arthritis.[4] For example, Nalven and O'Brien found that high scores of patients with rheumatoid arthritis on the hypochondriasis, depression, and hysteria scales of the Minnesota Multiphasic Personality Inventory were due largely to their responses to items that encompassed somatic symptoms;

for example, "I wake up fresh and rested most mornings; I hardly ever feel pain in the back of my neck; I am about as able to work as I ever was; I am in just as good physical health as most of my friends."[5] Thus research has failed to prove that psychological factors can cause rheumatoid arthritis. Rather, the patient's personality traits may represent responses to the disease. Evidence in support of this view has been provided by Spergel, Ehrlich, and Glass, who found that psychological test scores of a group of patients with rheumatoid arthritis did not differ from those of patients with other chronic illnesses.[3] As Spergel et al. have suggested, the rheumatoid personality is probably a "psychodiagnostic myth."

STRESS AND THE ONSET OF RHEUMATIC DISEASE

Some evidence supports the view that genetic and psychological factors (life stresses such as death of a spouse, conflict at work, family disruption) may interact to lead to the development of rheumatoid arthritis in some individuals.[6] Baker and Brewerton found that, in comparison with healthy matched controls, significantly more women with rheumatoid arthritis experienced an emotionally threatening event in the year prior to disease onset.[7] Rimon has suggested that patients with rheumatoid arthritis who manifest an acute onset of the disease with rapid progression of symptoms are more likely to have experienced a conflict situation and to lack an hereditary predisposition than patients whose disease is marked by a nonacute onset and slower progression.

PSYCHOLOGICAL ISSUES AND THE MANAGEMENT
OF RHEUMATIC DISEASE

Regardless of the role of personality factors in the etiology of rheumatoid arthritis, psychological issues should be taken into account in the management of patients with chronic rheumatic disease.[9] Kübler-Ross has described five sequential stages of emotional response to terminal illness: denial, anger, bargaining, depression, and acceptance.[10] Arthritis patients also exhibit these five stages, although there is an important difference between their emotional response and that of the dying patient. Because arthritis is commonly marked by flares and remissions, the fluidity between the stages of emotional response is more marked in individuals with arthritis than in most terminally ill people.[11] Thus the arthritis patient may partially or totally recapitulate indefinitely the series of emotional reactions.

Denial

Denial is a defense mechanism that serves as a buffer against threatening information. As such, denial is a healthy defense against a reality that could overwhelm the patient. However, denial may be detrimental if the patient cannot accept psychologically the need for treatment. While some patients may deny that they have arthritis, others can accept the diagnosis on an intellectual basis, but deny its potential seriousness or its chronicity.

How should one deal with the denying patient with arthritis? Confrontation—forcing the patient to "face reality"—may lead to resistance. Rather, these patients should be approached in a calm, supportive manner. Any questions they may have about their treatment or prognosis should be answered truthfully, but with optimism whenever possible. Since denial blocks satisfactory understanding of information, the health care professional must be willing to clarify treatment instructions more than once and to introduce a minimum of new ideas rather than extensive patient education.

Anger

Patients may become angry at the health care provider for not being able to alleviate their symptoms. They may be angry at the world in general and at the unjustice of their situation, saying, "Why me? I have done nothing to deserve this."

Anger is a normal part of coping with a chronic illness. When facing an angry patient, health care providers should not take the anger personally or believe that they are necessarily incompetent if the patient criticizes their behavior. Rather, creation of an atmosphere that implies that the professional understands and will not reject the patient is desirable; one might say to the patient, "You seem very frustrated today. Is that because you are discouraged about the results of your treatment?"

If anger is not expressed openly, it may be manifest by passive-aggressive, manipulative behavior. Manipulative patients express anger in socially acceptable ways. They may be always on the phone, watching television, or otherwise engaged when treatment sessions are scheduled. They may "forget" to do their exercises or to take their medication. It may be helpful to confront manipulative patients with their behavior and to encourage them to express anger in a more direct manner, saying for example: "You have missed several of your appointments with me. Are you trying to express your frustration with your disease in this way?"

Bargaining

In the bargaining stage, denial has lessened and the patient can accept part, if not, all of the situation. For example, the patient may state, "I believe I can cope with my arthritis if only I am able to work until I am 65 years old."

If the patient's bargain is realistic, the health care professional can use it as a goal. If the bargain is unrealistic, or, as is usually the case for arthritis, the outcome of treatment is difficult to predict, it may be helpful to encourage the patient to think through the bargain by asking a number of leading questions. For example, "You say you want to return to work in a few weeks? What can you do now? What activities does your job entail? How long can you stand or sit without tiring? The answers to these questions, along with a realistic opinion from the health care professional regarding the prognosis, may enable the patient to realize that renegotiation of an unrealistic bargain is necessary.

Depression

Evidence suggests that 30–60 percent of patients with rheumatoid arthritis are depressed.[8,12,13] Depression has been found to be associated with decreased independence in performance of activities of daily living and with the magnitude of joint involvement.[12] In patients with arthritis, depression may be considered a normal reaction to loss (loss of function, self-esteem, employment, mobility) or anticipated loss (loss of social contacts, marital dissolution).

When feelings of depression are held strongly by patients, it is difficult for them to see an opposite viewpoint. Thus cheerful clichés are apt to frustrate depressed patients further and cause them to feel that the health care professional views their feelings as unique or deviant. A more appropriate response is to allow such patients to express openly their feelings of grief.

Clarification of the basis for the patient's grief is often helpful. For example, the patient who says, "I am a burden," may be thinking, "I cannot cook for my family anymore." Such issues may then be dealt with directly by referral to an occupational therapist for discussion of ways to prepare meals with less expenditure of energy.

It is important for the health care professional to understand that, because of their attitude of hopelessness, depressed patients may be unable to respond to long-term gratification. They may not see the relevance of such statements as, "If you follow your exercise plan faithfully, you will probably notice strengthened muscles in several months." Immediate positive feedback may be more relevant: "Your sedimentation rate has gone down this month."

Acceptance

Patients who have accepted arthritis have come to terms with the situation, feel emotionally stable, and believe that they can manage the physical and emotional aspects of the illness. Patients who accept their illness may state, "I am not pleased that I have this disease, but I feel that I can live with it and make the best of things." At this point the patient can relate fully to care planning.

DEALING WITH UNCERTAINTY AND UNPREDICTABILITY

Patients with arthritis are frequently unable to predict how the disease will progress, how soon a response to treatment will be noted, which joints will be painful, and so on. The issue of not knowing what one will be asked to cope with complicates the process of emotional adjustment. In contrast, the person with a static disability, such as blindness or an amputated limb, knows what to expect in terms of future limitations and strengths.

Many patients with chronic rheumatic disease develop techniques to "normalize" their lives and keep their behaviors and interactions with others constant. Wiener has described two of these techniques as "covering up" and "keeping up."[14]

"Covering up" involves efforts to mask disability and pain. Patients often state, "I am fine," when anyone asks how they are, or they may attempt to walk as normally as possible in spite of discomfort. They may be unwilling to reveal symbols of their disability, such as canes or walkers, to the public. "Keeping up" involves maintaining whatever is perceived as a normal activity level despite the likelihood that increased joint pain may result. Some patients engage in frenzied activity on days of lessened pain, resulting in increased pain on the following day.

Patients who carefully hide their discomfort or disability may wonder why their families and friends are not more helpful or sympathetic. They may be "proud because no one knows, yet distressed because no one cares."[14] Because arthritis is not always a visible disease and because some people consider it trivial, lack of understanding from others can be a problem. Thus it may be useful to suggest to patients that by successfully concealing their disease they may be sacrificing potential support, help, and understanding from others.

THE FAMILY

Most patients live with families and patient-family interactions are obviously affected by arthritis. Patients commonly verbalize guilt because they are unable to fulfill their customary roles as family members. Mothers often feel that they are depriving their children of "a happy childhood" if they must rely on their family to perform a greater share of the household duties. Wives or husbands may state, "I think my spouse would be better off without me." The health care professional might encourage such patients to air their concerns openly with their family. In many instances the family does not perceive the patient a burden and can provide reassurance.

Family members may experience emotional reactions similar to those of the patient. Family members may deny the illness because it seems too threatening. They may react with anger toward the patient. Guilt may arise because of the anger, and family members may then deprive themselves of social and recreational activities because they feel obligated to remain at home with the patient. Their guilt may lead them to become overly solicitous, and this may lead to increased dependency by the patient. Family members too may experience depression. Ultimately, it is to be hoped, they too accept the reality of the situation.

To enhance family well-being and prevent family discord, intervening with family members regarding their own emotional reactions may be as important as intervention with the patient. In addition family members may require education regarding the common emotional reactions of patients. If they are aware that anger can be a normal reaction to arthritis, they may not feel as hurt as they would otherwise if the patient directs anger at them. Similarly, if family members recognize depression as a normal aspect of coping with chronic illness, they may be more willing to provide emotional support to the patient who expresses such feelings.

GROUP COUNSELING OF ARTHRITIS PATIENTS

Education or support groups for patients with arthritis may offer several benefits. Groups for patients with rheumatoid arthritis are reported to result in increased knowledge about the disease,[15,16] increased compliance, and improved communication with physicians and family members.[17] Participation in a group appeared to improve the self-image of people with systemic lupus erythematosus[18] and to increase knowledge about ankylosing spondylitis among patients with this disease.[19]

Education-support groups are provided by some local chapters of the Arthritis Foundation, or groups may be organized by physicians, psychologists, social workers, nurses, other health care professionals, or by patients themselves. Most mental health clinics and family service associations provide group counseling regarding interpersonal relationships and psychologic problems.

Forming a Group

Several issues should be considered in forming a group, including the purpose of the group, and its leadership, size, composition, and duration.[20] In addition group organizers should determine whether the group will be open (accept new members after its inception) or closed (have a fixed membership).

The purpose of the group should be determined at the outset. A group designed primarily to provide information about the illness should be led by an individual who is proficient in rheumatology. Although any group leader should be sensitive to emotional concerns and interpersonal dynamics, a group designed primarily to provide counseling regarding psychosocial issues should be led by an individual experienced in group work techniques.

The size of the group may depend on its purpose. Education groups often have as many as twenty participants. Groups designed primarily for emotional support typically consist of only five to ten members since larger numbers would reduce the opportunity for individuals to interact with one another and to discuss emotional concerns in depth. Also, cliques and subgroups are more likely to form in larger groups than in smaller ones.

As a rule support groups should be composed of patients who are homogenous enough to establish cohesiveness, but heterogeneous enough to allow for diversity of views and active exchange of ideas. This principle is difficult to translate into practical terms. However, most group therapists agree that groups should not include an "isolate"—one man among several women, one teenager among several adults. Evidence suggests that some group participants with rheumatoid arthritis may be fearful or depressed by the thought of meeting another patient with their disease who is more severely ill than they.[15] This indicates that leaders should facilitate open discussion of such feelings if groups are constituted of individuals who are highly heterogeneous with respect to disease severity.

The length of each group session should depend on the physical tolerance of participants. Breaks for standing and stretching are especially important in groups for patients with chronic rheumatic disease. Psychotherapy group sessions have been found to induce fatigue and to reach a point of diminishing efficiency if they last longer than 2 hours.[20]

Groups may be open or closed to new members after their inception. Most closed groups meet for a predetermined number of sessions and have the advantage of allowing members to deal intensively with individual concerns. The number of sessions typically varies from four to twelve. Participants may be unable to commit themselves to continued attendance at a group consisting of more than twelve meetings, and groups that meet for fewer than four sessions may fail to develop cohesiveness or resolve complicated psychosocial problems. Groups that are open usually continue to meet indefinitely. Open groups have the advantage of allowing a greater number of individuals to participate than is usually the case for closed groups. However, participants in open groups must acquaint themselves repeatedly with new members, so that cohesiveness may be reduced. In addition, educational content may need to be repeated. Open groups are often formed in in-patient settings, in which all patients with arthritis on the ward at a particular time are invited to participate.

The Role of the Leader

The group leader typically performs several functions. He organizes the group by enlisting participants and attending to logistic details such as time and place. During the initial meeting the leader should introduce group members to one another or ask them to introduce themselves. The leader should state the purpose of the group and discuss any ground rules such as confidentiality. It is desirable to ask group participants to express their expectations for the group and their views regarding what should be accomplished. The leader may arrange structured activities such as provision of educational content, demonstration of joint exercises, and role-playing.

During group discussions the group leader should attempt to maintain harmony and keep the group moving toward its goals. This may include clarification of points. For example, "When you say your doctor dropped your steroid dose, I do not believe you mean that you were taken off steroids abruptly." In addition, the leader may need to remind group participants that arthritis varies greatly from individual to individual and that the presence of a symptom in one participant does not necessarily mean that all participants will experience that symptom. Redirection of group discussion is often required. For example, "Everyone has mentioned that they have difficulty dealing with depression. What helps some of you to alleviate such feelings?" Group leaders may need to encourage reticent participants by asking them a direct question, or they may need to silence monopolizers in a tactful way. It is often helpful to summarize the content of the group discussion at the end of the meeting, and the group leader may wish to provide for continuity from session to session. The leader might conclude the session by saying, "We have discussed several methods of explaining arthritis to others who do not understand the disease. Before the next meeting, would everyone try to put one of these ideas into practice so that we can discuss the results next week?"

VOCATIONAL REHABILITATION COUNSELING

The self-concept of many people is related intimately to their employment, and the loss of employment can cause reduced self-esteem in addition to financial concerns. One goal of the health care professional should be to help patients maximize their potential for employment. This requires as an initial step the assessment of the functional capacity of the patient. In addition to the physician, occupational and physical therapists provide valuable input in determining whether the patient can work, and what kind of employment is feasible. The solution to employment problems may include self-modification of the patient's work style to allow the patient to take frequent rest breaks or utilize joint-protection principles. It may be helpful for the health care professional to contact the patient's employer to discuss the medical situation and the type of job modifications necessary. Patients may be referred to their state's department of vocational rehabilitation for job counseling, retraining, location of employment, aid in establishing an independent business, or assistance in seeking further formal education. (The role of the vocational counselor is discussed in chapter 6).

SUMMARY

Rheumatic diseases have various psychologic aspects. Whereas early findings suggested that patients with rheumatoid arthritis share a specific premorbid personality, later research indicates that the rheumatoid personality is a psychodiagnostic myth. Some evidence supports the view that genetic and psychological factors (stress or a conflict situation) may interact to lead to the development of rheumatoid arthritis. Finally, psychologic issues are involved in the management of patients with rheumatic disease. Patients and family members may exhibit emotional reactions (denial, anger, bargaining, depression, acceptance) that have implications for care planning and implementation. In addition patients may develop techniques (covering up and keeping up) to aid in dealing with the unpredictability of arthritis. Vocational counseling may be important for rheumatic disease patients in terms of both finances and self-esteem.

Education or support groups may help patients and family members learn about arthritis and deal more effectively with its psychosocial aspects. Factors that should be considered in forming and conducting a group include its purpose, leadership, size, composition, and duration; whether the group will be open or closed; and the functions of the group leader.

REFERENCES

1. Lowman EW, Lee PR, Miller S, King R, Stein H. The chronic rheumatoid arthritic: psychosocial factors in rehabilitation. Arch Phys Med Rehab 1954;15:643–647.

2. Ehrlich GE. Psychosomatic aspects of musculoskeletal disorders. Postgrad Med 1965; 38:614–619.

3. Spergel P, Ehrlich GE, Glass D. The rheumatoid arthritic personality: a psychodiagnostic myth. Psychosomatics 1978;19:79–86.

4. Polley HF, Swenson WM, Steinhilber RM. Personality characteristics of patients with rheumatoid arthritis. Psychosomatics 1970;11:45–49.

5. Nalven FB, O'Brien JF. Personality patterns of rheumatoid arthritic patients. Arth Rheum 1964;7:18–28.

6. Shochet BR, Lisansky ET, Schubart AF, Fiocco V, Kurland S, Pope M. A medical-psychiatric study of patients with rheumatoid arthritis. Psychosomatics 1969;10: 271–279.

7. Baker GHB, Brewerton DA. Rheumatoid arthritis: a psychiatric assessment. Brit Med J 1981;282:2014.

8. Rimon R. A psychosomatic approach to rheumatoid arthritis: a clinical study of 100 female patients. Acta Rheum Scand 1969;3(Suppl):1–154.

9. Zeitlin DJ. Psychological issues in the management of rheumatoid arthritis. Psychosomatics 1977;18:7–14.

10. Kübler-Ross E. On death and dying. New York: Macmillan, 1969.

11. Gross M. Psychosocial aspects of osteoarthritis: helping patients cope. Health Soc Work 1981;65:40–46.

12. Robinson, ET, Hernandez LA, Dick WC, Buchanan WW. Depression in rheumatoid arthritis. J R Coll Gen Pract 1977;27:423–427.

13. Zaphiropoulos G, Burry HC. Depression in rheumatoid disease. Ann Rheum Dis 1974;33:132–135.

14. Wiener CL. The burden of rheumatoid arthritis: tolerating the uncertainty. Soc Sci Med 1975;9:97–104.

15. Potts M, Brandt KD. An analysis of education-support groups for patients with rheumatoid arthritis. In press. Patient Couns Health Educ, 1983.

16. Udelman HD, Udelman DL. Group therapy with rheumatoid arthritis patients. Am J Psychotherapy 1978;32:288–299.

17. Schwartz LH, Marcus R, Condon R. Multidisciplinary group therapy for rheumatoid arthritis. Psychosomatics 1978;19:289–293.

18. Triche K. Group therapy with SLE patients. Fifth Interim Session, Allied Health Professions Section of the Arthritis Foundation, 1972.
19. Gross M, Brandt KD. Eductional support groups for patients with ankylosing spondylitis: a preliminary report. Patient Counseling Health Ed 1981;3:6–12.
20. Yalom ID. The theory and practice of group psychotherapy. New York: Basic Books, 1969.

28

Communications in Chronic Care

Gail Riggs, M.A.

The greatest problem in communication is the illusion that it has been accomplished.

George Bernard Shaw

Communication is a process by which senders and receivers of messages interact in given social contexts.[1] This process is polished, refined, and handled with delicacy in diplomacy, politics, and business. It has been elevated almost to a science in advertising and public relations.[2] Hospitals finding themselves in a competitive era are developing extensive internal and external communications with their many publics.[3] Communication is the basis and foundation for all psychosocial interaction, and it is written about almost as frequently as recipes for Swedish meatballs are published in the Sunday newspaper supplement. Yet nowhere is communication less perfected or abused more than in our health care system between provider and patient. It has been observed that "Much of what is currently labeled as noncooperative behavior may be involuntary, a result of incongruity between what the patient thinks he or she is supposed to do and what the provider thinks the patient is doing. To reduce errors attributable to involuntary noncooperation, health professionals need to better understand the process of communication."[4]

UNDERSTANDING THE BARRIERS TO COMMUNICATION

Many factors complicating the communications process are found to exist in the most extreme form in medical settings. "Every medical problem is in part a symbolic one. One cannot damage the physical self without injuring the symbolic self, nor can one inflict insult repeatedly on the same symbolic self without dam-

319

aging the physical self. Diagnosis and treatment are in large part symbolic problems, and to ignore this fact may distort or defeat their aims."*[5] These symbolic problems are the perceived malfunctions that bring patients to seek care and the persistence of such perceptions that keep them in treatment. "No illness lacks its semantic dimensions. The professional who feels involved exclusively in the maintenance of a physical mechanism and who dismisses the communicative aspect of this work operates on a simplistic and even dangerous premise."[5]

The study of communication focuses upon factors that hinder or help in the achievement of common meaning through an exchange of messages. (See table 28.1.) Barnlund[5] lists these factors as follows:

Ego involvement. If conversation is highly ego involving, such as when one is fearful of the matter under discussion, understanding is blocked. People rarely comprehend clearly when they are emotionally upset. "In the moments of shock after receiving a diagnosis for example, people frequently tune out what their physician is saying. Instead, their minds race over implications of the diagnosis on their lives, their careers, and their families. Patients may miss some important information, and may be too embarrassed to ask the doctor to repeat it later on."[6]

Differences in knowledge. "Where knowledge is unequal, where some people have access to the facts and others do not, equality of human relationships is impossible."[5] Incomplete and distorted communication results, a condition found often between specialists and lay people, resulting in communicative impotency on the part of the latter and a dependent state not tolerated well.

Social status. "The greater the disparity in education, income, and social standing, the less people are capable of learning, or of hearing what was said as it was intended."[5] When these distinctions are emphasized, people withhold information and distort the meanings intended.

Emotional distance. Communication is difficult unless both parties are totally present as persons. Often the patient is viewed as a problem, a disease, or an interesting curiosity rather than a human being. Martin Buber argues that the "I-it" relation is demeaning and frustrating, for it rests on perceptions of the other as no more than an object. This not only prevents sharing meanings but may arouse animosity.

One-way communication. Once communication was considered a linear process, but we know now that "receivers do not passively absorb the intentions of others (senders), but creatively interpret" what they hear in the light of their own perspectives, needs, their expectations, and beliefs.[5] The likelihood that a patient will understand or comply to an exercise program is based on the *value* that he places on it. Unless feedback is solicited or encouraged, it is unlikely that mutual understanding will result. Hayakawa suggests that communicants restate, clarify, and elaborate the meaning from the viewpoint of the other.[7]

Verbal manipulation. "Many efforts to communicate are prompted not by

---

*DD Barnlund. "The Mystification of Meaning: Doctor-Patient Encounter." J Med Educ 51 (September 1976):716–725. Reprinted with permission.

Table 28.1.   Solving Communication Problems

Communication Barriers	Eliminated by
Ego involvement	Helping the patient reduce anxiety and fear; humor
Differences in knowledge	Educating the patient; referring the patient to allied health personnel if time is a problem
Social status	Relating to the patient as a unique individual, not solely to the "arthritic"; not passing judgment
Emotional distance	Sharing responsibility, "power," or knowledge with patient; reducing the patient's diffidence
One-way communication	Listening actively; providing and asking for feedback
Verbal manipulation	Soliciting feedback; listening; surrendering communicative responsibility
Language ambiguity	Finding out what the *patient* means
Jargon	Not using medical terminology; speaking as if "on camera"
Pressures of time	Goal planning with patient; goal planning for the health professional

the desire to share or create new meanings but to maneuver the other person into a predetermined decision. From verbal seduction to verbal coercion, a moral superiority is assumed by one party."[5] Increasing the communicative responsibility of one person requires some surrender of responsibility by the other—a difficult task especially for the physician who has traditionally been perceived as a person who combines the "highest caring and authoritarian qualities."[8] The "Doctor is God" perception and the dominant-authoritarian role in the doctor/patient relationship results in a dependent patient relinquishing all responsibility for individual health to the physician, which in turn may result in inappropriate care.

Ambiguity of language. Language itself introduces barriers to mutual understanding. People share experiences through symbols with culturally sanctioned definitions. The word "illness" may have a hundred meanings. "Surgery" may have dozens.

Role of jargon. Every subculture, every trade, and every profession has a dialect and vocabulary of its own. "While contributing to communication within a group, the same dialects when turned outward confuse, frighten, and alienate."[5]

Pressures of time. Perhaps the greatest and most insurmountable barrier to communication is the health professional's belief that taking the time to explore the emotional context of the patient's life is an unaffordable luxury.[9] "In some ways our humanity seems threatened more by the pace of our lives than by any other single factor. There is no human relationship, no communicative act, that is enriched or improved by speeding it up. It takes time to explain, time to listen, time to dissipate fears, time to assimilate frightening facts, time to prepare for crisis, time to enter the experiental world of another person. The urge to hurry must be overcome if people are really serious about preserving the human community."[5]

Belsky identifies many of the same factors that block communication and in addition cites two crucial ones: poor listening skills on the part of the therapist or patient or both and failure to work out joint decisions (between provider and patient).[10] Myers and Myers list the worst listening habits:[11]

Calling subject "uninteresting"

Criticizing the speaker's delivery, personal appearance, and so on

Getting overstimulated and preparing rebuttal

Listening only for facts

Faking attention to the speaker

Tolerating distractions

ELIMINATING THE BARRIERS

Goal Planning

In *Working with People Called Patients*, a must for every health professional's library, Berger provides succinct hints for effective communication and how to avoid problems that occur when speaking, listening, understanding, interrupting, and interacting. In another chapter, five steps outline how patient and provider can work out joint decisions through goal planning.[12]

1. Involve the patient. This goes back to the patient's beliefs, needs, and concerns. Goals must be understood and accepted by the patient as being meaningful for him.
2. Set reasonable goals. Do not set goals that are beyond the patient's present level of functioning, life experiences, or resources.
3. Describe and explain the implications of the patient's behavior when the goal is reached.
4. Set a date of completion or deadline. This allows the patient to complete the goal and measure accomplishment.
5. Spell out the method of working procedure in detail. Clarify who does what, in which order, as clearly and specifically as possible so a third person can read and understand the intent and plan.

In this planning process it is necessary to praise patients for their efforts—a simple and effective communicative act. In fact, find something to praise in all or almost all the patients you have contact with and notice the results! If you dispense sincere praise for a week, you may be surprised to see what differences there are in your relationships to your patients, to your fellow employees, and to yourself.

Goal planning and patient education are essential in the care of the person with arthritis who will have it for the rest of his life. Neither is done efficiently or effectively without good communications. According to Bandler and Grinder in *Frogs into Princes*, one needs only three things to be an absolutely exquisite communicator: "to know what outcome you want, to have flexibility in your behavior, and enough sensory experience to notice when you get the responses."[13]

Use of Feedback

Feedback or active listening, a technique developed by Carl Rogers and others for psychologic interviewing, has been neglected in the medical field other than psychiatry.[14] It is especially relevant in the field of rheumatology, where dealing with the psychosocial impact of arthritis is considered by patient educators to be the most important part of patient education.[15] Feedback or active listening is listening to a person without passing judgment on what is being said, and mirroring back what has been said to indicate that you understood what feelings the speaker was putting across. In other words, put yourself in the shoes of the speaker. Feedback has several advantages. It lets patients know one is making an effort to really understand them. It can also clarify material that is not understood and prevent wording that might be interpreted as judgmental. Giving feedback can be hard work for physicians, as it requires that they make every effort to understand what their patients are trying to communicate rather than simply recording answers.

Feedback is most useful with information that is difficult for patients to present either because they do not clearly know what they are trying to express or because the subject is emotionally laden.[16] It can also be used in situations where the patient is resistant or diffident. For example, the health professional might say, "This is a complicated procedure and I'm sure it raises many questions in your mind. Let's see if I can answer all of your questions."

It has been widely found that patients are very diffident about asking for information from doctors.[17-19]

Because patients are diffident the clinician receives no feedback when he produces material which is too difficult, so his performance cannot improve, nor does he have the opportunity to learn the misconceptions his patients have. Indeed, a case could be made for maintaining that the reduction of patients' diffidence would go a long way to solving the communication problem. Reduction of patients' diffidence should produce not only more patient satisfaction, but also, by providing feedback to the clinician, improve his communication skills.[20]

Social Status, Verbal Manipulation, and the Role of Jargon

The following excerpt from *Alice in Wonderland* underscores, for those of us who use jargon, how language can be turned into "jabberwocky" and used to manipulate the other while maintaining a social barrier.

"I don't know what you mean by 'glory,'" Alice said.

Humpty Dumpty smiled contemptuously. "Of course you don't—till I tell you. I mean 'there is a nice knockdown argument for you.'"

"But glory does not mean 'a nice knockdown argument,'" Alice objected.

"When I use a word," Humpty Dumpty said in a rather scornful tone, "it means just what I choose it to mean—neither more nor less."

"The question is," said Alice, "whether you *can* make words mean so many different things."

"The question is," said Humpty Dumpty, "who is to be master, that's all."[21]

Listening

Isabel Hansen talks about her early experiences with rheumatoid arthritis in *Outwitting Arthritis*. Her main interest was the piano. She studied seriously, practiced hours every morning, accompanied singers, was part of a two-piano team, played with many chamber groups. Her arthritic foot trouble was bearable, but she awoke horrified one morning to find a finger on her right hand sharp with pain and within a week, fingers on both hands were stiff. Piano playing became almost impossible.

"So? Some days you won't be able to play the piano," was my doctor's comment. "Might as well get used to it. That's arthritis."

I still seethe at that response. How I wish I'd retorted, "You jerk! Would you get used to it if someone told you that some days you wouldn't be able to examine patients or operate?"[22]

This unempathetic response demonstrates the difference between listening just for the facts and listening for "meaning" or what the patient is really saying—in this case, "My world is being shattered." The meaning of a communication is the response it elicits, independent of the communicator's intention, and resistance is a comment upon the inflexibility of the communicator.

Some professionals really do not want to hear because of economic constraints; to really listen is impossible in a busy schedule, and a less busy schedule is not as profitable. But beyond that, listening to a complaining patient express negative feelings can be threatening and even cause stress to an "authority figure" resulting in silence, nonlistening, and escape from the examining room.

Doctors know arthritis hurts and bewilders, sure; they want resolution as badly as the patient does, not only for the patient's sake, but for their own egos. It's wonderful to be worshipped by eternally grateful patients, but when a sick person sings the blues, it comes too close to their own inner feelings. To acknowledge patients' anxieties might mean they would have to look at their own limits of effectiveness and hence, their own anxieties.[22]

Another form of not listening is when the health professional does all the talking. To communicate or solicit feedback from the patient means that both participants have to be willing to go forward and make verbal commitments. This entails sharing responsibility, sharing "power" or knowledge with the other, goal planning, and following through. The loquacious professional who believes that the patient can be convinced, persuaded, willed, or exhorted to change behavior is operating primarily to serve his own needs, time schedule, and ego. Increasing the time spent with a patient does not necessarily improve the quality of the encounter, nor patient compliance.

COMMUNICATION AND PATIENT INSTRUCTORS (PI)

At the University of Arizona patients with advanced, stable rheumatoid arthritis were taught to train and evaluate health professionals by using themselves as examination subjects. Because the PI functions as patient, teacher, and evaluator, a different communication pattern is established. The physician, who is usually the sender of information, becomes also the receiver. Open and complete communication lines with feedback are essential if the medical student or health professional is to be taught how to do the musculoskeletal examination and be evaluated. Learning this skill or behavior requires the professional to listen carefully, provide and ask for feedback, and share what he understands with the PI so skills can be improved. The patient or PI, because she is also the teacher and evaluator, ceases to be an "it," thereby removing social status differences and emotional distances. The PI, possessing all the jargon and terminology intrinsic to the musculoskeletal examination, ensures that the medical student understands them too so they can share common meanings. Beyond all this, the PI stays with the medical student or meets with him again in order to ensure improvement of the student's performance and competency.[23]

Such a training situation requires an investment of time and money and an understanding of educational principles and how to communicate. No sounder investment could be made than to ensure that beginning, life-long, physician careers are well founded. A similar investment seems appropriate for the many individuals who are to function and cope with the life-long problem of chronic illness.

SUMMARY

It is well documented that deficient physician-patient communication is one of the biggest complaints of patients[1,24,25] and possibly a major factor in patient noncompliance. Although barriers continue to exist in the communication process, they can be eliminated by learning a few simple techniques. The biggest barrier yet to be overcome is learning to appreciate that the patient is a unique human being and not simply a panoply of symptoms. Equally, it is incumbent upon the patient to actively pursue the improvement of communication between himself and the professional in order to ensure his own best health care. Health care, to be effective, must be an equal partnership.

REFERENCES

1. Bennett AE, ed. Communication between doctors and patients. London: Oxford University Press, 1976.
2. Lesly P, ed. Public relations handbook. Englewood Cliffs, N.J.: Prentice-Hall, 1978.
3. Riggs L. The health care facility's public relations handbook. Rockville, Md.: Aspen Systems Corporation, 1982.
4. Jette AM. Improving Patient Cooperation with Arthritis Treatment Regimens. Arth Rheum 1982;25(4):452.
5. Barnlund DD. The mystification of meaning: doctor-patient encounter. J Med Educ 1976;51:716–725.
6. McDuffie FC. Listen and ask questions. National Arth News (The Arthritis Foundation, Atlanta) Winter 1981.
7. Hayakawa SE. Language in thought and action. New York: Harcourt Brace Jovanovich, 1964.
8. DeArmond M. The dark side of medicine. Sombrero (Pima County Medical Society, Tuscon: Ariz.), 1982.
9. Jensen PS. The doctor-patient relationship: headed for impasse or improvement? Ann Intern Med 1981;95:769–771.
10. Belsky MS, Gross L. How to use and choose your doctor. Greenwich Conn.: Fawcett, 1975.
11. Myers GE, Myers MT. Listening—is anyone there? In: The dynamics of human communication. New York: McGraw-Hill 1980, p. 172.
12. Berger M. Working with people called patients. New York: Brunner/Mazel Publishers, 1977, p. 94.
13. Bandler R, Grinder L. Frogs into princes: neurolinguistic programming. Moab, Utah: Real People Press, 1979, p. 47.
14. Rogers C. Client-centered therapy. Boston: Houghton Mifflin, 1951.
15. Wade KJ. Rheumatoid arthritis patient education: a consensus on main topics. University of Alabama Multipurpose Arthritis Center, 1981.
16. Riffenburgh RS. Active listening in the medical interview. Post Grad Med 1974; 55(2):91–93.
17. Cartwright A. Human relations and hospital care. London: Routledge and Kegan Paul, 1964.
18. Ley P, Spelman MS. Communications in the outpatient setting. Brit J Soc Clin Psychol 1965;4:114–116.
19. Fletcher CM. Communication in medicine. London: Rock Carling Monograph, Nuffield Provincial Hospitals Trust, 1973.
20. Ley P. Towards better doctor-patient communications. In: Bennett AE, ed. Between doctors and patients. London: Oxford University Press, 1976.

21. Lewis Carroll. Alice's adventures in wonderland; Through the looking glass; and The hunting of the snark. New York: Modern Library Inc, 1925, pp. 246–247.

22. Hanson I. Outwitting arthritis. Berkeley: Creative Arts Book Company, 1981.

23. Riggs GE, Gall EP, Meredith KE, Boyer JT, Gooden A. Impact of intensive education and interaction with health professionals on patient instructors. J Med Educ 1982;57: 550–556.

24. Bird B. Talking with patients. 2nd ed. Philadelphia: JB Lippincott, 1973.

25. Ley P, Spelman MS. Communicating with the patient. London: Staple Press, 1967.

29

Sexuality

Mary P. Brassell, R.N., B.S.

Sexuality problems are associated with certain rheumatic diseases, including rheumatoid arthritis (RA), osteoarthritis (OA), systemic lupus erythematosus (SLE), ankylosing spondylitis (AS), polymyalgia rheumatica (PR), Behcet's syndrome, Sjogren's syndrome, and Raynaud's phenomenon. Sexual restrictions are associated as well with joint implants of the lower extremity, such as total hip and total knee replacement, in addition to medications such as long-term steroid therapy.

The health professional needs practical information in order to help patients and their sexual partners achieve solutions to some common sexual problems. Many clinical recommendations are made in this chapter. Family planning will be omitted since it is individualized for each patient.

FACTORS THAT INHIBIT SEXUAL ADVICE
BY HEALTH PROFESSIONALS

Sexuality is an area of health care that is often ignored by the medical profession. Studies have shown conclusively that physicians are most uncomfortable in dealing with sexual problems associated with any illness. Reciprocal embarrassment is probably the greatest contributing factor.[1] The physician assumes that to inquire about sexual problems is delving into personal, private sectors of the patient's life, which is tantamount to an invasion of privacy, while the patient fears that introducing the topic of sexuality is comparable to admitting to nymphomania or satyriasis.

Another contributing factor that is detrimental to the person with arthritis is the media. The 6-foot-tall Adonis sells sports cars and his female counterpart, the perfect bikini-clad blond touts cosmetics, whereas middle-aged people sell laxatives, sleep potions, and anal medication, and the elderly are portrayed as difficult and cantankerous. Sexuality is clearly presented as a privilege and pleasure of youth. Yet, over 60 percent of the arthritis population is over 45 years of age. Should health professionals assume that sexual activity is permitted for only those who conform to the media image?

Since the physician and other health professionals each bring to their own profession a personal moral, ethnic, religious, and cultural code, it essentially becomes the code of behavior and basis for value judgments, which is often applied to the patient whether deliberately, unconsciously, or inadvertently. Some physicians admit the need to counsel a married individual about sex but completely ignore the sexually active unmarried client.

APPROACHES TO SEXUAL COUNSELING

When should the health professional introduce the topic of sexuality?[2] The sexual history should be part of the admission work-up of the hospitalized client, or the physician may introduce the topic during an office consultation. Perhaps while performing the Faber maneuver, the physician might state, "I notice you have some restriction of motion and some pain when I bend your hip. Does it affect sexual activity? Intercourse?" Or, while reviewing the genitourinary system, he or she might ask about menses, dyspaurenia, and inquire, "Has arthritis affected your love life? How?" If the patient complains of fatigue, stiffness, restriction of motion, the physician might ask, "Have you noticed a decrease of interest in sex?" These queries are a natural lead into discussion and offering suggestions about sexual activity.

It is best for the health professional to assume the attitude that everyone is sexually active. Patients who are celibate or who do not wish sexual advice for other reasons will inform you. The sexual problems that are nonphysical or relationship-related may also be approached by other members of the team, such as the psychologist or social worker.

In the hospital or clinic setting the nurse is usually the first health professional to assess the patient. At Moss Rehabilitation Hospital, for example, the patient is asked how arthritis affects his job, housework, and sex life. The sequence of these questions leads to a logical inclusion of mentioning sex. When inquiring about pain, if the patient reveals lower extremity pain, the nurse may interpose, "Does it interfere with sexual activity?"

From the age of 16, all patients should be questioned about the sexual aspects related to arthritis, regardless of body build, appearance, age, or presence of deformities. Marital status should not be ascertained prior to asking about sexuality, since it would imply to the unmarried that sexual activity is only permissible for the married and would thereby inhibit unmarried patients from seeking sexual advice.

DO PATIENTS WANT SEXUAL ADVICE?

In a 1972 study thirty-five women, who ranged in age from 29 to 72, were asked if arthritis influenced sexuality.[3] All answered affirmatively. When asked to choose the health professional whom they would prefer to give them sexual advice, the majority chose the physician first, with the nurse as second choice, physical therapist third, and occupational therapist fourth. The women were also asked to state whether they would bring up the topic of sexuality. Thirty-four of thirty-five replied no. All the women who gave the negative reply rationalized that since physicians have had so much scientific exposure to the human body, physicians should be able to handle any and all questions related to sex and therefore introduce the topic. The group also postulated that they (patients) would not introduce the topic, lest the physician view them as "dirty old ladies."

When the health professional introduces the topic of sexuality to the patient, the professional is in essence saying to the patient, "It is normal, part of everyday life to include sexuality concerns into your treatment program." By asking about sexuality, the patient is asking for "permission" and seeking help regarding this aspect of care.

It must be noted that patients who are treated by a team in an arthritis center or rehabilitation center often perceive any member of the team as a potential source of sexual information. The patient will often ask the team member with whom he has good rapport, about sex. (Physical therapists and occupational therapists were also chosen by patients on a rheumatology unit, as sources of sexual information.)[3]

It has been my experience that the elderly are flattered rather than embarrassed when asked about sexual activity. Asking about sexuality reinforces their positive self-image of being a sexual and sexually desirable person. Many of the elderly who have been interviewed are sexually active but with a decrease in frequency of activity. Yet their needs are ignored or overlooked, since the mature population is commonly perceived as nonsexual.[4] With the increasing life span, it is unrealistic to assume or ignore the sexual needs of those over 60.[5] Numerous studies have illustrated that sexual activity continues well into the 80s.[7]

Arthritis clubs formed for clients with arthritis are further proof of the need to address sexuality concerns. Throughout the United States the topic of sexuality appears on their programs.

Another method of giving constructive practical advice is to have patient education handouts, illustrating positions.[8] Another approach for the health professional would be to use artist mannequins to demonstrate positions. The use of asexual mannequins allows both the professional and patient and/or partner to accept sexual advice without embarrassment. However, the lack or presence of discomfort is greatly dependent upon the attitude of the counselor. If the professional assumes a matter-of-fact tone yet displays empathy and understanding about the necessity for arriving at a solution to a sexual problem, the patient may be able to reach a solution to sexual problems without embarrassment.

Rheumatoid Arthritis (RA)

The patient with RA may exhibit significant stiffness, fatigue, joint pain or discomfort, and decreased mobility. All of these factors can adversely affect sexual performance of both patient and partner. It is imperative that the partner of the individual with RA understand the physical problems associated with the disease. For many patients sexual activity must be planned rather than spontaneous.[9] Mornings are often not suitable if significant stiffness is present, but the time of day or evening should coincide with when the person is feeling at his or her best. A warm bath and taking the nonsteroidal anti-inflammatory drug or nonnarcotic analgesic that does not lower libido approximately 45 minutes to an hour before sexual activity, may be of help. Communicating with the partner and asking the partner to ignore or overlook a few groans of discomfort can benefit both partners, since once sexual distraction takes place, painful symptoms may disappear or decrease.[8] Any position of comfort that is suitable for the patient is recommended. Couples should be encouraged to experiment with various positions and discover for themselves which is the most advantageous and comfortable.[10]

Women with Sjogren's syndrome, who have diminished vaginal lubrication, should be instructed to use a water-soluble lubricant, such as K-Y jelly.[11] This lubricant is aqueous and readily absorbed and does not require removal. Vaseline is contraindicated since it can predispose to infection.

If the patient with RA has no flexion contractures of the hip or knee, and experiences pain upon initiation of motion, the use of pillows under the knees is suggested, but with the proviso that the pillows be removed immediately after sexual activity has ceased, so as to prevent contractures.[12] Those who have adduction contractures of the lower extremity may use a side lying approach with either posterior or anterior entry, and the unaffected partner performing the most strenuous maneuvers. This enables the patient to participate more comfortably in the sexual activity. If the adduction contractures are severe enough to prohibit intercourse, however, alternate forms of sexual expression may be employed. Hip surgery may help such patients resume more normal sexual function. References 8, 9, 12, 22, 23, and 25 are publications written explicitly for patients to which health professionals may wish to refer their clients.

Individuals who have significant cervical spine problems, that is, subluxation, should specifically be advised by their physicians regarding contraindications of any activity that may compromise the spinal cord during sexual activity. These patients may have to resort to modes of sexual expression other than intercourse. The client with C-1, C-2 subluxation may have to take a passive role and/or be advised to wear a cervical collar during sexual activity.[13] Neck flexion should be avoided.

Sometimes the man or woman with RA gives body language signals of disinterest if they are experiencing pain. The presence of pain can cause either partner to withdraw from sexual encounters fearing inadequacy and rejection. A partner can become impotent if he fears causing injury to his partner. It is best if the woman with RA buffers her expressions of pain with positive encouragement. If the body language of the client says, "Let's get this over with," both participants may find the episode distressing. A woman with RA can become frigid if she fears pain, being an inadequate partner, or becoming pregnant. Understanding the influence of pain and attempting to work through its problems can lead to a less traumatic and more satisfying sex life. It is important for the health professional who advises about sexual activity to stress the positive effects of sexual activity. In a study conducted with patients who had arthritis it was found that patients who had had orgasms after sexual activity were pain-free for approximately 6 hours.[14] Whether this finding was psychological or physiological in origin, sexual activity seemed to have aided in decreasing painful symptoms of arthritis.

The woman with decreased hand function because of ulnar drift or swan-neck deformities may have difficulty in removing or inserting a diaphragm, or the man with hand problems may have difficulty with condoms. It is wise to suggest that the patient place a foam hair curler or other substitute grip builder on the diaphragm inserter to get a better grip or else to consider alternate forms of contraception.

The problems associated with RA are not insurmountable but require practice and at times a bit of ingenuity. Most of all, patients with RA need to be assured that sexual advice is available.

System Lupus Erythematosus (SLE)

Just as RA is a chronic disease that can lower self-esteem, body image perception, and produce depression, so too can SLE induce the same responses. In a relationship the unaffected partner must be aware of the implications of SLE so as not to interpret a change of sexual attitude as diminished love or affection. The physician or nurse should, if possible, counsel both patient and partner together, so that the healthy partner will understand the need for adjustment of sexual activity.

Since SLE is a rheumatic disease that may be accompanied by joint pain, fatigue, fevers, dermatological problems, or vascular, pulmonary, and renal complications, a variety of sexual problems can occur. But these difficulties are not insurmountable.

Vaginal ulcers may be present and painful, but both patient and partner need to be reassured that they will resolve. Their resolution is aided by prescriptions for topical steroid application.[15] When the ulcers are present, the couple may wish to use other forms of sexual expression.

Mouth ulcers may be present in a small percentage (10–15 percent) of individuals with SLE. If oral expressions of sexuality are used, the ulcers may be painful. Steroid mouthwash, with or without antibiotics, may be prescribed. If Sjogren's syndrome is present, the use of K-Y jelly should be recommended in facilitating intercourse and relieving dryness of the vaginal mucous membranes. If generalized joint pain is present, recommending a warm bath an hour prior to relations can help alleviate discomfort and stiffness, since the modality of wet heat relaxes muscular tension. The effects of pregnancy on SLE are controversial and should be discussed with a knowledgeable physician.

Raynaud's Phenomenon

If the patient with RA or SLE has Raynaud's phenomenon, sexual activity can be severely impaired as well as produce pain. Pain can occur because of decreased blood flow to the extremities, since during sexual activity much of the blood is directed to the genital area.[15] If the patient is experiencing cyanosis of the toes or fingers, during sexual encounters, the pain can increase if the client is in a cool room. Again, a warm bath prior to activity will dilate the blood vessels. As unromantic as it may seem, it may help the client to wear socks. The patient should not bear weight on the hands and feet during sexual activity since blood flow is further compromised, therefore producing pain. Finding a position that will diminish or prevent constriction of blood vessels is most advantageous, for example, lying supine or on the side.

Osteoarthritis (OA)

Since OA is not a systemic disease, the sexuality problems associated with it are primarily mechanical. Lower extremity OA usually involves either the hip or knee, or both.[16] Very often pain is elicited during initiation of movement in the hip joint. The health professional should suggest to the patient that using pillows under the knees during intercourse, while lying supine, may relieve the pressure or pain that is experienced in the hip or knee. Pillows under the knee transfer some of the weight borne by the hip joint to the pillow and minimize pain. If the person has OA in the hips or knees, flexion positions such as kneeling are painful. Side-lying positions, with the partner bearing part of the body weight of the affected partner, can minimize pain or discomfort. Any position is permissible if both partners find it comfortable and painless.

Ankylosing Spondylitis (AS)

Ankylosing spondylitis has a greater predilection for young men. The sexual problems associated with it include fatigue, back pain, stiffness, and decrease in endurance.[17] Back pain and stiffness can be decreased considerably if the patient adheres to his regime of anti-inflammatory drugs. Timing of the sexual activity should revolve around time of day or night that the patient is least fatigued. The use of hot baths or showers prior to sexual activity will also help. Since back pain can be the major focus for pain, it is wise to recommend to the patient that he take the bottom position. The partner with AS may need back support with pillows if side-lying positions are used, to prevent initiating or antagonizing preexisting back pain. Any position that does not aggravate back pain is suitable.

Polymyalgia Rheumatica (PR)

One of the greatest difficulties the patient with PR may have at the height of disease activity is the inability to initiate position change because of pain and stiffness, even prior to sexual activity. The detriment to sexual expression may be that the partner of the patient misconstrues the lack of mobility as sexual disinterest. The physician or health professional who counsels the patient with PR should make certain to inform the patient and partner that, during severe phases of PR, mobility will be decreased and impaired, and therefore the patient will need help in assuming the desired position. Once again, during the acute phase of PR, other forms of sexual expression may be necessary, until the pain is under control and the patient more comfortable.

Behcet's Syndrome

There are varying descriptions and definitions of Behcet's syndrome. However, most authorities agree that a triad of oral and genital ulcerations, and iritis (or other eye lesions) is requisite for diagnosis. It is the sexual implications of two members of the triad that concern the physician or nurse who will be involved in offering sexual advice.

The recurrent ulcers of the mouth and pharynx resemble an aphthous stomatitis and are quite painful. However, the vaginal and labial ulcers may be asymptomatic. Therefore, while oral-genital sex is often difficult, sexual intercourse may be painless. If the male has penile ulcerations, the lesions can be quite painful, and wearing a condom may help decrease pain during intercourse. The lesions can also occur on the scrotum. If the lesions are severe, intercourse is contraindicated. Usually the ulcerations are reversible and episodic.

TOTAL HIP REPLACEMENT, TOTAL HIP RESURFACING

The patient who undergoes total hip replacement (THR) or resurfacing is particularly jeopardized by a lack of information concerning sexual positioning. There have been documented cases of patients who dislocated or fractured either hip or prosthesis during intercourse, during the first 3 months postoperatively. Since the patient is given abduction precautions related to activities of daily living, certainly abduction precautions related to sexual activity should be included. While the individual with THR may understand that stooping to retrieve an object is contraindicated, he may not visualize that a flexion during posterior entry may increase flexion to a dangerous level. The approach used in counseling about sexual activity at the Arthritis Center at Moss Rehabilitation Hospital has been to strongly advise against intercourse for 6 to 8 weeks after surgery.[18] This is to allow the healing of the internal capsule and musculature. Intercourse can be safely engaged in after the first 6 to 8 weeks post surgery, but using a supine position.[19] Posterior-entry or side-lying positions are unadvisable since they promote adduction. After the 3 month recuperation the patient is then evaluated by the surgeon regarding the assumption of other positions. Patients who have undergone total hip replacement or resurfacing must also be advised to prevent the partner from falling onto the operated hip. The impact of a fall onto the operated limb can cause either a bone or prosthetic fracture, especially if the bone is severely osteoporotic.

Total Knee Replacement

The patient who has undergone either partial or total knee arthroplasty (TKR) must be advised that repetitive, weight-bearing flexion of the operated knee or knees is to be avoided during coitus. Weakening of the prosthesis, prosthetic fracture, and fracture of any of the bones of the knee joint can occur. The patient and partner should be advised to prevent falls onto the operated extremity. Kneeling positions are to be avoided during coitus.

After discharge from the hospital following joint replacement, the patient may require the use of a pillow under the knee during sexual activity. However, the pillow should be removed immediately after sexual activity so as to prevent flexion contractures.

Long-Term Corticosteroids

Unfortunately some patients with arthritis may be on long-term corticosteroids. The fragile, friable, tissue-paper skin, accompanied by petchiae and varying degrees of ecchymosis, is at best extremely vulnerable to pressure injuries. Gentleness during sex play is important. If intercourse is too strenuous, alternate forms of sexual expression can be recommended. Since the body automatically splints against pain, it is important to take measures to prevent pain from occurring. Support of the trunk upon a firm mattress and the use of pillows under the vulnerable joints such as the knees can minimize discomfort. Side-lying positions must be accompanied by pillow support or partner support. Since patients on long-term corticosteroids may have significant osteoporosis, undue stress on unsupported joints may induce a fracture. Especially prone to fractures are those patients who, in addition to being on steroids, have had previous surgery such as an osteotomy of the femur or joint implant of the lower extremities.

OTHER IMPORTANT CONSIDERATIONS

Sexuality is a multifaceted psychological and physiological mass of characteristics that begin at birth. Masters and Johnson have stated that at delivery vaginal secretions are present in the female infant and the male infant may experience his first erection as he draws his first breath.[20] Infants learn quickly the security, warmth, and affection associated with parental cuddling. Tots explore the genitalia and are aware of the pleasurable sensations and toddlers' cuts are often best healed by a mother's kiss rather than the surgeon's sutures. The child, adolescent, and adult is aware of and may employ masturbation according to personal or religious perogatives. By adulthood, the individual is aware of the preference for homosexuality, heterosexuality, or bisexuality.

Advising, counseling, or helping patients achieve solutions to arthritis sexual problems is an obligation of the health professional who treats the person, not merely the disease. Patients who had undergone total hip replacement were asked to respond to a questionnaire regarding sexual adjustment after discharge from the hospital. The results of the study were startling. A respondent who had been recently widowed 8 months prior to receiving the questionnaire stated that sexual activity declined in his marriage when his wife was forced to wear dentures! A woman in her 70s stated that when she went into the hospital for bilateral THR, her husband installed another woman in her marital bed! And a 25-year-old unmarried woman explained that she was denied advice about sexual intercourse by her surgeon because, he said, she was "unmarried and wouldn't need that kind of advice." And the respondent who admitted that she suffered a linear fracture of the femur on her first day home asked, "Should I have avoided sexual activity?" This study clearly supported mounting evidence that sexuality is a major concern of patients and partners and an issue that must be addressed. The withholding of sexual advice may lead to legal implications.

Patients without partners are often neglected because of embarrassment or conflicting values. There are professional and appropriate sources of literature that will help the health professional to advise and the patient to achieve fulfillment. While alternate methods of sexual expression may be anathema to many health professionals, they do have an obligation to refer the patient to sources or to others who can best aid them.[23]

People without arthritis may have sexual problems because of stature, weight, body build, and so on. When it is recommended that one partner assume the superior position, if that partner is obese or short, the person superiorly may have difficulty assuming the position for the desired time span. While both hard and soft core pornography abound, practical, safe advice is lacking from the people whom patients assume to be the experts! However, the bank of sexual information is increasing, and it is hoped that physicians, nurses, physical therapists, occupational therapists, social workers, and other health care professionals will avail themselves of the information and pass it along to their clients.[24] Becoming aware and admitting that sexuality is a health care issue for every patient is the first step to delivering total health care.

SUMMARY

Creating an atmosphere of privacy and empathy for patients is the first thing the professional must do who wishes to counsel patients on sexual matters. A nonjudgmental attitude is essential in dealing with both married and unmarried patients. The primary obligation of the professional is to inquire about sexual problems in order to give the patient a chance to cope comfortably with the topic of sexual needs. Publications specifically for patients, written in lay, rather than medical language, and accompanied by illustrations are recommended. These publications can serve as positive reinforcement as well as a source of reference for both patients and professionals.

REFERENCES

1. Ehrlich GE, ed. Sexual problems of the arthritic patient. In: Total management of the arthritic patient. Philadelphia: JB Lippincott, 1973.
2. Ehrlich GE. Arthritis and sexuality: a specialist's view. Medical Tribune, November 1973.
3. Brassell MP. Who should mention sex? Unpublished paper, Moss Rehabilitation Hospital. Philadelphia, 1973.
4. Fox N. Sexuality among the aging. J Prac Nurs 1978;41 (August):16-18.
5. Falk G., ed. Sexuality and the aged. Nurs Outlook 1980;28(1):51-55.
6. Palmore E, ed. Normal aging, I: Report from Duke University Longitudinal Studies 1955-1969. Durham, 1970.
7. Palmore E, ed. Normal aging, II: Report from Duke University Longitudinal Studies 1970-1973. Durham, 1974.
*8. Lachniet D, Onder J. Sex, arthritis and women. Allied Health Professions Section of the Arthritis Foundation Newsletter. New York, 1975.
*9. Blau S, Schultz D. How to cope with the question of sex and arthritis. In: Arthritis: complete up to date facts for patients and families. Garden City, N.Y.: Doubleday, 1974.
10. Comfort A. Sexual consequences of disability. Philadelphia: George F. Stickley, 1978.
11. Wallace R, Heiss ML, Bautch JC. Psychosocial issues. In: Staff manual for teaching patients about rheumatoid arthritis. Chicago: American Hospital Association, 1979.
*12. Shaul S, Bogle J, Hale J., Norman AD. Towards intimacy, family planning and sexuality concerns of disabled women. Washington Planned Parenthood of Snohomish County, 1977.
13. Rubin D. The NO!—or yes and the how of sex for patients with neck, back, and radicular pain syndromes. Calif Med 1970;6:113.
14. Sadoughi W, Leshner M, Fine HL. Sexual adjustment in the chronically disabled population, a pilot study. Arch Phys Med Rehab 1971;52:311.
15. Blau S, Blau B. Sex and systemic lupus erythematosus. Med Aspects Human Sexuality 1976 (Nov.).
16. Currey HL. Osteoarthritis of the hip joint and sexual activity. Ann Rheum Dis 1970;29:448.
17. Katz WA. Sexuality and arthritis. In: Rheumatic diseases diagnosis and management. Philadelphia: JP Lippincott, 1977.
18. Brassell MP. Rehabilitation nursing and the surgical patient. In: Ehrlich GE, ed. Rehabilitation management of rheumatic conditions. Baltimore: Williams and Wilkins, 1980.
19. Bleyberg LS. Sexuality and the rehabilitation process. Med Aspects Human Sexuality, 1982; 16(3):34L-34U.

---

*References for patients.

20. Masters WH, Johnson V. Human sexual response. Boston: Little, Brown, 1966.
21. Brassell MP, Kauffman M. Sexual adjustment of patients with THR. Unpublished paper, Moss Rehabilitation Hospital, Philadelphia, 1974.
*22. Boggs J. Living and loving with arthritis. Arthritis Center, University of Hawaii, 1977.
*23. Heslinga K. Not made of stone. Springfield, Ill.: Charles C Thomas, 1974.
24. Kaplan HS. The new sex therapy. New York: Brunner Mazel, 1974.
*25. Arthritis Foundation. Arthritis, living and loving: information about sex. Atlanta, 1982.

Rehabilitation Techniques for Regional Disorders and Specific Diseases

Now that the roles of the health professionals caring for arthritis patients and the techniques that they employ have been explained, it will be of interest to try to apply some of these principles to specific diseases and regional disorders. Representative disorders have been chosen, including inflammatory arthritis, noninflammatory arthritis, nonarticular diseases, and the "collagen vascular" disorders. It is impossible within the confines of space to include all rheumatologic and arthritic diseases with more complete discussion. Even the disorders chosen for this section are not discussed in great detail; however, we have tried to apply the most salient principles that have been discussed in the previous two sections. Entire books have been written about each of these individual disorders or regional syndromes. The reader is referred to major textbooks of arthritis for more detailed discussions of each.

30

Painful Cervical and Low Back Syndromes

Marjorie C. Becker, P.T., Ph.D.

According to the epidemiologic work of Kelsey et al.[1] a U.S. population of 18.9 million has musculoskeletal impairments. Eight million of this number suffer disorders of the spine and back; this represents a back complaint rate of 18/1,000 with 4/1,000 population on disability.

During the course of various rheumatic diseases many patients experience acute or chronic pain syndromes of the cervical, lumbar, or lumbosacral spine. The primary complaint of pain may be integral to the rheumatic disease process, as in ankylosing spondylitis or degenerative joint diseases; secondary to the disease process, as in root compression from osteophyte formation; or an independent event, as in traumatic strains or subluxations.

Although patients present with varying degrees and specificity of pain, there is no correlation between the degree of pain and the presence or severity of other clinical signs or symptoms.[2] Therefore observation, an in-depth history, thorough physical examination, and an understanding of the patient's life-style are of utmost importance in managing cervical and lower back syndromes.

THE SPINE

The cervical, thoracic, and lumbar vertabrae are a series of diarthrodial joints and subject to disease processes and symptomatology of other such joints (knee, ankle, wrist, phalangeal).[3] Figure 30.1, from Finneson,[4] provides a lateral view of the normal vertebral column showing the natural curves and relative size of the bodies. The design of the cervical spine permits flexion, hyperextension, rotation, and lateral bending. The elasticity and tensile properties of the ligamentous structures contribute to normal functioning of the multijointed cervical spine. Laxity of the joint structures allows subluxations, abnormal ranges of motion, or slipping between the articular surfaces.[5]

The thoracic spine is less mobile in all planes than either the cervical or

343

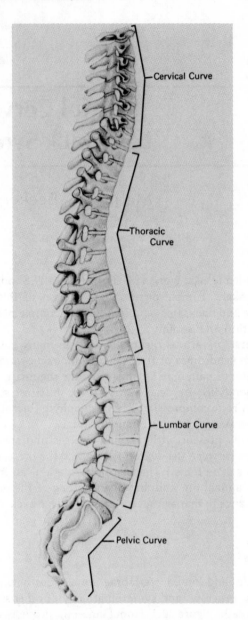

Source: BE Finneson, Low back pain. Philadelphia: JB Lippincott, 1973. Reprinted with permission.
Figure 30.1.   Lateral view of the vertebral column.

lumbar spine, in part due to the rib cage being attached. Lumbar spine motion is primarily in flexion-extension and, except for the thoracolumbar junction, the lumbar spine has little lateral or rotational motion. The lumbar vertebrae are more massive and heavier than the other vertebrae, which is consistent with their

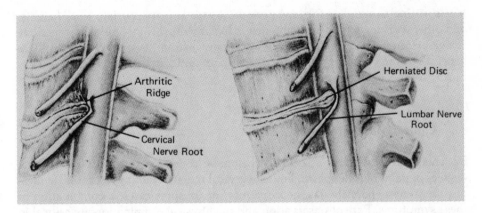

Source: BE Finneson, Low back pain. Philadelphia: JB Lippincott, 1973. Reprinted with permission.
Figure 30.2.   The difference in bone-disc ratio between the cervical and the lumbar spines accounts for the different types of root compression lesions found in these two different areas. Most lumbar disc lesions are "soft-tissue" in nature, in contrast to the primarily bony lesions seen in the cervical spine.

weight-bearing function.[6] The intervertebral disc is thicker and contributes a greater amount to the length of the lumbar spine than in either the cervical or thoracic areas. Similarly, root compression related to lumbar disc protrusion is due to soft tissue whereas cervical root compression syndromes are either from bony spur impingement or spurs in association with some soft disc protrusion, as shown in figure 30.2, from Finneson.[4]

Finally, figure 30.1 shows an acute lumbosacral angle at the articulation of L-5 with the triangular sacrum. Normal motion in this area is quite limited. At the same time, mechanical forces and the upper-body weight on this joint are significant.

PAINFUL CERVICAL SPINE

Cervical spondylosis or osteoarthritis of the lateral interbody joints as described by Jackson[5] is the most common cause of cervical pain. Most of these patients also have osteoarthritis elsewhere.[7] Rheumatoid arthritis is also a significant source of neck pain since 86 percent of rheumatoid arthritis patients have involvement of the cervical spine.[7] Other sources to be considered in the differential diagnosis of cervical pain include juvenile polyarthritis, ankylosing spondylitis, fibrositis, hyperextension-flexion injuries (sprains), torticollis, and postural deviations resulting from congenital or idiopathic structural defects of the spine. Infections and neoplasms can also produce such pain and should be considered during evaluation.

Functional causes should not be overlooked or underestimated in assessing cervical pain. Often these causes can be dealt with more successfully.[8] They include poor posture, environmental conditions of poor lighting and high noise levels, sitting or standing for long periods of time at inappropriate work heights, and other working habits or requirements like moving heavy objects or repetitive upper extremity motions. Shoulder or upper extremity weakness as well as general tension can also produce cervical pain and can be identified as sources during a thorough assessment.

Clinical Manifestations

Patients with or without associated rheumatic conditions present with varying degrees of pain, muscle spasm, limited cervical range of motion, stiffness, tenderness, weakness, paresthesias, neuropathies, or, in some cases, a combination of these symptoms. Patient observation and the physical examination are critical in identifying the nature of the pain and the existence of nerve root compression. A thorough understanding of these patient complaints more rapidly leads to appropriate diagnostic tests and treatment.

Assessment

Reference to normal spinal anatomy, an accurate history regarding trauma, and knowledge of the pathophysiology of rheumatic diseases are integral to establishing an accurate diagnosis as well as short- and long-term treatment plans. Physical examination of the cervical area is discussed in chapter 11. A description of the onset and recurrence of the problem should be obtained. A thorough understanding of the patient's environment and life-style at home, at work, and at play is useful not only in establishing an accurate diagnosis but in developing an appropriate long-term management plan, especially in the presence of a rheumatic disease.

Laboratory and radiography studies are needed in order to diagnose the cause(s) or the presenting complaints, but treatment of the symptoms is quite similar regardless of their etiology. Depending on the ultimate diagnosis, additional therapy may also be indicated. This is especially true in the case of infection or neoplastic disorders.

Treatment

The general goals of treatment are to relieve pain by use of appropriate drugs and physical measures, to optimize physical function, and to prevent or minimize the recurrence of the problem diagnosed.

An individually designed physical therapy program should also reduce inflammation, relax muscle spasm, protect injured parts, restore any lost strength, and restore any lost range of motion. A 2-week course of professionally administered physical therapy incorporating these goals provides relief in most cases.

Acute cervical root compression resulting from trauma, disc prolapse, or impingement of spurs produces immediate symptoms. In these cases application of cold for relief of pain may initially produce best results. In most other cases of acute cervical pain, moist heat pads followed by intermittent graded cervical traction up to 35 lbs applied at an angle of 30° of forward flexion for a short time generally produces maximal relief of inflammation, pain, and muscle spasm.[5,9] Patients can be instructed in home use of a Hydrocollator pack or heating pad over moist terry cloth for 20–30 minutes. Various home traction units are also commercially available.[10] The patient can safely initiate this procedure at home for maintenance or with recurrence of acute symptoms.

For chronic or recurrent cervical pain, especially in degenerative joint disease, treatment with ultrasound over the cervical area for 10 minutes at 0.8 to 1.5 watts/cm^2 in conjunction with intermittent traction often provides good results. The modality to produce analgesia and relief of muscle spasm should be selected more on the basis of comfort of the patient during the treatment. For example, if the patient is more comfortable in a supine position, moist heat is preferred followed by traction. If greater comfort is experienced in a sitting position with the thorax flexed and head resting on a pillow at a table, then ultrasound may be the modality of choice. Obviously ultrasound treatment cannot be carried out on a home basis.

Not infrequently cervical pain is a symptom secondary to neuromuscular pathology elsewhere, especially the shoulder and upper extremity. While physical treatment of the secondary cervical muscle spasm or decreased range of motion may be indicated, diagnosis and treatment of the primary pathology is the key to longer term relief.

Manipulation or "thrust" mobilization of the cervical spine in the presence of rheumatic disease, especially spondylolysis, as described by Paris is contraindicated.[11] Soft-tissue injections particularly when muscle spasm is present are sometimes helpful. Surgical intervention in cervical spine management is indicated only when more conservative management fails or when instability, disc extrusion, or spur formation produces root or cord compression.[5,9] In this situation, when subluxation causes cord compression, rigid fixation in a four-poster cervical brace, halo traction, or similar device is indicated. Prompt neurologic consultation for a determination of the need for surgical decompression is required.

A strategy of long-term management of the traumatized or degenerative cervical spine should be worked out with the patient and the assistance or guidance of the various health team members. The plan should include home use of heat and cervical traction when pain recurs as well as organization of the home and work environment to minimize physical stresses and excessive energy consumption. Patient education should incorporate protection of the cervical spine and reduction of activities or environmental barriers that produce excessive motion or cervical strain. A soft or semi-rigid cervical collar provides desirable head positioning, helps immobilize or rest the cervical spine, but does not necessarily protect the cervical spine from trauma, especially while the wearer is riding in a car.

PAINFUL LOWER BACK

Low back complaints account for a significant number of visits to physicians. The sources of low back pain are musculoskeletal, neurological, and (less commonly) visceral. While many rheumatic disease patients present with back pain caused by inflammatory or degenerative joint processes, other causes should not be disregarded in the differential diagnosis. The etiology includes traumatic (acute and chronic), congenital, developmental, degenerative, neoplastic, metabolic, toxic, neurologic, and vascular causes.[3]

Clinical Manifestations

Mixter and Barr in 1934 first described pain of lumbar root entrapment resulting from herniation of the nucleus pulposa.[12] Recent work adds disc degeneration, secondary anatomical changes, and lumbar root entrapment to the general category of spinal stenosis.[13] Narrowing of the spinal canal, then, is the focus of attention. Inflammatory diseases of the low back are discussed elsewhere (see chapter 38).

The degenerative disease process produces instability and allows abnormal intervertebral motion. Osteophytes may develop. These two phenomenon in combination or separately may produce back pain with or without root pressure. Root entrapment from degenerative spinal stenosis is frequently related to aging and treated conservatively.[13] Spondylolesthesis can result secondarily in degenerative disc disease. Its appearance is usually after 50 years of age. The slippage of L-4 on L-5 occurs most frequently with L-5 on S-1 less frequently and L-3 on L-4 least frequently. The disc and ligaments degenerate allowing excessive motion, facet degeneration, and forward slippage.[14] Pain is acute and may or may not relate to root pressure. Table 30.1, from Lipson,[13] summarizes the characteristics of low back pain.

The patient's presentation and description help in differentiating root compression or root entrapment from pain of musculoskeletal origin secondary to a rheumatic disease process. Disc herniation or prolapse generally produces pain of sudden and severe onset and is aggravated by positions or activities that increase intradiscal pressure. Therefore the patient prefers being supine or standing to sitting. There may be a list to the symptomatic side if the disc extrusion is medial to the root and away from the symptomatic side when lateral to the root.[13] A positive straight-leg raising test is an accurate diagnostic tool for disc herniation 75 to 80 percent of the time. Myelography raises accuracy to 90 to 95 percent[13] but should be utilized only if surgical decompression is being considered or in

Table 30.1. Summary of the Characteristics of Low Back Pain of Various Origins

Source of Pain	Distribution	Nature	Aggravating Factors	Neurologic Changes
Spinal pain	Sclerotomal Local	Sharp Dull	Motion	None
Discogenic pain	Sclerotomal	Deep Aching	Increased intradiscal pressure, e.g., bending, sitting, Valsalva maneuver	None
Nerve root pain	Radicular	Paraesthesias Numbness	Root stretching	Present
Multilevel lumbar spinal stenosis pain	Radicular Sclerotomal	Paraesthesias Spinal claudication pattern	Lumbar extension Walking	Present
Referred visceral pain	Dermatomal	Deep Aching	Related to affected organ	None

Source: Reference 13. Reprinted with permission.

certain other special instances. Body scans using computer tomography have also been helpful in localizing disc abnormalities.

Laboratory and radiographic baseline studies are indicated to confirm or aid in the clinical diagnosis. In cases of questionable nerve root compression, an electromyogram (EMG) showing fibrillations of muscles innervated by the involved root provides confirmation of neurologic involvement.

Assessment

Since low back pain can be integral to rheumatic disease pathology, a secondary symptom, or independent of rheumatic disease involvement, an accurate history, and systematic examination are of utmost importance. Depicting the onset and chronology of symptoms is the first important step. Noting the character of the pain regarding severity, duration, quality, localization, radiation, alleviation, reduplication, and aggravating circumstances is imperative in diagnosis as well as in establishing the short-term and long-range management plan.[3]

Observation of the patient's posture and demeanor as he or she approaches the examination area can be quite informative. One can observe splinting, listing, gait deviations, and a preference to stand or lie down rather than sit during the initial history-taking. The manner in which the patient removes clothing in preparation for the examination can also help localize the problem. Observation of barefoot gait should note any foot slap, unequal heel rise from the floor, or other lower extremity weakness indicative of possible neurologic deficit. Discrepancies in leg lengths as well as contractures at the hip, knee, or ankle should be ruled out as the cause of any observed gait deviations, postural deviations, and potential cause of the back pain.

Paraspinous and interspinous tenderness and muscle spasm can be palpated. The presence or absence of the lumbar lordotic curve should be noted. Range of motion is assessed by manually stabilizing the pelvis and having the patient flex forward as far as possible and then noting the distance from hands to floor. One can also observe compensated or uncompensated scoliotic curves in this position. With the patient standing upright and the pelvis still stabilized, lateral rotation can also be assessed.

Mobility and strength of the upper and lower extremities should be assessed in a sitting or supine position. Muscle-bulk changes, especially in the lower extremities, should be noted by circumferential measurements taken bilaterally. With the knee flexed, the flexion, abduction, external rotation (Faber) maneuver of the hip should be done.

The patient should be queried in detail as to any trauma or strain in the immediate or remote past as well as the constancy or frequency of the pain. Lightening-like pain elicited with a sneeze or cough is more typical of nerve root compression and often related to disc prolapse or herniation. Progressive and constant pain causing awakening in the night may be symptomatic of a neoplasm.[6] Weakness, decreased sensation, and absent reflexes are further neurologic indicators.

Urinary retention, saddle anesthesia, and inability to ambulate are symptoms of cauda equina syndrome and represent a surgical emergency. In these cases postoperative recovery of function correlates with the preoperative neurologic insult but is usually less than normal.[15] For completeness a rectal exam should be done to rule out a mass or prostate disease as well as to assess rectal sphincter tone. At the same time palpation of the coccyx may also identify a source of pain.

Treatment

Treatment of back pain without associated neurologic signs or symptoms is directed toward relief of pain and muscle spasm, reduction of inflammation, strengthening of abdominal musculature, increase in range of motion, and minimization of recurrence.

Acute pain is managed by use of analgesics, short-term bed rest, and application of moist heat for 20–30 minutes. Muscle spasm can be reduced by massage. Soft tissue injection may help. Hip flexors, hamstrings, and heel cords should be maintained at normal lengths and isometric exercises taught so the patient can regain a normal pelvic tilt and lower extremity strength, especially in extension. Frequently support of the lumbar spine is helpful both immediately and in the long range. Application of a corset may reduce pain from excessive motion produced by instability.

In cases of nerve involvement, initial treatment of up to 2–3 weeks' bed rest and application of pelvic traction is indicated in addition to the use of analgesics and a graded exercise program. Patients tolerate constant traction of 35–40 lbs or intermittent traction of 65–70 lbs. One should note that many hyperactive patients often do not tolerate constant traction.

The physical therapy program has its greatest benefit if the patient is hospitalized or if treatment can be provided in a setting where the patient's transit to and from the treatment does not cancel the positive effects of the treatment given. Patient education in body mechanics, posture, and organization of the work and home environment is integral to the treatment so as to minimize mechanical stress on the back. As with other degenerative processes, the patient's life-style must be considered and adaptations suggested to maximize function and coping behaviors. In intolerable cases of spinal stenosis, surgical intervention provides good relief.[13]

Long-Term Management

Long-term back care must be incorporated into the rheumatic disease patient's life-style to minimize the recurrence and disability of chronic low back pain. Musculoskeletal models are helpful in teaching good back care. In addition many illustrative back care pamphlets are available to aid in patient education.

The patient should be instructed to sleep on an extra firm mattress or insert a ¾-inch-thick to 1-inch thick plywood bed board between the mattress and the springs. A small head pillow is recommended. The use of the water bed is controversial and should be considered on an individual basis. Weight loss may also be indicated to reduce stress on the spine.

Range of motion and muscle strength should be maintained to the extent possible in upper and lower extremities. While corsets and cervical collars serve as supportive or protective devices for the unstable hypermobile spine, especially for riding in automobiles and other vehicles, these devices will not correct or prevent further deformity.

Patients should be instructed to assess and organize their homes so as to protect and minimize stress on the back. The installation of grab bars in a bathtub is recommended, as is using chairs and table or countertop work space of a height to encourage optimal posture. Wearing comfortable shoes other than sandals or scuffs and eliminating loose throw rugs and slick surfaces prevent falls and unnecessary trauma to the back.

The use of hand trucks, a dolly, or grocery cart is preferred to carrying unwieldy or heavy items. Use of a backpack prevents the unilateral upper extremity and back strain produced by carrying a heavy purse or shopping bag.

Recreational activities should be reviewed and adaptations suggested. Trauma to the back experienced in contact sports or strenuous demands such as digging with a shovel over a long period should be avoided. Moderate and regular exercise of swimming or golfing is tolerated quite well once a suitable level of muscular strength is attained.

SUMMARY

The natural course of several of the rheumatic diseases frequently involves acute and chronic cervical spine and low back syndromes. This chapter has presented a brief structural description of the spine as well as the clinical manifestations, assessment, and treatment of cervical and low back syndromes as they relate to the rheumatic diseases. Establishing an accurate diagnosis is always the first goal. Treating the recurrent symptomology is often much more difficult. Long-term management is especially important. Health team members can teach the patient appropriate care of the spine and home treatment for intercurrent episodes. Knowledge of the patient's life-style must be incorporated into this education so that feasible adaptations that maximize function and minimize disability can be effective. As there is still much to be learned about pain, health team members who listen carefully and incorporate the patient's goals and needs into a long-range treatment plan are likely to better serve the patient who must cope with pain when its alleviation may not be possible.

REFERENCES

1. Kelsey JL, White AA 3rd, Pastides H, Bisbee GE Jr. The impact of musculoskeletal disorders on the population of the United States. J Bone Joint Surg (A) 1979;61(7): 959–964.

2. Bandilla KK. Back pain: osteoarthritis. J Am Geriatr Soc 1977;25(2):62–66.
3. Levine DB. The painful low back. In: McCarty DJ Jr, ed., Arthritis and allied conditions. 9th ed. Philadelphia: Lea and Febiger, 1979, ch. 69, pp. 1044–1079.
4. Finneson BE. Low back pain. Philadelphia: JB Lippincott, 1973, pp. 6 and 11.
5. Jackson R. Syndrome of cervical nerve root compression. In: McCarty DJ Jr, ed., Arthritis and allied conditions. 9th ed. Philadelphia: Lea and Febiger, 1979, ch. 67, pp. 1023–1037.
6. Finneson BE. Lower back in the diagnosis of rheumatic diseases. In: Katz W, ed., Rheumatic disease diagnosis and management. Philadelphia: JB Lippincott, 1977; 7:114–135.
7. Bland JH, Nakano KK. Neck pain. In: Kelley WN, Harris ED, Ruddy S, Sledge CB, eds. Textbook of rheumatology. Philadelphia: WB Saunders, 1981, ch. 28, pp. 411–436.
8. Ehrlich GE. The physicians' headaches: syndromes of the back, neck and shoulder: the rheumatologist. Pa Med 1969;72(7):89–91.
9. Katz WA. Cervical spondylosis. In: Katz W, ed. Rheumatic disease diagnosis and management. Philadelphia: JB Lippincott, 1977;29:629–641.
10. Waylonis GW, Denhart C, Pope Grattan M, Wapenski JA. Home cervical traction: evaluation of alternate equipment. Arch Phys Med Rehab 1982;63:388–391.
11. Paris SV. Mobilization of the spine. Phys Ther 1979;59(8):988–995.
12. Mixter WJ, Barr JS. Rupture of the intervertebral disc with involvement of the spinal canal. New Eng J Med 1934;211:210–215.
13. Lipson SJ. Low back pain. In: Kelley WN, Harris ED, Ruddy S, Sledge CB, eds. Textbook of rheumatology. Philadelphia: WB Saunders, 1981;pt. I, ch. 30, pp. 451–471.
14. Rosenberg NJ. Degenerative spondylolesthesis. J Bone Joint Surg (A) 1975;57(4): 467–474.
15. Scott RJ. Bladder paralysis in cauda equina lesions from disc prolapse. J Bone Joint Surg (B) 1965;47:224–235.

31

Disorders of the Shoulder

Terence W. Starz, M.D.

Shoulder pain is one of the most common musculoskeletal problems encountered in daily medical practice. The most common shoulder disorders are the following:

Degenerative rotator cuff tendinitis

Calcific rotator cuff tendinitis (acute and chronic)

Bicipital tendinitis

Adhesive capsulitis (frozen shoulder)

Reflex sympathetic dystrophy (shoulder-hand syndrome)

Glenohumeral arthritis (with generalized inflammatory arthritis)

In the majority of cases the problem arises in the soft-tissue structures around the shoulder and not in the joints themselves. The clinical approach to shoulder pain must begin with a clear understanding of the anatomy of the shoulder region (see figure 31.1).

The shoulder girdle consists of an intricate interrelationship among bony ligamentous, muscular, and articular structures. There are three joints (the glenohumeral, the acromioclavicular, and the sternoclavicular joints) that function synchronously throughout the arc of shoulder motion. The *glenohumeral joint*, the primary one, is formed by the proximal end of the humerus and the shallow glenoid fossa of the scapula. This joint has little inherent structural stability and depends on the surrounding muscles, ligaments, and joint capsule for its support. The spine of the scapula ends laterally in the bony acromion, which overlies the glenohumeral joint.

The upper anterior lateral portion of the humerus, called the lesser and greater tuberosities, is the site of attachment of the *rotator cuff muscles*. Included in this group of muscles are the supraspinatus, infraspinatus, teres minor, and subcapularis, which insert on the tuberosities by a common conjoined tendon. The combined actions of the rotator cuff muscles are external rotation and elevation of the arm, in addition to stabilization and depression of the humeral head in the glenoid fossa.

355

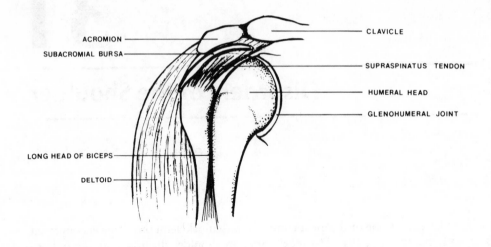

ACROMION

SUBACROMIAL BURSA

CLAVICLE

SUPRASPINATUS TENDON

HUMERAL HEAD

GLENOHUMERAL JOINT

LONG HEAD OF BICEPS

DELTOID

Figure 31.1.   Major anatomic structures of the shoulder.

The anterior portion of the rotator cuff is known as the "critical zone." This area has a reduced blood supply, making it more susceptible to injury. Calcification of the cuff tendons with hydroxyapatite crystals in the critical zone may be found radiographically in 3 to 8 percent of persons over 30 and may be bilateral. As many as one-third of individuals with tendon calcification manifest shoulder pain. Also within the critical zone, degenerative changes of the cuff tendons consisting of fissuring and tearing develop with age. These changes can also be related to shoulder pain.

The long head of the biceps muscle courses through the bicipital groove between the two tuberosities and attaches to the superior margin of the glenoid fossa. The major function of the biceps is to supinate and flex the forearm; a minor function is assisting in forward flexion of the arm. The deltoid muscle arises from the scapular spine and the distal clavicle and inserts on the deltoid tuberosity at the lateral upper humeral shaft. The deltoid abducts the arm with the assistance of the supraspinatus.

The shoulder capsule encircles the humeral head and is quite redundant, especially inferiorily, to permit the great range of shoulder motion. The conjoined tendon of the rotator cuff blends into the upper portion of the capsule, while the long head of the biceps invaginates it. Between the rotator cuff tendons and the overlying acromion is the subacromial (subdeltoid) bursa, which cushions the tendons as they impinge on the acromion during abduction of the arm.

Elevation of the arm from the side to overhead requires the integrated movement of the humeral head within the glenoid fossa, coupled with upward rotation of the scapula on the posterior chest wall, thereby elevating the glenoid. Of the 180° of shoulder abduction (circumduction), 120° occurs at the glenohumeral area, while 60° is the result of scapular rotation. Movement of the clavicle that accompanies shoulder abduction occurs at the acromioclavicular and sternoclavicular joints.

The most common shoulder problems involve the periarticular soft tissues and are collectively referred to as **periarthritis of the shoulder**. These disorders primarily affect the rotator cuff tendons and the subacromial bursa. They are best considered as a spectrum rather than separate entities. Included in this group are tendinitis of the rotator cuff (degenerative and calcific), bicipital tendinitis, and adhesive capsulitis (frozen shoulder). Codman proposed that the primary abnormality in periarthritis of the shoulder is a localized rotator cuff tendinitis, usually of the supraspinatus tendon, which can extend to the other cuff tendons, the subacromial bursa, and the biceps tendon. The periarthritis spectrum is most severe when the joint capsule and the other intra- and extra-articular structures become involved leading to a frozen shoulder. Subacromial bursitis does not commonly occur as an isolated process. Usually it is related to inflammation of the adjacent rotator cuff tendons.

Degenerative tendinitis of the rotator cuff is most frequent after the age of 45, in persons whose occupation or other activity involves significant shoulder stress. (See table 31.1) The onset is often gradual and intermittent, with the pain described over the humeral head and deltoid muscle. Night discomfort is a prominent feature, especially when the person lies on the affected side. On examination, palpation over the tuberosities at the cuff insertion usually elicits tenderness. Furthermore, abduction of the arm past 60° results in considerable pain because of rotator cuff impingement on the acromion. The range of motion of the shoulder may be normal although scapulohumeral rhythm is reversed with abduction of the arm, beginning with shrugging of the shoulder (scapular rotation) in order to minimize glenohumeral movement. X-rays of the shoulder may be normal or show sclerotic and cystic changes of the tuberosities. Degenerative tendinitis must be distinguished from tears of the rotator cuff tendons, which affect the same age group. Tears most frequently involve the supraspinatus tendon. The onset usually accompanies a sudden shoulder strain or a fall, and a snap may be heard. Severe pain is present over the deltoid area and, depending on the extent of the tear, abduction of the arm is weak and incomplete. With

Table 31.1.   Stages of Rotator Cuff Tendinitis

Degenerative	Calcific
1. Asymptomatic	1. Asymptomatic
2. Acute and subacute	2. Acute crystal-induced inflammation
3. Rotator cuff tear	3. Chronic—like degenerative tendinitis

Note: Both forms of tendinitis often have an associated subacromial bursitis and may also have bicipital tendinitis.

complete tears, the arm falls to the side when support is removed after passive elevation.

The next disorder on the periarthritis spectrum is **calcific tendinitis**, which usually affects younger persons in sedentary occupations. The onset is often abrupt and may follow vigorous shoulder activity or mild trauma. The shoulder is diffusely tender, and all motions are quite painful. Rotator cuff calcification is present on x-ray, but the size of the calcific deposit correlates poorly with the clinical picture. The course is limited, in most cases lasting 1 to 2 weeks. Occasionally the "calcium boil" ruptures into the subacromial bursa. Pathophysiologically the hydroxyapatite crystals are able to evoke an active inflammatory response. Less commonly this disorder may be more insidious and resemble the course of degenerative rotator cuff tendinitis. In this chronic stage the calcium deposits are less hydrated and do not cause much inflammation.

In association with rotator cuff tendinitis or at times as an isolated finding, **tendinitis of the long head of the biceps** muscle may develop. Considerable variation in the width and length of the bicipital groove occurs, which may be a predisposing factor. Tenderness is present over the biceps tendon and may be intensified by supination of the hand against resistance thereby contracting the biceps muscle (Yerason sign).

The treatment of degenerative and calcific tendinitis and bicipital tendinitis is quite similar and is directed toward pain relief and maintenance of shoulder motion:

1.   Resting the shoulder during the acute stage
2.   Physical therapy modalities—heat and cold
3.   Analgesic and nonsteroidal anti-inflammatory drugs
4.   Local anesthetic and corticosteroid injection
5.   Shoulder exercise program to maintain range of motion

Rest is essential in the acute stage and should be coupled with adequate doses of analgesic and nonsteroidal anti-inflammatory drugs such as salicylates and indomethacin. Physical therapy modalities, including moist heat or ultrasound, provide additional benefit; however, cold packs may be preferred with acute calcific tendinitis. Local anesthetic and corticosteroid injections into the subacromial bursa and rotator cuff or biceps tendon region (not directly into the tendons) may be useful if symptoms do not readily resolve. Last, an adequate shoulder exercise program should be initiated early in the course to ensure preservation of shoulder motion. In most cases considerable improvement occurs within 1 to 6 weeks of treatment. Persistence beyond this time suggests a rotator cuff tear and reevaluation including arthrography of the shoulder is indicated.

The last periarthritic disorder of the shoulder is **adhesive capsulitis** or **frozen shoulder**, which is a pathologic problem unique to the shoulder girdle. In this condition increasing restriction of shoulder motion is accompanied by pain and stiffness. Individuals in the fifth and sixth decades, especially females, are most often affected. The common denominator for adhesive capsulitis is prolonged reduced mobility of the shoulder. Conditions frequently associated with a frozen shoulder include shoulder tendinitis, trauma (including humeral fractures), cervical discogenic disease, rheumatoid arthritis, stroke, and myocardial infarction. The clinical spectrum ranges from a mild limitation of motion in one plane to total loss of active and passive glenohumeral joint motion. Shoulder pain is often quite intense, especially at night, and may radiate either to the neck or down the arm. As shoulder motion is lost, the discomfort usually diminishes. Pathologic changes include a thickened contracted joint capsule, which may be adherent to the humeral head, as well as chronic inflammation and fibrosis of the other periarticular soft tissues. X-ray of the shoulder may show osteoporosis of the humeral head related to the immobilization, and an arthogram may show loss of joint space volume.

Early recognition and treatment of the frozen shoulder is essential in order to limit its progression. A regimen similar to the one for shoulder tendinitis is employed; however, local anesthetic and corticosteroid injections should be used initially. Alternatively a tapering course of prednisone over several weeks, starting with 40 mg daily, may be employed. In all cases a vigorous exercise program must be initiated. An overhead pulley may be quite helpful. At times careful manipulation of the shoulder under general anesthesia is necessary to restore shoulder motion. The long-term prognosis is generally favorable, though it may take 18 to 30 months for recovery. With certain associated disorders, including rheumatoid arthritis and stroke, range of motion of the shoulder may remain limited.

In evaluating a patient with shoulder pain, causes other than periarthritis of the shoulder must be considered. Isolated osteoarthritis of the glenohumeral joint is uncommon and is usually associated with a predisposing condition such as aseptic necrosis of the humeral head or a humeral fracture. In the acromioclavicular joint radiographic changes of osteoarthritis occur with increasing age, but symptoms referable to the joint are not often present. The clinical picture is pain directly over the acromioclavicular joint, which increases with shoulder elevation (shrugging). Treatment of acromioclavicular osteoarthritis is with local measures, including heat and injecting the joint with corticosteroids.

Reflex sympathetic dystrophy (shoulder-hand syndrome) consists of pain and limitation of shoulder motion, much like adhesive capsulitis, accompanied by discomfort in the hands and fingers. Other features are related to vasomotor instability and include swelling of the hand, trophic changes, hyperesthesia of the skin, and hand coolness or warmth. In this disorder finger motion is painful and reduced. Very often a precipitating factor such as trauma, myocardial infarction, stroke, or cervical discogenic disease can be identified. Bilateral upper extremity involvement is commonly present. The etiology of this disorder is unclear; however, abnormal neurogenic reflexes appear to be important. Early recognition is essential and significantly improves the prognosis. Treatment consists of vigorous physical therapy, systemic or local corticosteroids, and at times a stellate ganglion blockade with local anesthetics.

SUMMARY

Shoulder involvement occurs as a frequent manifestation of inflammatory arthritis, such as rheumatoid arthritis or ankylosing spondylitis. Other joints are almost invariably affected in these disorders as well. In persons past 50, bilateral shoulder pain and stiffness with normal shoulder motion should suggest a diagnosis of polymyalgia rheumatica. Rapid sedimentation rate, morning stiffness, and associated temporal arteritis in some cases are additional clues to the diagnosis. Last, the shoulder may be the site of pain referred from other structures, including the lungs (especially with apical tumors), the heart, and the abdomen (diaphragmatic irritation).

Disorders of the shoulder most commonly originate in the periarticular soft tissues and can result in considerable pain and functional impairment. They are best understood as a periarthritis spectrum with the initial abnormality beginning in the rotator cuff tendons.

REFERENCES

1. Codman EA. The shoulder. Boston: Todd, 1934.
2. Bland JH, Merritt JA, Boushey DR. The painful shoulder. Semin Arth Rheum 1977; 7:21–47.
3. Rizk TE, Pinals RS. Frozen shoulder. Semin Arth Rheum 1982;11:440–452.
4. Bateman JE. The shoulder and neck. Philadelphia: WB Saunders, 1978.

32

Hand Dysfunction Associated with Arthritis

Jeanne L. Melvin, O.T.R., M.S.Ed., F.A.O.T.A.

Many of the complications and limitations of arthritis hand involvement can be prevented, particularly those related to tendon impairment. This chapter reviews criteria for evaluation and treatment of the hand conditions associated with arthritis, with an emphasis on early detection and preventive intervention.

Clinical experience over the past 10 years makes it clear that the time-honored practice of waiting for patients to develop limitations before sending them for therapy is no longer valid. To be most effective, precise assessment and range-of-motion (ROM) instruction needs to be instituted early before joint contractures occur, thus allowing the patient's normal mobility to be the baseline and goal for therapeutic processes. The occupational therapist is a specialized health professional who has the knowledge and training to apply the principles noted in this chapter.

NECK, SHOULDER, AND ELBOW INVOLVEMENT

Several conditions in the upper extremity can produce symptoms in the hands. Some of the more common conditions are briefly reviewed to encourage their consideration in a full hand assessment. All hand assessments should include evaluation of the neck and proximal extremity before the clinical diagnosis is made. Comparison to a normal contralateral extremity is also advised wherever possible.

Cervical arthritis can produce nerve root compression with paresthesias, sensory loss, and motor loss along nerve root patterns in the hand.[1] For example, C-6, C-7 compression may result in sensory loss in the thumb and index finger that can be easily confused with carpal tunnel syndrome.

It is not uncommon to find cervical nerve root compression concomitant with distal nerve entrapment of the median or ulnar nerve. This is typically referred to as the "double-crush syndrome."[2] It is believed that the proximal

361

lesion alters the physiology of the nerve, rendering the nerve more susceptible to compression at a lower level.[2]

Shoulder synovitis may possibly refer pain down the lateral border of the arm into the forearm and occasionally refer pain into the palm. Whenever pain in the hand or forearm does not correlate with either anatomic structures or specific pathology, referred pain from the shoulder should be considered a possible source.[3]

Although this syndrome usually occurs by itself, shoulder-hand syndrome can also occur in people with arthritis. It initially presents as diffuse unilateral hand pain that does not correlate with joint or tendon involvement. The condition can also be bilateral. In fact minor involvement of the contralateral extremity often goes undetected.[4]

Elbow synovitis may affect the hand by causing pressure entrapment of the ulnar nerve as it passes through the ulnar groove of the medial epicondyle.[5] It is also possible to get entrapment of the radial nerve in the forearm due to elbow synovitis.

When evaluating forearm rotation, it is important to keep in mind that rotation may be limited by synovitis at either the distal or proximal radial-ulnar joint or both.[6] The site causing the limitation is determined by the site of pain at the end of rotation. The median nerve can also become trapped in the forearm. Although this is rare, it should be considered in patients who have paresthesias in the median distribution but who have a negative Tinel or Phalen's test and no obvious wrist involvement.[5,7]

HAND AND WRIST INVOLVEMENT

Joint and Soft-Tissue Involvement

Pain

When joint inflammation is suspected, the assessment of joint pain and synovitis are one and the same. Synovitis can be reflected in pain in three different ways. First, patients with severe inflammation often experience pain "at rest" when the joint is not being used due to excessive intra-articular pressure. Second, patients with mild or moderate inflammation may report pain only with motion or functional use. And third, patients with very mild synovitis may deny pain during motion but experience pain when specific medial-lateral compression is applied to the joint.[6]

For people with osteoarthritis, pain typically occurs during motion or functional use and is attributed to osteophyte formation or cartilage damage creating a mechanical derangement pressure on the subchondal bone and capsule producing pain. The pain mechanism in osteoarthritis is not clearly understood. Some patients can progress to marked joint deformity without any pain, whereas others are limited by pain and have minimal radiographic changes. It is common for patients with osteoarthritis to develop localized inflammation that results in pain at rest. Usually other features, such as osteophyte formation, help distinguish this from other forms of inflammatory arthritis.

When pain is felt over a tendon at the site of a tendon sheath, it is usually indicative of tenosynovitis. But pain is not essential for diagnosing this problem. It is possible, in fact common, to have severe flexor or extensor tenosynovitis without any symptoms of pain.[7]

Pain can inhibit muscle function. This may be sudden, for example when wrist pain inhibits supporting muscles and the joint "gives way." It may also be subtle and only reduce rather than completely stop muscle function. This may manifest as a sense of subjective weakness, for example when a patient reports "weak hands because he can no longer open jars or apply hard pressure." It is possible for true muscle weakness to present with the same symptom, but for patients with painful hands, pain inhibition of muscle strength is the most common cause of subjective weakness during functional activities. Thus whenever a patient reports "weakness," it is important to determine if there is true muscle weakness, which will be clearly evident on a manual or Dynamometer grip test, or if pain during the activity is the limiting factor. The latter is usually the case if a patient experiences marked hand or wrist pain during a grip strength test. When pain is the limiting factor, the treatment is joint-protection instruction or training in adaptive methods to eliminate pain during the activity. When muscle weakness is present, strengthening exercises are indicated.[7] (See figure 32.1)

Synovitis

Understanding the synovitis process forms the basis for prescribing hand exercises. The most successful hand therapy prevails when the patient as well as the physician and therapist recognize this.

The synovial tissue is responsible for both producing synovial fluid that lubricates the joint and for removing or draining the fluid. When the synovial membrane becomes inflamed, it produces an excessive amount of fluid. The resorptive mechanism becomes ineffective and the fluid becomes trapped inside the joint capsule (an effusion). The joint capsule is a tight-fitting structure leaving little room for expansion. Excess fluid inside the joint greatly increases the intra-articular pressure and stretches the capsule and the surrounding structures to their limit.

When there is an effusion, exercise must be gentle, because forceful external pressure to increase range of motion only traumatizes the expanded capsule and ligaments further. Patients with active synovitis should have a gentle range-of-motion exercise program and a plan for regaining motion once swelling has subsided.[7] The more acute the synovitis, the greater the degree of warmth, swelling, and possibly redness. These signs diminish as the inflammation subsides.

In the early phases of synovitis, when the joint is filled with fluid, it feels boggy to the touch. If the inflammation becomes chronic, the synovial membrane proliferates, forming pannus, filling the joint with tissue, and becoming firm to

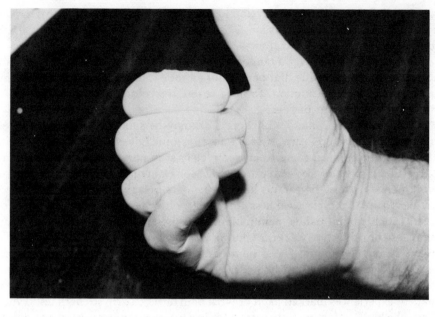

(a)

Figure 32.1a.   Right hand of man with severe painless flexor tenosynovitis of all digits of 1½ years duration. Full active flexion at the beginning of therapy (passive flexion was near normal). At this point he was considered a surgical candidate for a flexor tenosynovectomy.

the touch.[6] Occasionally the synovium may herniate through the capsule, forming a focal mass.[8]

Swelling

In rheumatoid arthritis swelling is typically seen with the following conditions: (1) synovitis, which produces a characteristic fusiform enlargement of the joint; (2) extensor tenosynovitis, which produces a puffy swelling and is easily detectable through the thin skin over the sheath or sheaths; (3) wrist flexor tenosynovitis, although this is less obvious since it is deep to the carpal ligament and palmar fascia; and (4) digital tenosynovitis with swelling along the volar aspect of the digit, most notably over the proximal phalanx.

Patients with psoriatic arthritis or other spondyloarthropathies often develop a characteristic "sausage" swelling throughout the entire digit, which is attributed to a combination of joint synovitis and severe flexor digital tenosynovitis.[9]

One method for determining the degree of swelling is to compare the dorsal skin folds of the edematous hand with the nonedematous hand. The skin folds

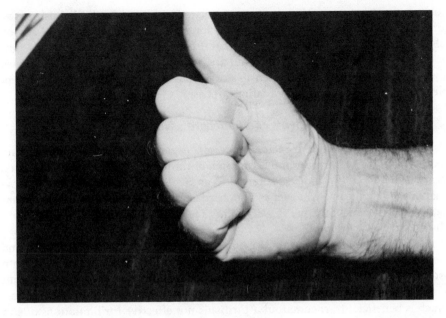

(b)

Figure 32.1b.   Active flexion following 6 weeks of diligent hand therapy (the degree of swelling had not changed), including contrast baths, deep tissue massage, and a host of active ROM exercises. For many patients with complex tendon involvement, the value of therapy cannot be determined until it is tried.

will be diminished if there is swelling. If the swelling is unilateral, it is helpful to compare side views of the digit with the contralateral digit by placing the palms together. Swelling of the digits can be quantitated by measuring their circumference with a regular tape measure, a circumference arthrometer, or a jeweler's ring sizer.[10] Swelling denotes something that is changing rather than a fixed enlargement such as osteophyte formation.

Subcutaneous (Rheumatoid) Nodules

These modules are discrete subcutaneous masses of fibrous and granulomatous tissue, typically found over bony prominences exposed to pressure, for example along the ulnar ridge of the forearm or hand.[6] Occasionally they occur on the dorsum of the finger joints and less commonly on the palmar surface of the hand. Nodules may arise over the bony prominence created by a subluxed joint such as the thumb interphalangeal (IP) joint. Generally they are not painful, but they can become tender if irritated by pressure.[8,11]

Some nodules appear to occur in response to pressure (microtrauma) or are aggravated and enlarged by pressure. For other nodules, however, pressure does not seem to be a factor. Nodules that are related to pressure will diminish in size (or disappear) if the pressure source is eliminated. The new commercial slip-on elbow-protector sleeves (Heelbo, Diamond) can be very effective for this purpose. Nodules on the palm of the hand are particularly disabling and are almost always sensitive to pressure. Utensil/surface padding techniques should be implemented early to reduce aggravating stresses.[7]

Osteophytes (Heberden's and Bouchard's Nodes)

Osteoarthritis involves two major processes: degeneration of the cartilage and proliferation of the bone around the margin of the joint. Osteophytes at the distal interphalangeal (DIP) joint are referred to as Heberden's nodes and at the proximal interphalangeal (PIP) level as Bouchard's nodes. Osteophytes are also common at the carpometacarpal (CMC) joint. They rarely occur at the metacarpophalangeal (MCP) joints.[12]

Osteophytes are important because they are diagnostic of osteoarthritis and are indicative of cartilage damage. It is common to find patients who have both osteoarthritis and rheumatoid arthritis. In a patient with the latter, it is important to clarify any limitations due to osteoarthritis because range-of-motion exercise, which is beneficial to rheumatoid arthritis, is not effective for limitations due to the osteophyte formation.[7]

Osteoarthritis is common in the CMC joint and is often the first symptomatic joint. Diagnosis is facilitated by a positive "grind test," a procedure that involves compression and rotation of the metacarpal into the CMC joint.[13] The test is positive if it elicits CMC pain or crepitus. CMC arthritis may radiate pain up the forearm or into the palm. It is frequently confused with de Quervain's tenosynovitis. Symptoms of CMC joint pain and mild inflammation are usually episodic and aggravated by motion or functional use. A simple solution is a short slip-on thumb (opponens) splint that blocks CMC motion with a C-bar over the web space, but allows wrist and thumb interphalangeal joint motion.[7] Most patients are very pleased to have something to use during functional activities that stops the pain. This splint has greater acceptance if it is made of a thin thermoplastic material such as 1/16-inch-wide Aquaplast.[35] If the pain becomes constant and nonresponsive to conservative measures, the patient is a candidate for surgical CMC arthroplasty.

Joint Contractures

The term *contracture* is used to describe a fixed limitation as compared to a temporary limitation due to transitory edema, inflammation, or pain. A joint contracture is generally due to capsular and ligamentous fibrosis, secondary to partial or complete immobility. Common conditions that reduce mobility and consequently can lead to contracture include the following:[7]

Chronic synovitis and synovial hypertrophy

Ineffective tendon motion due to tenosynovitis

Shortening of the collateral ligaments due to chronic malpositioning and inappropriate splinting

Periarticular edema, which compresses the joint structures

Subluxation, which blocks or prevents motion, as when radioulnar subluxation prevents supination

Muscle weakness

When a muscle is not able to hold against slight resistance (less than 3.5/5), it is no longer able to balance antagonistic forces, which results in chronic malpositioning and immobility. A typical example would be weakness of the wrist extensors leading to a wrist-drop (flexion) contracture.[7] This type of weakness is not restricted to myopathies but can occur during severe systemic illness.

A large percentage of the contractures seen in patients with arthritis is either preventable or correctable if treatment is initiated early (from 1 to 2 months from the onset). The majority of hand contractures could be prevented if patients received instruction in precise range-of-motion techniques before they developed any limitations as well as guidelines for being able to recognize the contracture, how to reduce it if it occurs, and where or how to seek assistance from a therapist if they are unable to reduce the contracture on their own.[7]

The most effective technique, perhaps the only effective one for reducing contractures, is sustained, gentle, passive range-of-motion exercise carried out *without* pain over prolonged periods of time (hours or days). A sustained gentle stretch can be applied in several different ways: (1) manually, using the non-affected hand; (2) with the use of splints, either dynamic or static; (3) the use of Coban® wrapping techniques (Coban is a stretchable self-adhering tape made by 3M); (4) with serial casting, a technique similar to that used with serial casting of the knee.[14] In addition mobilization techniques in both lateral-medial and volar-dorsal planes can facilitate mobility in the capsule and ligaments.

In patients with rheumatoid arthritis or other inflammatory conditions, these *techniques should be applied only when there is no inflammation present in the joints.* The pressure applied during the sustained stretch should not cause pain but should create tension in the tissues under pressure and be tolerable for prolonged periods. If the tension is so intense that the patient cannot tolerate the splint or technique more than 10 minutes, it is too strong. The tension should be tolerable over the desired length of treatment—30 minutes, 2 hours, or more.[7]

Generally the foregoing treatments are not effective for contractures that have been present for longer than 3 months. But this is a generalization and for some people with a tendency for stiffness, 1 month is too long. Another exception to this is for wrist flexion contractures, which may be amenable to serial casting even after 3 months have elapsed. If the joint is completely immobile (ankylosed), before attempting any treatment, it is important to determine whether the joint is immobile due to soft-tissue or capsular changes (fibrous ankylosis) or whether the immobility is due to ossification of the joint (bony ankylosis). Sustained stretch may be effective on fibrous ankylosis, but no conservative treatment is effective in changing bony ankylosis.

Tendon Involvement

The hand tendons pass through synovial sheaths at four locations: the dorsum of the wrist, volar aspect of the wrist, volar aspect of the fingers, and the entire volar aspect of the thumb.[15] The purpose of the sheath is in part to provide nutrition and lubrication to tendons and to facilitate gliding, particularly where the tendons slide over several bones. The sheaths have a double-wall construction. Thus inflammation of the synovial lining results in excessive fluid being trapped within the walls of the sheath.[15] If the inflammation becomes chronic, synovial and granulation tissue can proliferate. Tenosynovitis impedes the gliding of the tendons and through an enzymatic process diminishes tendon integrity.[8]

The symptoms of tenosynovitis differ from joint synovitis, in that pain and warmth may be absent. Even in severe cases, swelling and impaired tendon function (producing a difference between active and passive motion) may be the only symptoms. Adults with volar wrist tenosynovitis often have wrist pain, but this is usually due to coexistent radiocarpal joint involvement. One exception to this rule is tenosynovitis of the first wrist compartment (de Quervain's tenosynovitis). This area is almost always painful, possibly because of close approximation to superficial nerves or the fact that it is often due to trauma.

The presence of pain has an effect on therapy. *Painful* tenosynovitis is generally very responsive to ice compresses, splinting, and steroid injections. *Nonpainful* tenosynovitis is often responsive to ice and contrast baths but is generally unresponsive to splinting. In fact splinting can frequently make it worse by eliminating muscle action as a means of decreasing swelling.[7] The thermal modality of choice for tenosynovitis is ice compresses (for 15–20 minutes) because of its effectiveness in reducing swelling when there is both digit and wrist involvement.[16] Contrast baths (alternate submersion in hot and cold water) are also very effective and more comfortable for the patient. Hot whirlpool water should *not* be used, since the heat applied in a dependent position *increases* swelling.[17]

Dorsal Wrist Tenosynovitis

Twelve wrist and digit extensor tendons pass through six separate tendon sheaths in the dorsal wrist compartment.[15] Tendon sheath effusions are fairly easily detected under the thin dorsal skin and frequently delineate the shape or length of the involved sheath. Inflammation of the first compartment is usually painful. The sixth also frequently hurts, whereas compartments 2 to 5 are rarely symptomatic. In the adult patient with rheumatoid arthritis it may be difficult to tell if the tenosynovitis is painful because they usually have concurrent painful radiocarpal synovitis.

Inflammation of the sixth compartment is of special concern, because it contains the extensor carpi ulnaris tendon. Damage or displacement of this tendon contributes to subluxation of the wrist.[8] Every effort should be made to protect this tendon in the early stages of development.

Another major consequence of dorsal tenosynovitis is rupture of the digital extensor tendons. (See figure 32.2.) Chronic tenosynovitis compromises the integrity of the tendons, rendering them vulnerable to fraying over subluxed or eroded carpal bones. The finger extensor tendons usually rupture over the distal end of the ulna, and the extensor pollicis longus ruptures over Lister's tubercle where it turns radially toward the thumb.[18]

The extensor digital quinti (EDQ) is frequently the first tendon to rupture. This tendon, though of little functional significance, is the most important tendon to evaluate, because if it has ruptured, the extensor communis to the fifth and fourth digits are also in danger of rupture, leaving the patient without extensor power in the ulnar digits.[18] To test the integrity of the EDQ tendon, have the patient flex the MCP joints (to rule out communis function) and then actively extend only the little-finger MCP joint. Inability to extend the MCP joint or palpate tendon function is indicative of rupture. (PIP joint extension is a function of the intrinsic muscles.)

In addition to rupture of the extensor tendons mentioned above, rupture of the extensor pollicis longus (EPL) is common. The EPL is a prime extensor of the

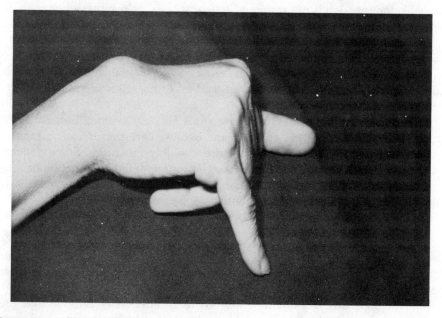

Figure 32.2. For evaluation of ruptured extensor tendons, the extensor digiti quinti should be routinely tested, for it is often the first to rupture and its loss, though not functionally significant, indicates the extensor communis is also in danger of rupture. To test, have the patient make a fist to rule out extensor communis function; then have the patient actively extend the fifth MCP. The patient in the photograph is unable to perform this motion and has a rupture of the EDQ.

distal thumb joint; the thumb intrinsic muscles can also extend the distal joint through their action on the extensor hood mechanism. Determination of EPL rupture should be based on inability to palpate tendon function during active thumb extension, not motion alone.[18] Rupture of the flexor tendons to the index finger can also occur but is fairly uncommon.

Volar Wrist Tenosynovitis

In contrast to dorsal tenosynovitis, the consequences of volar tenosynovitis are primarily due to compression. The volar wrist compartment forms a narrow, rigid tunnel that contains nine flexor tendons, the flexor sheaths, and median nerve.[15] The roof of the tunnel formed by the strong transverse carpal ligament does not readily yield to swelling. Thus tenosynovitis results in compression of the structures within the carpal tunnel. This can affect hand function in three major ways. The first is compression of the median nerve, which results in pain, paresthesias, or possibly sensory and motor loss (carpal tunnel syndrome). Second, swelling may impede gliding of the profundus tendons, resulting in inability to fully flex the DIP joints, in mild cases, or inability to fully flex or extend the digits, in severe cases.[19] If this occurs, daily passive range-of-motion exercises are needed to prevent contractures of the DIP joints. In severe cases patients can develop marked MCP and PIP contractures in a matter of weeks if active tendon function is not restored.[7] In many cases ice compresses or contrast baths are sufficient to reduce swelling to allow tendon gliding.[7] If this fails, steroid injections or surgical tenosynovectomy is indicated. Third, excessive tenosynovium in a compressed area can compromise the blood supply to the tendons, reducing their integrity and rendering them vulnerable to rupture. This most commonly occurs in the profundus tendons to the index and middle fingers at the level of the scaphoid.[19]

Tenosynovitis in the volar compartment is not easy to detect because of the strong rigid transverse carpal ligament and because each person can accommodate a different amount of swelling before it visibly protrudes. Some patients have barely detectable swelling but marked limitation of tendon function or conversely severe swelling yet normal tendon excursion. If the tenosynovitis is painless, it may go undetected for months (see figure 32.3).

Digital Flexor Tenosynovitis

The finger sheaths begin at the level of the MCP joint and extend to the DIP joint. The flexor pollicis longus tendon has its own sheath, which is continuous from the IP joint to approximately 3 cm proximal of the wrist.[15]

In the digits swelling due to tenosynovitis is most easily detected over the proximal phalanx. It should be possible to pinch the skin in this area, whereas tension or fullness is indicative of tenosynovitis.[6] Again, pain or warmth may or may not be present.

The most common consequence of digital tenosynovitis is "triggering" of the digit, where a granulomatous plaque, nodules, or thickening of the tendon

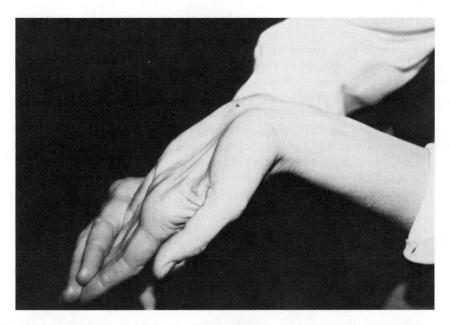

Figure 32.3   To determine if the long flexor tendons can achieve full distal excursion through the carpal tunnel, gently passively extend the wrist and fingers as shown. If the fingers flex as the wrist is extended, the tendons are binding in the carpal tunnel. To check proximal excursion, the patient should be able to make a complete fist (finger tips to palmar crease) with the wrist in a neutral position. Active and passive motion should be equal.

can catch on the annular ligaments (pulleys) that maintain the alignment of the tendon on the volar aspect of each joint.[20] It is most common for triggering to occur at the MCP or PIP level. Severity may range from feeling an inconsequential lump during flexion or extension to complete painful blockage of motion.[20] If there is a great deal of swelling, ice may be helpful on a temporary basis. Many times steroid injections alone can reduce inflammation sufficiently. Generally, if steroid injections are not effective, surgery is indicated.[19]

Similar to volar wrist tenosynovitis, swelling in the digital sheath can prevent gliding of the flexor tendons resulting in limited active DIP or PIP flexion or extension.[19] For this situation passive ROM exercises are essential for maintaining joint mobility until tendon function is restored. Chronic tenosynovitis can also result in rupture of the profundus or sublimus tendons, although this is uncommon compared to the frequency of extensor tendon ruptures.[19]

MUSCLE INVOLVEMENT

In the hand the intrinsic muscles demonstrate the greatest degree of involvement with inflammatory arthritis. The intrinsic muscles should be evaluated for atrophy, weakness, and tightness.[7]

Atrophy of muscles can occur fairly rapidly in patients with systemic arthritis. It appears to occur at a faster rate than might be expected from simple disuse, although no specific myopathy has been identified.[6] Atrophy of the intrinsic muscles is usually gauged by the loss of muscle bulk in the first dorsal interosseous muscle. Atrophy of this muscle indicates similar changes in the other intrinsic muscles. It is important to keep in mind that in the absence of neurologic impairment, there is not a direct correlation between atrophy and weakness. A person can have marked atrophy and still score 4 out of 5 on a muscle test.[7] (This fact is often comforting to patients who associate atrophy with disability.)

Evaluation of intrinsic muscle strength is a critical aspect of an arthritis hand assessment. Weakness can occur due to peripheral nerve entrapment, cervical radiculopathy, and disuse.[21] These must be distinguished from *inability to apply* strength due to pain.

In a routine hand assessment it is generally sufficient to test selected muscles in order to screen for neurologic impairment or disuse weakness. Testing the abduction pollicis brevis, dorsal and volar interossei, the abductor digit quinti, and abductor pollicis can be done quickly and easily, and it can provide key information about ulnar and median innervated muscles.[7] Specific testing procedures are described in detail in several publications.[22-24]

Weakness of the abductor pollicis brevis is generally indicative of carpal tunnel syndrome. This is an important muscle, for it provides abduction for grasp. Chronic weakness typically results in limited abduction and a CMC joint adduction contracture, a limitation that cannot be reduced even if median nerve function is regained.[7] Patients with marked abductor pollicis weakness of 3.5/5 or less should wear a CMC splint at night to maintain the web space until surgery can be scheduled to restore nerve function.[7]

The dorsal and volar intrinsic muscles are prime MCP joint flexors.[23] In some patients strengthening the intrinsic muscles can help compensate for extrinsic flexors that are not working effectively due to tenosynovitis, attenuation, or contractures.[7] The dorsal muscles can be tested by applying resistance to finger abduction in a standard fashion.[24] The volar muscles are tested by having the person adduct the digits in full extension, then applying quick passive abduction to the little finger, then the index. If the digit snaps back strongly, it is graded as 5/5.[7]

Intrinsic muscle tightness can create a major deforming force, particularly for the person with incipient swan-neck deformities. The assessment and treatment of this condition is discussed under treatment of the MCP joints.

Common Deformity Patterns

The major hand deformities associated with the rheumatic diseases are wrist (radiocarpal) and radioulnar subluxation; swan-neck, boutonniere, and mallet deformities; MCP joint subluxation and ulnar drift; and the various thumb deformities.[8] Anatomically these are a complex group of aberrations, because they are dynamic deformities that literally involve every anatomical structure of the hand and wrist.

In a person with a rheumatic disease, all of these are essentially imbalance deformities. That is, chronic synovitis stretches and weakens the joint capsule and supporting ligaments, altering the mechanical alignment, and consequently the forces exerted by the tendons produce an imbalance between opposing forces.[8]

There is a normal synchronous balance and interplay between all of the joints and tendons in the hand. Consequently, chronic synovitis or beginning deformity in a single joint can create an imbalance and deformity in adjacent joints. Likewise treatment to a specific joint can alter the stresses to adjacent joints, creating either a positive or negative effect. For example, a splint that immobilizes the MCP joints can create compensatory stress that can exacerbate synovitis in the PIP joints. Professionals responsible for hand evaluations and treatment planning must therefore be cognizant of the influences treatment can have on adjacent joints.[7] This section identifies pathodynamics that can be influenced by preventive and therapeutic interventions and those that alter forces on adjacent joints.

Wrist Joint

The wrist should not be treated as a separate joint but viewed as an integral, functional unit with the hand. The wrist provides the stability essential for hand function. Its integrity and alignment can have a major impact on the digital tendons and the deforming forces applied to the digital joints.[8]

Clinical Goal 1.   To reduce pain and stress to the wrist in order to protect (preserve) integrity. One of the most effective means of accomplishing this goal is with the use of a flexible elastic or leather wrist gauntlet splint with a volar reinforcement; these are commercially available. (See figure 32.4.) These splints allow approximately 50° of wrist flexion and extension to allow hand function, but they prevent circumduction. With this splint on, a patient *must* use the wrist in neutral alignment. It cannot be twisted or deviated from neutral alignment during functional activities. This restriction allows function but eliminates a considerable amount of stress to the wrist tendons and carpal joints. For moderate to severe wrist synovitis, a combination of a flexible wrist splint during the day and a thermoplastic wrist splint at night is the most effective treatment protocol. Some patients who do not need to wear a splint throughout the entire day often find it particularly valuable to use one during specific stressful activities such as grocery shopping.[7]

Wrist splints of all types have the potential to cause compensatory stress to the MCP joints, exacerbating MCP synovitis. Rigid wrist splints tend to create the greatest stress to the MCP joints. The more flexible the wrist splint, the less functional forces are transferred to the distal joints. Patients should be taught to monitor MCP inflammation and to alter the flexible splint by removing the support bar if the splint aggravates MCP synovitis.[7]

Clinical Goal 2.   To preserve ulnar motion. The most common sequelae of the wrist synovitis are ulnar-volar subluxation of the proximal carpal bone on the

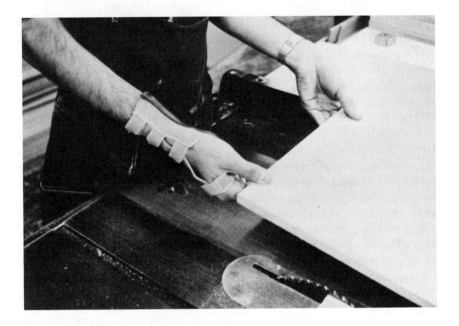

Photo courtesy of AHP Teaching Slide Collection. Reprinted with permission.
Figure 32.4.　The flexible wrist gauntlet splint with a metal volar support (Futuro brand) on this patient's right wrist allows approximately 50° of flexion or extension but prevents circumduction and consequently reduces considerable stress to the wrist. Compare the angles of both wrists in this picture.

radius and rotation of the distal carpal bone resulting in the hand being radially deviated on the forearm.[8,25] The rotation distorts functional alignment of the finger and necessitates MCP ulnar deviation to compensate (this is the zigzag phenomenon).[25] Thus radial deviation of the wrist creates a dynamic force that encourages MCP ulnar drift deformity. To help minimize this process, rigid wrist splints should be fabricated to position the wrist in 10° of ulnar deviation (the functional position of the wrist).[7]

Occasionally a patient will develop radiocarpal subluxation without carpal rotation, and the wrist will be *ulnarly* deviated on the forearm. This is ideal, for these patients typically have less MCP drift than those with radial deviation of the wrist.[7,25]

Clinical Goal 3.　To protect the extensor carpi ulnaris tendon. This tendon has a unique insertion into the base of the fifth metacarpal. It allows the tendon to slide over the ulnar styloid during supination. If the ligament securing this insertion is damaged by tenosynovitis, the tendon can displace volarward, preventing it from functioning as an extensor tendon and creating a flexor force that contributes to volar subluxation of the wrist.[8] Splinting can be an effective means of protecting the tendon.

The extensor carpi ulnaris tendon travels through the sixth dorsal wrist compartment.[15] For the occasional patient with severe or isolated tenosynovitis of this compartment, a steroid injection may be necessary to protect this tendon.

Clinical Goal 4.   Prevention of digital tendon ruptures. The digital extensor tendons typically rupture due to tenosynovitis and attrition over roughened subluxed carpal bones. If one tendon ruptures, it is likely that other tendons may also rupture.[18] After the first rupture a rigid wrist support may protect remaining tendons until a tenosynovectomy and repair can be carried out.

MCP Joints

Clinical Goal 1.   Elimination or reduction of strong grip or flexion during periods of inflammation. Chronic synovitis of the MCP joints typically results in volar and ulnar subluxation, often referred to as "ulnar drift" deformity. Until 1960 it was believed that displacement of the extensor tendons into the ulnar valleys was a major causal factor in ulnar drift deformity. Smith's work has demonstrated that it is the flexor tendons that create the damage, not the extensor tendons, and has provided the theoretical basis for joint-protection instruction.[26]

In a normal joint the strong flexor tendons exert force directly over the metacarpal head during flexion, without consequence. If the ligaments supporting the flexor sheath are damaged and lengthened by synovitis, the mechanical forces are altered and the fulcrum of the force is displaced over the proximal phalanx instead of the metacarpal. Thus strong grasp and pinch creates a flexor force that subluxes the phalanx in a volar and ulnar direction.[26] For every 1 lb of pinch or grip force exerted, 4 lbs of force is displaced over the proximal phalanx.[8,26,27]

Instruction in joint-protection methods for avoiding power grip during active synovitis can be very effective in reducing the stress and pain and consequently the inflammation in these joints.[28] But in order for this treatment to work, patients must comply with the process. Teaching joint protection in a manner that elicits patient compliance is one of the true challenges in arthritis patient education.

Three factors seem to influence joint-protection compliance the most. The first includes having the patient clearly understand the rationale for the process. Second, one must demonstrate the effectiveness of the procedure. This may be as simple as having the patient perform a task such as lifting a frying pan the regular way, which is usually painful, and then performing the same task using a joint-protection method *without* pain. However, it may require something more involved, such as creating a contract with the patient to use specific procedures for a limited time period such as 3 days or 1 week. Most patients can comply with a limited regimen. When the benefits of joint protection, such as less inflammation, less pain, greater comfort, become obvious, the patients are more likely to use the procedures in daily life. Third, one must let patients know that the joint-protection techniques are necessary only during period of inflammation or swelling. When these symptoms subside, they can use their hands normally.

Clinical Goal 2.   Prevention of intrinsic muscle contractures. The "intrinsic plus" hand deformity is rarely discussed in the rheumatologic literature but should be because this deformity can usually be prevented. It is theorized that pain and swelling in the MCP joints elicits spasm in the associated interossei muscles, which are prime flexors of the MCP joints and extensors of the PIP joints. Chronic spasm of these muscles can eventually lead to MCP flexion contractures and loss of PIP flexion.[29] If a person has natural hyperextension or joint damage of the PIP joint, intrinsic contractures can lead to a swan-neck deformity. Intrinsic muscle tightness also reduces dexterity and diminished PIP flexion strength when the MCPs are in extension, as in grasping large objects.[7] The intrinsic muscles can also become shortened secondary to MCP subluxation; this allows the intrinsic muscles to rest in a shortened position and thus become contracted.[30]

All patients with MCP joint involvement should be tested for intrinsic tightness. If the muscles are normal, it should be possible passively to flex fully the PIP joint with the MCP point in full (neutral) extension. If the muscles are shortened, there will be less PIP flexion with the MCP joint extended in contrast to the MCP joint being flexed (Bunnell test).[31] A 5° difference in PIP flexion in these two positions can be considered significant.

Patients with intrinsic tightness should be given instruction in intrinsic stretching exercises, which include any activity or exercise that involves flexion of the PIP joint with the MCP joint in extension, e.g., using a Bunnell block.[31] For some patients it may be easier to make a slip-on MCP extension splint to use during exercise or functional activities.[7] These patients should also be cautioned against using their hands in activities that require an intrinsic-plus position (MCP flexion and PIP extension) for prolonged periods such as holding a book, crocheting, or sketching.

Clinical Goal 3. Maintaining the length of the collateral ligaments. The collateral ligaments are the structures that provide lateral stability to the digital joints, and the length of these ligaments determines the degree of flexion and extension possible.[31] Synovitis can result in these ligaments being lengthened, allowing joint instability, or it can result in fibrosis and shortening of the ligaments, limiting flexion and extension mobility.[31,32] In addition to synovitis, improper positioning can result in fibrosis and shortening of the ligaments.[31] Because of this, all hand splints must be designed to preserve the integrity of the collateral ligaments.

The collateral ligaments reinforce the joint capsule on either side of the joint. Each is composed of two sections: the *cord portion* that extends from the dorsal lateral side of the proximal bone to the volar lateral side of the distal bone and the *accessory portion* that attaches into the volar plate. The two portions have reciprocal roles.[32,33]

In the MCP joint the cord portion predominates in determining stability and the ligaments have variable length depending on the position of the joint. When the joint is flexed, the full length of the cord portion is required to accommodate the wide lateral condyles of the metacarpal head, limiting lateral mobility. When the joint is in extension, the full length is not required and the cord portion is slack.[31-33] This has two clinical implications. First, to evaluate laxity of the MCP ligaments, the joint must be positioned in full flexion. Second, if positioning during bedrest or a hand splint maintains the MCP joints in extension for a prolonged period (say 2 days), the cord portion can become shortened in its slack position and not have sufficient length to allow MCP joint flexion. Static splints should maintain the MCP joints in at least 45° of flexion to preserve the length of the ligament, and range-of-motion exercises should be done daily.[7,33]

Clinical Goal 4. Preservation of wrist ulnar deviation. The prescription described earlier under wrist synovitis maintaining wrist alignment and ulnar deviation is a key factor in reducing MCP ulnar drift forces.

Finger Joints

Most discussions about rheumatoid finger deformities review the swan-neck, boutonniere, and mallet deformities. Contractures of the PIP joints and DIP joints are also common and can limit functional abilities.

Clinical Goal 1. Daily range-of-motion exercises to ensure full flexion and extension. If a patient can make a complete fist with full DIP flexion, that is, touch the tips of his or her fingers to the palmar crease, then daily active flexion is sufficient exercise. But patients with mild tenosynovitis or any limitation to full mobility should be instructed in gentle *passive* range-of-motion techniques to maintain mobility.[7]

Many patients develop DIP contractures because the profundus tendon is not sliding its full excursion due to mild tenosynovitis. These patients often do daily active flexion exercises but are not aware that their DIP joints are not flexing fully.[7]

Clinical Goal 2. To regain motion loss as soon as possible. Many joint contractures can be reduced or eliminated if patients are taught what to look for and guidelines for applying therapeutic measures after the inflammation subsides. If they are unable to reduce the contracture themselves, a therapist's intervention should be sought. Having a therapist evaluate and instruct a patient in range-of-motion exercise early, before deformities occur, connects the patient with the therapy department and encourages patients to seek professional therapy promptly. Specific measures for reducing joint limitations are discussed under "joint contractures."

Clinical Goal 3. Maintain the length of the collateral ligaments. In the PIP and DIP joints, the two portions of the collateral ligament play an equal role. When the joint is in extension, the cord portion is slack and the accessory portion is taut. When the joint is flexed, the reverse occurs; the cord portion becomes taut and the accessory slack.[32,33] This reciprocal process ensures stability in any position, but unfortunately it also makes the PIP joints very prone to stiffness during immobilization. When the joint is splinted in extension, the cord portion becomes fibrosed in a shortened position, and when the joint is splinted in flexion, the accessory portion can become contracted in a shortened position. Either ligament can prevent mobility.[32,33] In order to maintain mobility, splinting must be combined with daily range-of-motion exercise. In the PIP and DIP joints, collateral ligament laxity is typically determined with the joint positioned in extension. It is possible to rupture only one portion of the ligament, however, in which case it is necessary to test the ligament in both flexion and extension. (Ligamentous laxity is highly variable. Compare laxity to a normal contralateral joint whenever possible.)

Clinical Goal 4.   Specific therapeutic measures. (a) Swan-neck deformity is a deformity that involves flexion of the MCP joint, hyperextension of the PIP joint, and flexion of the DIP joint. (See figure 32.5.) This deformity most frequently occurs in rheumatoid arthritis due to inflammation of the MCP joint, causing spasm of the intrinsic muscles and excessive pull on the lateral bands—hyperextending a vulnerable PIP joint. However, a swan-neck deformity can also result from DIP synovitis damaging the distal attachment of the extensor communis tendon.[30] Less frequently it occurs from PIP synovitis damaging the volar plate, which provides volar joint stability, or the attachment of the sublimus tendon.[30] The severity of this deformity is determined by the loss of PIP joint flexion; for it is the loss of flexion that interferes the most with functional ability.[34]

The first therapeutic measure for this condition is to rule out or eliminate intrinsic muscle tightness as a deforming force (as described earlier). If the condition is due to MCP synovitis and the PIP joints are not inflamed, splinting to control MCP inflammation and to counter intrinsic tightness may be effective for preventing progression of the deformity.[7]

Early splinting of the PIP joint to block hyperextension but allow full flexion (using a slip-on tripoint Aquaplast splint)[35] may encourage tightening of the volar structures in selected patients. However, this type of splinting is still experimental. There are several surgical options available for this condition including soft-tissue reconstructive arthroplasty or fusion in a functional position.[30]

(b) Boutonniere deformity in its early stages involves flexion of the PIP joint and hyperextension of the DIP joint. As the condition becomes established, hyperextension of the MCP joint occurs secondary to extending or clearing the fingertips during functional activities. Unlike the swan-neck deformity, which has three possible causes, the boutonniere only has one—synovitis of the PIP joint causing stretching of the central slip and volar slippage of the lateral bands.[8]

There have been informal reports of early splinting with a tripoint splint being effective in reducing incipient deformities. However, it is difficult to catch patients in the very early stages. In addition to routine range-of-motion exercises, antideformity exercises are beneficial in maintaining mobility. For the boutonniere deformity, these involve manually stabilizing the PIP joint in extension and actively flexing the DIP joint. Maintaining mobility is important for being able to don gloves and facilitates surgical repair and outcome.

(c) The mallet-finger deformity solely involves flexion of the DIP joint secondary to disruption of the distal attachment of the extensor communis tendon.[8] It is common in psoriatic arthritis due to synovitis and in osteoarthritis due to osteophyte formation. It is also possible to incur this condition secondary to trauma.[8]

In the treatment of this abnormality, splinting is rarely effective. Therapy

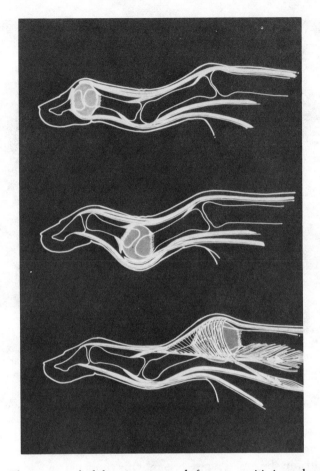

Figure 32.5.   The swan-neck deformity can result from synovitis in each of the digit joints. In rheumatoid arthritis the most common cause is synovitis of the MCP joints. Involvement of the DIP joint may either be synovitis, as in psoriatic arthritis, or osteophytes in osteoarthritis rupturing the distal attachment of the extensor communis tendon. Swan-neck deformity due to PIP synovitis is rare, since inflammation in this joint usually produces a flexion contracture, but it can produce a swan neck if the synovitis damages the volar plate.

primarily involves maintaining mobility. If the mallet deformity is beginning to contribute to swan-neck deformity, surgical intervention is prudent. The surgical procedure of choice is usually a DIP fusion in about 5° flexion.

Thumb Joints

Thumb deformities have been classified by Nalebuff into four general patterns and they result from either synovitis of the MCP or CMC joints.[36] Type I, the most common in rheumatoid arthritis, involves MCP synovitis leading to MCP

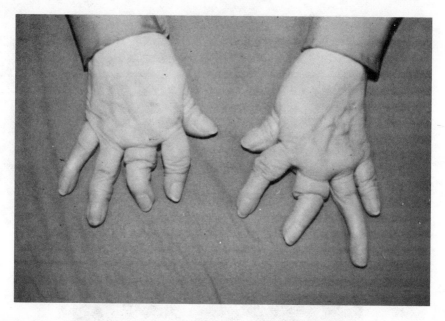

Figure 32.6. This patient has mutilans deformity (resorption of the ends of the phalanges) creating gross instability and shortening of all the digits except the left ring finger. This digit is unaffected because it has ankylosed spontaneously prior to mutilans. In the early stages of bone loss and instability, surgical fusion in a functional position can prevent progression of the mutilans.

flexion, IP hyperextension, and secondary CMC abduction. Type II and type III are due to synovitis of the CMC joint and therefore are far less common in rheumatoid arthritis. In these two types the synovitis results in an adduction contracture of the CMC joint. During hand function, the patient actively attempts to clear the thumb from the palm. If there is laxity of the IP joint, it will go into hyperextension, creating a type II pattern. If the MCP is lax, it will hyperextend, creating a type III deformity. (Although uncommon in rheumatoid arthritis, the type III is frequently seen in osteoarthritis.) The fourth type involves CMC adduction and lateral deviation of the MCP joint.

Mutilans Deformity

Fortunately this condition (figure 32.6), which involves resorption of the ends of the phalanges, producing floppy, unstable, short digits, is uncommon. There is no specific therapy for mutilans beyond adaptive equipment and medical attempts to arrest the inflammation. However, surgical fusion of a joint before digital length is lost can prevent progression of the resorption.[36] This can preserve functional ability, particularly in the index and thumb, where fusion in a functional position can provide stability for strong pinch.

SUMMARY

Patients with inflammatory arthritis of the hands tend to fall into three categories. First are patients with isolated joint or tendon involvement, in which it is easy to determine that all structures except the involved area are normal. Second are people with multiple joint and tendon involvement, for whom a cursory hand evaluation is not sufficient for revealing all nuances of hand pathodynamics necessary for planning treatment. And third are people with severe stage IV arthritis with fixed contractures, for whom therapy must be adaptive rather than corrective in nature.

It is the second group that requires some type of systematic assessment, reviewing the intricate interplay between the joints, tendons, ligaments, and muscles and providing objective measurements for maintaining function and determining the effectiveness of treatment. This type of assessment is documented in the literature[7] and is available in most occupational therapy departments as well as hand therapy centers throughout the United States. Physicians interested in providing preventive therapy for their arthritis patients with early hand involvement are encouraged to meet with therapists, who are skilled in hand therapy, in their community to set up a mechanism for providing comprehensive hand assessments and treatment.

REFERENCES

1. Jackson R. The cervical syndrome, 4th ed. Springfield, Ill.: Charles C Thomas, 1978.
2. Upton ARM, McComas AJ. The double crush in nerve entrapment syndromes. Lancet 1973;2:359–362.
3. Cailliet R. Neck and arm pain. Philadelphia: FA Davis, 1964.
4. Kozin F. Painful shoulder and the reflex sympathetic dystrophy syndrome. In: McCarthy DJ, ed. Arthritis and allied conditions, 9th ed. Philadelphia: Lea and Febiger, 1978, pp. 1091–1120.
5. Nakano KK. Entrapment neuropathies. In: Kelley WN, Harris ED, Ruddy S, Sledge CB, eds. Textbook of rheumatology. Philadelphia: WB Saunders, 1981.
6. Polley HF, Hunder GG. Rheumatological interviewing and physical examination of the joints, 2nd ed. Philadelphia: WB Saunders, 1978.
7. Melvin JL. Rheumatic disease: occupational therapy and rehabilitation, 2nd ed. Philadelphia: FA Davis, 1982.
8. Flatt AE. The care of the arthritis hand, 4th ed. St. Louis, Mo.: CV Mosby, 1982.
9. Wright V. Psoriatic arthritis. In: Kelley WN, Harris ED, Ruddy S, Sledge CB, eds. Textbook of rheumatology. Philadelphia: WB Saunders, 1981.
10. Hunter JM, Macklin EJ. Edema and bandaging. In: Hunter JM, Schneider LH, Macklin EJ, Bell CB. Rehabilitation of the hand. St. Louis, Mo.: CV Mosby, 1978.
11. Harris ED. Rheumatoid arthritis: the clinical spectrum. In: Kelley WN, Harris ED, Ruddy S, Sledge CB, eds. Textbook of rheumatology. Philadelphia: WB Saunders, 1981, p. 951.
12. Calabro J. Rheumatoid arthritis. Clin Symposia (CIBA) 1971;23(1).
13. Swanson AB. Flexible implant resection arthroplasty in the hand and extremities. St. Louis, Mo.: CV Mosby, 1973.

14. Bell JA. Plaster cylinder casting for contractures of the interphalangeal joints. In: Hunter JM, Schneider LH, Macklin EJ, Bell JA, eds. Rehabilitation of the hand. St. Louis, Mo.: CV Mosby, 1978.

15. Lampe E. Surgical anatomy of the hand. CIBA Pharmaceutical Company, Summit, N.J. 1969 (still available in 1981).

16. Lehmann JF, Warren CG, Scham SM. Therapeutic heat and cold. Clin Orthoped 1974;99:207–245.

17. Magness JL, Garrett TR, Erickson DJ. Swelling of the upper extremity during whirlpool baths. Arch Phys Med Rehab 1970;297–299.

18. Nalebuff EA. The recognition and treatment of tendon ruptures in the rheumatoid hand. In: American Association of Orthopedic Surgery symposium on tendon surgery in the hand. St. Louis, Mo.: CV Mosby, 1975.

19. Millender LH, Nalebuff EA. Preventative surgery-tenosynovectomy and synovectomy. Ortho Clin N Am 1975;6(3):765–792.

20. Medl WT. Tendonitis, tenosynovitis, "trigger finger," and de Quervain's disease. Ortho Clin N Am 1970;1:375–382.

21. Nakano KK. Entrapment neuropathies. In: Kelley WN, Harris ED, Ruddy S, Sledge CB, eds. Textbook of rheumatology. Philadelphia: WB Saunders, 1981.

22. Guide for muscle testing of the upper extremity. OT Department, Professional Staff Association of RLAH, Rancho Los Amigos Hospital, Downey, California, 1976.

23. Kendall HO, Kendall FP, Wadsworth GE. Muscles—testing and function, 2nd ed. Baltimore: Williams and Wilkins, 1971.

24. Daniels L, Worthingham C. Muscle testing: techniques of manual examination. Philadelphia: WB Saunders, 1972.

25. Pahle JA, Raunio P. The influence of wrist position on finger deviation in the rheumatoid hand. J Bone Joint Surg (B) 1969;51:664.

26. Smith EM, Juvinall R, Vender L, Pearson J. Role of finger flexors in rheumatoid deformities of the MCP joints. Arth Rheum 1964;7:467–480.

27. Smith RJ, Kaplan EB. Rheumatoid deformities of the MCP joints. J Bone Joint Surg (A) 1967;49:31.

28. Cordery JC. Joint protection: a responsibility of the OT. Am J Occup Ther 1965;19: 285–294.

29. Swezey RL, Fiegenberg DS. Inappropriate intrinsic muscle action in the rheumatoid hand. Ann Rheum Dis 1971;30:619–625.

30. Nalebuff EA, Millender LH. Surgical treatment of swan neck deformities in rheumatoid arthritis. Ortho Clin N Am 1975;6(3):733–752.

31. Boyes JH. Bunnell's surgery of the hand. 5th ed. Philadelphia: JB Lippincott, 1970.

32. Eaton RG. Joint injuries of the hand. Springfield, Ill.: Charles C Thomas, 1971.

33. Fess EE, Gettle KS, Strickland JW. Hand splinting—principles and methods. St. Louis, Mo.: CV Mosby, 1981.

34. Swanson AB. Flexible implant resection arthroplasty in the hand and extremities. St. Louis, Mo.: CV Mosby, 1973, p. 109.

35. WFR/Aquaplast Corporation, P.O. Box 215, Ramsey, N.J. 07446-0215.

36. Nalebuff EA, Garrett J. Opera glass hand in rheumatoid arthritis. J Hand Surg 1976; 1(3):210.

33

Knee Pain and Quadriceps Atrophy

Anneli H. Navarro, R.P.T., M.Ed.

The knee is frequently a major site of involvement in inflammatory, infectious, and degenerative forms of arthritis. Additional causes of impairment include trauma to the knee with resultant internal derangements, as well as a variety of metabolic, hematologic, neurologic, and neoplastic disorders. One must be aware that knee pain can be referred from the hip and patients without knee pathology will sometimes have knee effusion secondary to hip pathology. Thus the entire lower extremity must be examined even though signs and symptoms may suggest knee pathology. A common feature of most disorders affecting the knee is pain, which when ongoing characteristically results in quadriceps atrophy and knee flexion contracture.

The primary functions of this, the largest joint in the body, are weight-bearing and propulsion. In level walking alone, forces equal to 3 to 4 times body weight are transmitted through the articular surfaces of each knee upon each step taken.[1] Such forces are further increased in stair climbing and in sitting down and raising up to standing from low surfaces. Logically, disorders of the knee account for much of the disability associated with standing and walking. Although knee pain and quadriceps atrophy associated with rheumatoid arthritis are the subject of discussion in this chapter, the principles of management proposed apply also to other disorders of the knee with the same basic symptomatology.

MECHANISMS OF QUADRICEPS ATROPHY AND KNEE FLEXION CONTRACTURE

It has been shown that experimentally induced distension of the human knee joint using plasma is associated with an inability to contract the quadriceps muscle voluntarily.[2] Subjects with rheumatoid arthritis demonstrate less tolerance with earlier onset of pain on gradual distension of the knee joint, as compared to normal subjects. It has also been demonstrated that a strong quadriceps contraction increases the intra-articular pressure, and likewise the intra-articular pressure was found to be lowest with the knee in a position of slight flexion.

These findings suggest that increases in intra-articular pressure and pain are important factors in the development of both quadriceps atrophy and flexion contracture of the knee in rheumatoid arthritis.

General inactivity and cautiousness toward physical activity in the setting of joint disease probably further contribute to gradual disuse atrophy of muscle and limitation of motion in the affected joint. These processes often occur with alarming rapidity, with up to 5 percent loss of strength per day in the total absence of muscle contraction.[3]

MANAGEMENT

Muscle Strength

Since elevation of intra-articular pressure in the knee causes an apparent reflex inhibition of the quadriceps muscle, efforts to control knee joint distension are of primary importance in rheumatoid arthritis. Medical management with systemic or local drug therapy can be augmented with temporary immobilization of the knee using a cylinder splint, which has been shown to be effective in reducing pain and swelling without loss of range of motion or muscle strength.[4] Only after distension has been reduced can exercises to maintain or improve quadriceps strength be instituted without causing further reflex inhibition of the extensor mechanism. To minimize further the undesirable increases in joint pressure, the quadriceps muscle is strengthened with the knee maintained in a partially flexed position while any evidence of joint distension remains.

Maximal isometric contractions of the quadriceps muscle carried out on a regular basis are effective in increasing the strength of this muscle group.[5] Such isometric exercises need to be carried out with the knee also fully extended to strengthen the vastus medialis component of the quadriceps muscles, the former being responsible for the last 10° of knee extension.[6]

Weakening of the extensor mechanism leads to an imbalance between the extensor and flexor muscles of the knee. Persons with weak quadriceps muscles typically walk with stiff legs, locking the knees into a straight position to avoid buckling of the knees and falling. Repetitive stresses of this kind cause abnormal wear and hasten the development of deformity. With close medical and physical therapy monitoring and intervention, however, quadriceps atrophy connected with knee disorders is preventable, and if present, it can be effectively reversed.

Examples of isometric quadriceps exercises performed lying down are as follows:

Acute phase. With slightly bent knee, raise entire leg until heel is approximately 5 inches off the surface. Hold for 5 seconds. Return. Repeat 5 times.

Subacute phase. "Quad sets": stiffen the knee by pressing it firmly into the surface. Hold this contraction as strongly as possible for 5 seconds. Relax. Repeat 5 times.

Subacute and inactive phase. "Leg bounces": with straight stiff knee and strongly bent up foot, lightly and rapidly bounce the leg against the surface until *tired*. Relax. Perform once daily. Once weekly record the number of bounces to measure progress.

Range of Motion

Disorders to the knee, particularly chronic inflammatory processes, also predispose the knee to flexion contracture. Among causative factors can be identified the intra-articular pressure being lowest with the knee in partial flexion, increased discomfort when the knee is held in any other position, and the resultant protective muscle spasm to maintain the joint partially bent at all times. Soft-tissue adaptation will lead to eventual flexion contracture. A simple, daily program of exercises to improve the active range-of-motion program of the involved joint to prevent soft-tissue contracture must be instituted at the time of diagnosis and initiation of medical management. Gentle bending and straightening of the knee through its full range of motion a few times each day usually suffices as a preventive measure.

In the setting of recent-onset flexion contracture caused by soft-tissue shortening, permanent reelongation of these tissues is most effectively achieved through prolonged low-intensity stretching at elevated tissue temperatures, with stretching continued during the cooling-off period.[7,8] This technique can readily be applied to the knee with the patient lying on his stomach. A Hydrocollator pack on the posterior aspect of the knee and gravity dependent position with no weight or only little added weight at the ankle can be used to achieve the desired stretching.

The longer the duration of flexion contracture, the less likely it is to respond to the stretching regimen. As a last resort serial casting and traction to reduce long-standing flexion contractures are sometimes effective but not always recommended as these methods tend to cause undesirable compression of articular surfaces.[9] Thus prevention and early intervention are essential components of nonsurgical management of knee flexion contracture.

Locomotion

Increases in flexion contracture and decreases in total available range of motion at the knee correlate with increases in knee pain.[10] The greater the degree of weight-bearing pain, the less loading of the knee can be tolerated. This leads to characteristic alterations of gait, with delay in loading and premature unloading on the affected side, as well as decreased walking speed, shorter steps, and fewer steps per minute. Such changes in gait correlate not only with walking pain and night pain, but inversely also with quadriceps strength.[11]

Thus knee pain, the availability of adequate range of motion in the knee, and quadriceps strength all are important determinants of locomotion and ultimately of many activities of daily life for the person with knee disorder. Each of these potentially disabling factors can be dealt with preventively.

Patient Education

A specified exercise program designed to maintain or increase joint range of motion and quadriceps strength must be accompanied by instruction in methods to reduce undue stresses on the compromised knee joint.

Particularly stressful activities include deep knee bends and stair-climbing. Knee bends should be avoided altogether, and stair-climbing may need to be reduced as much as possible or modified, leading with the better leg going up, and with the more involved leg going down each step.

Raising to standing from a chair and sitting down frequently aggravate knee pain. The following method to raise to standing reduces the time and magnitude of abnormal forces to the knee:

1. Move forward in the chair.
2. Place feet under the knees.
3. Keep knees separated throughout procedure.
4. Place palms on arm rests or on seat next to thighs.
5. Lean forward and push up with hands until knees are straight (figure 33.1).
6. When stable on the feet, let go with hands and straighten up the back.

This process is reversed for sitting down. Strong quadriceps muscles are required for patient confidence and best possible stability while raising to standing or sitting down.

Canes or crutches may be used to reduce weight-bearing stresses on the knee. The physical therapist fits the device to the patient and teaches its proper and safe usage.

To lessen the risk of insidious onset flexion contracture in the knee, prone lying on a regular daily basis is recommended. A small pillow under the lower abdomen with feet hanging freely over the edge of the bed assures maximum comfort and efficacy of stretching. It must be clearly understood by the patient that a pillow or any other support under the knee used on a regular basis increases the risk for flexion contracture.

The fact that there is a threefold body weight loading of the knee on level normal walking suggests that weight control is an important factor in joint protection. For the same reason swimming is a particularly beneficial form of activity permitting vigorous muscle-strengthening, range-of-motion, and cardiovascular conditioning exercises without undue stress on vulnerable joints.[12]

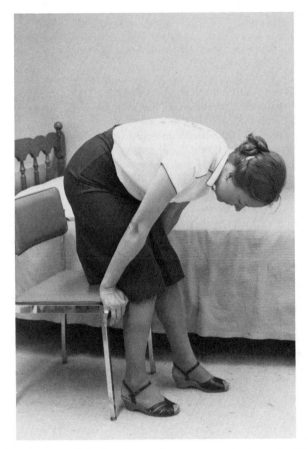

Figure 33.1   Pushing up with the hands to reduce stress on the knees in rising from a seat.

Interestingly, research currently underway suggests the stationary bicycle can be used by persons with rheumatoid arthritis to improve physical capacity as measured by exercise tolerance, aerobic capacity, and cardiac response without causing increase in joint symptoms or other disease manifestations.[13]

SUMMARY

Pain, quadriceps atrophy, and limitation of motion are serious threats to knee function—that is, weight-bearing and propulsion. Suppression of inflammation is essential for successful rehabilitation of the knee. Additionally a program of isometric and range-of-motion exercises designed to maintain quadriceps strength and for the particular needs of the patient should be part of early intervention. Patient education, including instruction in joint-protection measures, is another valuable component of early management.

REFERENCES

1. Morrison JB. The forces transmitted by the human knee joint during activity. Thesis, University of Strathclyde, Scotland, 1967.
2. deAndrade JR, Grant C, Dixon A St. L. Joint distension and reflex muscle inhibition in the knee. J Bone and Joint Surg (A) 1965;47(2):313–322.
3. Müller EA. Influence of training and of inactivity on muscle strength. Arch Phys Med Rehab 1970;(8):449–462.
4. Nicholas JJ, Ziegler G. Cylinder splints: their use in the treatment of arthritis of the knee. Arch Phys Rehab 1977;58 (June):264–267.
5. Machover S, Sapecky AJ. Effect of isometric exercise on the quadriceps muscle in patients with rheumatoid arthritis. Arch Phys Med Rehab 1966;47 (Nov.):737–741.
6. Lieb FJ, Perry J. Quadriceps function: an electromyographic study under isometric conditions. J Bone Joint Surg (A) 1971;53(3):749–758.
7. Lehmann JF, et al. Effect of therepeutic temperatures on tendon extensibility. Arch Phys Med Rehab 1970;51(Aug.):481–487.
8. Sapega AA, Quedenfeld TC, Moyer RA, et al. Biophysical factors in range-of-motion exercise. Physician Sports Med 1981;9(12):57–65.
9. Marmor L. Arthritis surgery. Philadelphia: Lea and Febiger, 1976.
10. Kettlekamp DB, Leaverton PE, Misol S. Gait characteristics of the rheumatoid knee. Arch Surg 1972;104 (Jan.):30–34.
11. Györy AN, Chao EYG, Stauffer RN. Functional evaluation of normal and pathologic knees during gait. Arch Phys Med Rehab 1976;57 (Dec.):571–577.
12. Scott FE. Arthritis: a patient's view. Phys Ther 1969;49:373–376.
13. Beals C. A case for aerobic conditioning exercise in rheumatoid arthritis. Clin Res 1981;29(4):780A.

34

Rheumatic Conditions Causing Hip Pain

Anneli H. Navarro, R.P.T., M.Ed.

The most common cause of hip pain in older persons is degenerative joint disease. Hip pain with resultant disability may occur at any age, however, when caused by inflammatory arthritis, as in juvenile chronic polyarthritis, rheumatoid arthritis, and the spondyloarthropathies. Furthermore, in ankylosing spondylitis a less than optimal spinal posture must be compensated for by flexion of hips and knees to enable the patient to see in front of him while upright. This flexion posture of hips and knees may cause soft-tissue shortening with resultant flexion contractures of those joints.

Other causes of hip pain include inflammation of the adjacent bursae as well as referred pain from the lumbosacral spine. Ischemic necrosis of bone, most commonly seen in the femoral head, has been associated with many causes including alcoholism, collagen diseases and with the use of steroid therapy. An early sign of ischemic necrosis of the femoral head, prior to discernible x-ray change, is hip pain on ambulation.[1]

Clinical Manifestations

Degenerative joint disease is perhaps the most common problem seen by physicians and allied health practitioners. Like rheumatoid arthritis degenerative joint disease is also associated with morning stiffness and stiffness after stationary positions. However, the stiffness of degenerative joint disease usually lasts only a brief period of time. Characteristically the hip pain is worsened by activity and tends to increase as the day progresses; in the advanced stage of disease it may interfere with the patient's ability to sleep. In early disease the patient exhibits an antalgic gait, in which the stance phase of the involved extremity is characterized by delayed loading and premature unloading of the limb.

Other early findings include loss of internal rotation and extension, which may progress to a classical triad of flexion, adduction, and external rotation deformities of the involved hip. Loss of hip flexion is also characteristic. Pelvic tilt with the involved side elevated adds to a functional shortening of the limb. The discrepancy in leg length must be compensated for by flexion of the opposite knee on walking, which may lead to a long-leg arthropathy of that knee. Problems with locomotion and other aspects of function will increase if the degenerative process is allowed to continue without intervention.

TREATMENT

Heat Therapy

In early disease superficial heat is used with success to relieve stiffness and to reduce pain, which is thought to be aggravated by secondary spasm of muscles surrounding the joint. Hydrocollator packs wrapped around the hip joint, immersion into a whirlpool, Hubbard tank or heated pool may be selected in an institutional setting. The advantage of immersion therapy is a major one, in that quite vigorous joint range-of-motion and muscle-strengthening exercises can be performed with minimal stress on the compromised joint. A warm bath or shower is a good source of moist heat for regular use at home. Heat is generally used in preparation for exercise and activity but may also be enjoyed as a means of relaxation after activity.

Deep heating by ultrasound is often prescribed in chronic disease processes for treatment of joint contractures caused by scarring of the capsule and other periarticular soft tissues. With as yet many unanswered questions regarding thermal as well as nonthermal effects of deep heating,[2] coupled with mounting evidence pointing to cartilage degeneration caused by local hyperthermia in inflamed joints,[3,4] the use of deep heating for inflammatory and degenerative joint disease must be seriously questioned. The latter concern arises from the fact that secondary synovitis is not an infrequent finding in degenerative joint disease.[5]

Prescribed Exercise

Heat therapy is normally accompanied or followed by prescribed exercise. Three major aims of exercise can be identified in degenerative disease of the hip. One aim is to maintain—or if already reduced, to increase—joint range of motion. Special emphasis needs to be placed on the preservation of motion in flexion, extension, abduction, and internal rotation of the hip. This is preferably worked on in hydrotherapy, especially if such exercises would cause increased joint symptoms when performed out of the water. Progression to exercise out of water may include sling suspension exercise with regulation of gravity, active exercise, and stretching exercises combining gravity and local moist heat.

A second aim of exercise is to maintain optimal strength of muscles surrounding the joint. Potential disuse atrophy combined with muscle imbalance as a result of protective muscle spasm add to the instability of the joint and may lead to decreased safety in transfers, standing, and walking. Particular attention needs to be given to the strength of hip extensors and abductors and the quadriceps muscle groups bilaterally. The methods of choice to build up muscle strength are isometric exercises or pool therapy, as mechanical stresses on a joint afflicted by degenerative changes may cause secondary synovitis and further deterioration of the articular cartilage.[6]

A third aim of exercise is to restore optimal cardiorespiratory condition. Studies have shown that the oxygen requirement for walking a defined distance in patients with unilateral degenerative joint disease of the hip is approximately twice the normal requirement.[7] Slower walking speed and use of ambulation devices are contributing factors to the increased energy cost. Aerobic conditioning exercises that are well tolerated by the patient with joint disease may be difficult to find, however. By trying different activities, such as swimming, walking, dancing, and calisthenics, patients often find out what works best for them.

When a patient is referred to a physical therapist for exercise, the actual treatment is selected on the basis of physician's prescription, findings from a thorough clinical evaluation performed by the therapist, patient tolerance and response to therapy, as well as resources available to the therapist.

Every patient with hip disease should know how to use heat at home and what to do to preserve best possible joint range of motion, muscle strength, and general fitness. A home program of heat and exercise may include the following:

Generalized heat in form of bath or shower. Hydrocollator packs or electric heating pad may be used for local heat directly over the joint.

Range-of-motion exercise lying flat on top of bed.
1. Raise knee as high up toward chest as possible. Return. Repeat 3–5 times.
2. Slide leg as far out to the side as possible. Return. Repeat 3–5 times.
3. With legs slightly apart, roll legs inward. Relax. Repeat 3–5 times.

Strengthening exercise lying flat and supine on top of bed.
1. "Quad sets": make the knee stiff by pressing it down into the bed. This will tighten the muscle in front of the thigh. Hold this contraction as strongly as possible for 5 seconds. Relax. Repeat 5 times.
2. "Gluteal sets": squeeze the buttocks together as firmly as possible. Hold this contraction for 5 seconds. Relax. Repeat 5 times.
3. Thread a loop over the ankles (insert feet into a pillow case or use elastic webbing or bath towel tied into a loop). As strongly as possible press the legs apart inside the loop. Hold this contraction for 5 seconds. Relax. Repeat 5 times.

Conditioning exercise chosen on the basis of acceptability and availability to the patient.
1. Swimming, walking, or exercising in a heated pool.
2. Stationary bicycle with no or minimal resistance, walking, and dancing, as tolerated.

3. Physical fitness type exercises for the upper extremities and the trunk.
4. Continue customary activities of daily life, as tolerated.

Functional Training

Given hip pain as the primary complaint, a clinical assessment should include a thorough evaluation of not only articular and muscular status, but also the patient's ability to perform needed activities of daily life. To compensate for losses in the hip, exaggerated demands will be placed on the ipsilateral knee and ankle[8] and the contralateral limb. Gait[9] and posture will be altered and patient may experience difficulty in sitting, rising to standing, ascending and descending stairs. Reaching to the feet for cleaning and manipulation of lower extremity clothing and shoes may be difficult, especially if knee flexion is also impaired.

With early institution of therapy combining heat and prescribed exercise to optimize joint mobility, muscle strength, and overall fitness, functional impairment should remain at a minimum. However, when normalcy in function can no longer be obtained, functional training is aimed at safety and independence in any given task. Thus alternate methods for performing a task need to be developed when the usual method is no longer possible or safe. Since a great number of falls in the home take place on stairs and in the bathroom, special emphasis needs to be placed on safety training in these areas.[10]

Using bathing as an example, the sequence of goals and therapy may flow as follows:

1. Try to restore independence and safety in tub bathing. Use exercise to improve or maintain joint range of motion and muscle strength. Practice difficult components of tasks such as lowering into the tub or rising from the tub. Employ assistive devices such as nonskid mats and bathtub safety rails.
2. Find an alternative method of bathing, such as the shower. Exercise and practice alternate methods. Use assistive devices such as a tub seat for seated transfer into tub, grab bars, shower stool, and hand shower.
3. Find a substitute, such as sponge bathing. Exercise; practice the substitute method; employ assistive devices (a scrub sponge or sponge wash mit).

Assistive Devices

An ever-increasing number of assistive devices designed specifically for persons with arthritis can be found.[11] Such devices offer safety, independence, and joint protection. (See chapter 23.) Each device must be individually prescribed and personally fitted, and the patient must be taught its proper use. The person with hip pain and associated losses may benefit from some of the devices described in the following paragraphs.

Canes and crutches. A cane or crutch is used on the side opposite to the involved hip. As the ambulation device is to be moved simultaneously with the involved leg, this will allow for normal, reciprocal arm and leg movements during gait. (See chapter 20.) A functional handle cane or platform crutch may be preferable if hands and wrists are also involved. Two crutches may be required to assure safety and adequate protection of the joint. Steps and curbs are negotiated leading with the "good" leg going up and with the involved leg going down when the normal method is not possible or desirable.

Raised surfaces. Pain with limitations of motion in the hip makes it particularly difficult to use low surfaces for sitting. Raised toilet seats and high chairs with one side cut down to accommodate a stiff hip are available through local surgical supply houses or through mail order companies specializing in self-help aids.

Self-care devices. A bath sponge with a long handle may be needed to clean the feet. Useful dressing aids include sock and stockings pusher/pullers, dressing sticks, long-handled shoe horns, and elastic shoe laces (figure 34.1). A reacher to pick up items from the floor is helpful when bending down is not possible or safe.

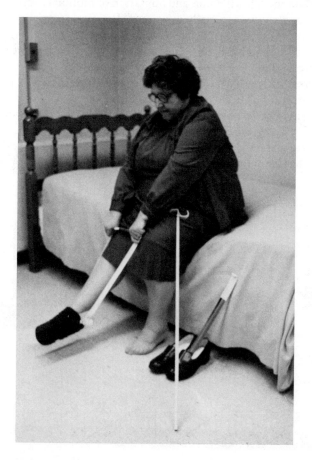

Figure 34.1. A stocking donner is being used by the woman in the photograph; also shown are a dressing stick and long shoe horn.

Patient Education

An understanding of the disease process and effects of drug therapy, heat, prescribed exercise, rest, and activity should be complemented with specific skills in joint protection. Since mechanical stresses accelerate the degenerative process, the patient needs to find ways to reduce weight-bearing on the hip.[12] Reduction in the amount of walking and especially stair-climbing as well as sitting to perform an activity rather than prolonged standing are helpful. This can be planned with the therapist and physician depending on patient tolerance. Weight reduction in the obese patient is generally considered advisable, although frequently difficult to attain. Daily prone positioning, if tolerated, may be helpful in early disease to prevent flexion contracture of the hip. (See figure 34.2.) Attention to the alignment of the leg in bed avoiding habitual posturing of the leg, especially propped up with pillows, is also important. Pillows under the knee lead to hip and knee flexion contractures.

Arthritis in the hip with pain and limitation of motion is very likely to interfere with sexual activity, especially in women. Practical suggestions can be given to circumvent some of the problems experienced by the patient.[13-15] (See chapter 29.) Planning sexual activity for the time of day when the patient feels best and most energetic is wise. The use of moist heat, range-of-motion exercises, relaxation procedures, and perhaps some analgesics or muscle relaxants prior to sexual activity are helpful. Positioning of the affected partner as comfortably as possible is helpful. Trying out new positions that put less strain on painful joints as well as propping with pillows are simple measures to improve comfort. Communication between the partners about physical limitations, fears of pain, and sexual preferences helps to eliminate many unnecessary problems.

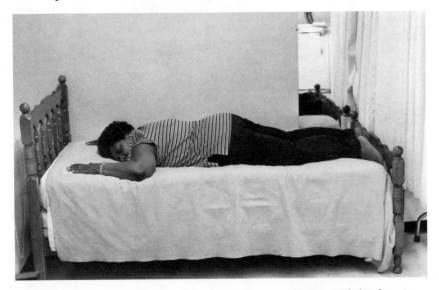

Figure 34.2. Patient in early stage of disease lies in prone position with feet hanging over the edge of the bed daily to prevent flexion contracture of the hip.

SUMMARY

Much can be done to help the patient with hip pain remain comfortable and able to continue needed activities of daily life, as listed in table 34.1. Early intervention should include close attention to the particular needs of the patient with regard to application of heat, specific exercises, posture, gait, necessary functional skills, and patient education. As the disease progresses, periodic reevaluations must be undertaken to update and modify the patient's home therapy program. Carefully selected assistive devices may be prescribed to provide joint protection and improved safety or to compensate for specific losses of function that may appear with time. Finally, great advances in joint-replacement surgery, particularly of the hips, have made such a procedure a viable option for most people with severe joint disease.

Table 34.1.   Treatment Summary

- Superficial heat application
- Prescribed exercise
  - Range of motion
  - Muscle strength
  - General fitness
- Functional skills training
  - Mobility
  - Self-care
- Assistive devices
  - Ambulation
  - Self-care
  - Joint protection
- Patient education
  - Disease process
  - Medical management
  - Patient's own role in managing the disease

REFERENCES

1. Zizik TM, Hungerford DS, Stevens MB. Ischemic bone necrosis in systemic lupus erythematosus. I: The early diagnosis of ischemic necrosis of bone. Med 1980;59(2): 134–142.
2. Lehmann JF, Warren CG, Schan SM. Therapeutic heat and cold. Clin Orthoped Related Res 1974;99 (March–April):207–245.
3. Feibel A, Fast A. Deep heating of joints: a reconsideration. Arch Phys Med Rehab 1976;57(11):513–514.
4. Mitrovic DR, Gruson M, Ryckewaert A. Local hyperthermia and cartilage breakdown. J Rheum 1981;8(2):193–203.
5. Howell DS, Woessner JF, Jimenez S, et al. A view of the pathogenesis of osteoarthritis. Bull Rheum Dis 1978–79;29(8):996–1001.

6. Radin EL. Mechanical aspects of osteoarthrosis. Bull Rheum Dis 1975–76; 26(7):862–865.

7. Macnicol MF, Mettardy R, Chalmers J. Exercise testing before and after hip arthroplasty. J Bone Joint Surg 1980;62-B(3):326–331.

8. Saunders M, Inman VT, Eberhart HD. Major determinants in normal and pathological gait. J Bone Joint Surg (A) 1953;35:543–558.

9. Murray MP. Gait as a total pattern of movement. Am J Phys Med 1967; 46(1):290–333.

10. Rodstein M. Accidents among the aged: incidence, causes and prevention. J Chron Dis 1964;17:515–526.

11. Self-help manual for patients with arthritis. Atlanta: Arthritis Foundation, 1979.

12. Moskowitz RW. Management of osteoarthritis. Hosp Prac 1979;14(7): 75–87.

13. Boggs J. Living and loving with arthritis: information on sex and arthritis. 1975. Arthritis Center of Hawaii. 347 North Kuakini Street, Honolulu, 96817.

14. Zimmerman D. Sex can help arthritis. Penthouse Forum Magazine, November 1975. (available from Arthritis Foundation, Atlanta.)

15. Richards JS. Sex and arthritis. Sexual Disabil 1980;3:97–104.

35

Disorders of the Foot

Martin Snyder, D.P.M.

HEEL PAIN

The human foot consists of twenty-six bones. The articulating surfaces between these bones along with the supportive soft-tissue elements are prone to the complications of arthritis. Many rheumatic diseases affect the feet either primarily or secondarily. Factors producing pain in the heel are many. The complaint may be at the attachment of the plantar aponeurosis on the bottom of the heel, or it may be felt at the rear of the calcaneous where the achilles tendon inserts.[1] Primary conditions that cause pain in the heel would include some of the inflammatory arthritidies such as rheumatoid arthritis (see figure 35.1) as well as primary bone disorders and infections.[2] Secondary causes of painful heels are due in part to the biomechanical dysfunction of proximal components of the musculoskeletal system (see table 35.1). Prime examples include arthritis of the hips or knees. In each instance abnormal stance or swing phase of the gait cycle is the genesis of improper foot function. Tarsal coalitions and neurologic diseases may also cause such pain. Differences in leg length can produce unilateral heel pain and should always be considered.

Pain and stiffness are the symptoms most frequently noted by the patient. The discomfort can range from mild transient aching to severe unremitting pain. The pain may be present whether the patient is at rest or ambulating. Objective signs include edema, color changes, and temperature variations. Palpation of the area often reveals the precise location of the pathology. Radiographs may delineate not only osseous changes but also the soft-tissue abnormalities.

The treatment of heel pain is discussed from a conservative viewpoint. Semantics are important in accurately describing to the orthotist the exact device that will best serve the patient. Since primary goals include restoration of function and reduction of pain and disability, the various appliances and devices that may be fabricated are important.[3] (See table 35.2.)

The orthoses that reduce heel pain may be classified into two major categories: (1) soft, yielding, and accommodative or (2) firm, restrictive, and con-

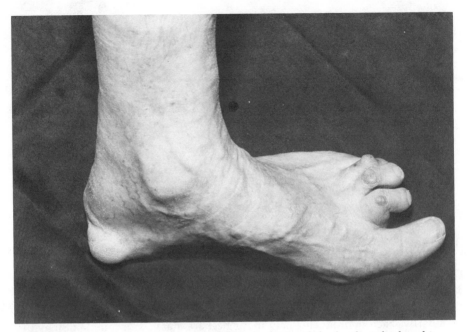

Figure 35.1.   Various foot pathologies both at the heel and the forefoot displayed in a 60-year-old man with rheumatoid arthritis. A rheumatoid nodule is very evident at the heel.

Table 35.1.   Heel Pain—Primary and Secondary Causes

Primary Causes	Secondary Causes
Ankylosing spondylitis	Tarsal coalitions
Reiter's disease	Limb length differentials
Psoriatic arthritis	Arthritidies of proximal skeletal components
Inflammatory bowel disease	Pes cavus
Rheumatoid arthritis	Neurotrophic subtalar joint
Gout	Pes planovalgus
Scleroderma	
Paget's disease	
Xanthoma of the Achilles tendon	
Osteomyelitis	
Primary bone tumors	
Avascular necrosis	
Subtalar arthritis	
Achilles tenosynovitis	
Metastatic neoplasms	

Table 35.2.   Etiology of Midtarsal Joint Pain

Primary Causes	Secondary Causes
Degenerative joint disease	Subtalar joint arthritis
Severe pes planus	Ehlers Danlos disease
Dorsal tendonitis	Marfan's syndrome
Cruciate ligament rupture	Rear-foot valgus
Tarsal coalitions (calcaneonavicular bar)	Talipes adductus
Rheumatoid arthritis	Neurotrophic joint
Gout	
Hyperparathyroidism	
Pseudohyperparathyroidism	

trolling. The first class includes Spenco®[a], Reston®[b], polyurethane, soft sponge rubber, Plastizote®[c], MOLO®[d], and latex devices made to the casts of the heels with protective or cut-out areas. All of these materials can be used to cushion the heel. Soft felt may be placed in the heel of the shoe to relieve pressure at the top of the counter area. This is very effective, if, for example, a rheumatoid nodule is located just above the attachment of the achilles tendon. (See figure 35.2.)

More rigid materials are employed when control of the foot is mandatory. Orthoses made from leather reinforced with fiberglass, Celastic®[e], or metal springs can be made over a cast of the foot. The same is true for appliances fabricated from a variety of thermoplastic materials, such as Rhoadur®[f], polyethylene, or similar substances.[4] Control of the rear foot is a prime reason for using these rigid devices. Since the calcaneus comprises the lower half of the subtalar joint, the talus being the superior component, and this articulation is vital to normal foot function, one must consider the total effect of this orthosis. The control that a rigid appliance places upon the rear foot may result in stress or torque to the entire lower limb. The rotation of the lower leg (or lack of rotation) influences the talus through the action of the mortise formed by the lower ends of the tibia and fibula.[4] The reverse action of the talus through the control of the calcaneus may inhibit or increase the lower limb torque. Overcorrection at the subtalar joint may force a lateral rotary force that could create stresses applied to the knee joint in particular. It would be wise to caution patients with rear-foot control appliances that are rigid to look for possible discomfort at the knee level.

®[a]   Spenco Medical Products, 603 Imperial Drive, Waco, Texas 76710.
®[b]   3M Center, St. Paul, Minn. 55144.
®[c]   Alimed Corp., 168 Harrison Avenue, Boston, Mass. 02111
®[d]   Molo Products, 4500 Old Vestal Road, Binghamton, N.Y. 13903
®[e]   XLO Products, New York, N.Y. 10001
®[f]   Teltscher Corp., Mt. Kisco, N.Y. 10549

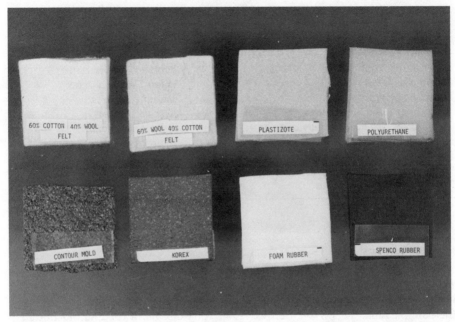

Figure 35.2. Materials that are used for support and cushioning of painful plantar lesions are shown. Clockwise from upper left corner there is felt that is 60 percent cotton and 40 percent wool for firmness, and felt that is 60 percent wool and 40 percent cotton for softness; Plastizote®, which has a giving quality for relief of severe plantar lesions; polyurethane, a compound that is extra soft and lightweight; Spenco® rubber, designed to absorb torque as well as shock; foam rubber for cushioning; korex, a firm compound to add to various appliances for balance; contour mold, a material that has compressibility yet memory.

The footgear that a patient uses is either soft or firm. Crepe-soled shoes or shoes with Spenco® insoles will reduce shearing forces. Foam rubber inside footwear can reduce the impact of the heels upon contact with the ground. Soft-counter shoes such as tennis or running shoes can eliminate or reduce counter pressure on the back of the heel. Shoes that are made over casts of the feet or that have extra-depth inlays are designed to accommodate areas of tenderness. Orthopedic footwear features elongated medial counters as well as heavy ribbed steel shanks and Thomas heels. A Thomas heel is slightly higher on the medial side and is extended forward approximately 1 to 2 inches. Heel valgus may be reduced by the extra support and firmness found in these shoes.[5] Furthermore, when orthoses are used in this type of footwear, the effect of control by the device is enhanced. (See table 35.2.)

In summary, management of heel pain requires accurate diagnosis, podiatric evaluation of the biomechanical function of the foot, and fabrication of an appliance by an orthotist. Knowing what is needed, how it should be made, and the best material for maximum results is best facilitated by teamwork.

MIDTARSAL FOOT PAIN

As the weight of the body moves forward and applies pressure upon the more distal part of the foot, the midtarsal joint becomes a prime area for distress. This joint encompasses three articulations of four bones: the talocalcaneal (or subtalar joint), the talonavicular, and the calcaneocuboid.[6] When alignment of these articulations is disturbed, excess wear of the opposing cartilagenous surfaces may eventually lead to osteophyte proliferation. Patients will complain of midfoot pain on ambulation especially when they are not wearing shoes. The dorsum may appear edematous. If there is concomitant plantar fascial strain, a buckling effect is produced on the dorsal joint surfaces. Tenderness of palpation or crepitus with motion may be elicited, but such patients do not have discomfort at rest. Passive motion of the toes may produce pain in the area of the midtarsal joint. Radiographic findings include narrowed joint spaces, osteophytes, and midtarsal joint subluxation.[7] This pathology may cause pain but also can be secondary to joint laxity. The hyperelasticity and increased motion seen as a result of joint injury, aging, or the primary collagen disorders weaken the supportive fascial structures and cause pinching of the dorsal surfaces of the tarsal bones. Pain at the midtarsal joint may have numerous causes. (See table 35.3).

Conservative treatment of midtarsal pain consists of either external or internal shoe modifications as well as orthoses. Firm sponge-rubber scaphoid pads can be used to relieve pain. Medial heel wedges in the heel seat or as an addition to the heel will further enhance the effect of the pads for the longitudinal arch. The wedges thus employed cause an inversion pressure applied to the heel and arch supporting the midtarsal joint and preventing the buckling effect. (See chapter 8 on role of the podiatrist, prosthetist, and orthotist.)

Orthoses fabricated from rigid material will control the rear foot and prevent dorsal squeezing of the midtarsal joint bones. Side-laced shoes made to a cast of the foot or Plastizote shoes® c with Velcro closures will reduce dorsal pressure. Any device must be accurate as to elevation, grade of material to be used, and the location of pressure from the appliance itself. For these one must choose a competent podiatrist to order the proper orthosis and an orthotist to complete the fabrication. Some devices may require a Morton syndrome extension, which is an extension to include the first metatarsophalangeal joint. These should be of sufficient size and thickness. With all rigid orthoses, patients should be given complete instructions regarding the wearing of such appliances. Instructions in writing are acceptable. Knee or thigh discomfort may result from prolonged wear initially and patients must be alerted to this possibility. It is

Table 35.3. Materials and Orthoses to Relieve Midtarsal and Forefoot Pain

	Pain in Dorsum of Foot	Pain in First mpj	Longitudinal Arch Pain	Forefoot Valgus	Hammer Toes	Bunions	Pain Area Mpj Areas
Scaphoid pads	B	C	A	C	C	B	B
Metatarsal pads	B	C	C	C	B	B	A
Metatarsal bars	B	B	C	B	B	C	A
Orthopedic shoes including Thomas heels, steel shanks, and long counters	C	B	B	B	C	A	A
Custom-molded shoes	A	A	A	B	A	A	A
Spenco insoles	A	A	B	C	A	A	A
Plastizote	B	A	B	C	B	B	A
Soft cushioning materials, e.g., foam rubber or polyurethane	B	B	B	C	B	B	A
Morton syndrome pads	B	A	C	A	C	B	A
Leather orthoses	A	B	A	A	A	B	B
Soft orthoses, e.g., sponge rubber or grindable rubber	A	B	B	A	C	C	B

A—usually effective; B—may be effective; C—not effective.

incumbent upon the prescribing professional to check the appliances when they are obtained by the patient.

FOREFOOT

When the heel leaves the plane of support, all body weight is transmitted to the metatarsal heads and the digits. Any pathology present in the rear foot and midfoot is translated to the metatarsals. The variety of pain and deformity develops according to the disease. The osseous changes in osteoarthritis are usually not as severe as those found in the inflammatory diseases. The osteoarthritic patient may have reduced motion at the first metatarsophalangeal joint. Often a large spur may be visualized on radiographs or palpated at the head of the first metatarsal. When osseous erosions occur as with rheumatoid arthritis, advanced hallux valgus may exist along with fibular deviation of the lesser digits. Hammer toes and overlapping digits are also common with the destructive process of the rheumatoid patient.[8] (See figure 35.3.) Gout may also cause erosion or even tophi in advanced cases. Patients with psoriatic arthritis may exhibit destruction of the joints, including bony resorption, subluxation, and even dislocation in later stages.

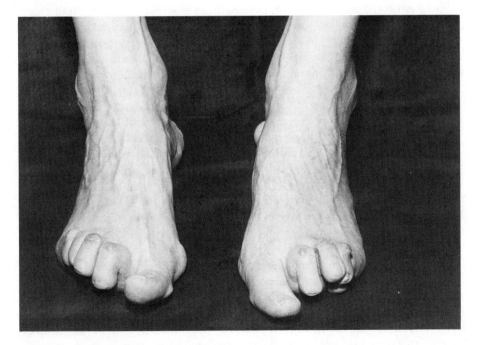

Figure 35.3.   Digital deformities including overlapping toes and hammer toes exhibited in a rheumatoid arthritis patient. Note the corn formation on several proximal interphalangeal joints.

Therapy in the early stages of all of the forefoot deformities is conservative. Prevention of hallux valgus may be accomplished by the use of commercial slings or nighttime braces. These are available in podiatric offices or pharmacies. Exercise and manipulation under supervision of trained professionals can be very helpful. If acute bursitis accompanies the enlarged bunion joint, careful padding with felt, Reston®, or foam rubber will allay shoe irritation. Advanced hallux valgus with digital rotation of the great toe and underlapping an adjacent toe is generally unresponsive to conservative care. The podiatric or orthopedic surgeon must be consulted in these end-stage cases of severe and complicated bunion deformities. After surgical correction postoperative management is essential and should be carried out by a skilled specialist trained in that field. The use of some orthotic often is used to prevent further changes in the structures involved.

Hammer-toe deformities can be commonly encountered[9] and can be treated in several ways. Metatarsal pads in the shoes or bars placed on the outside can distribute weight away from painful areas. These are located plantarly and result from the subluxation of the proximal phalanx upon the metatarsal head. The elevation of the proximal bone of the digit and the resultant flexion of the middle phalanx are the hallmark of the hammer-toe deformity. Pressure on the proximal interphalangeal joint can be relieved by shoes with high toe boxes. Digital crest pads can be used. These are employed in the sulcus area under the toes to encourage intrinsic foot muscles to plantar flex the proximal phalanx and reduce the subluxation at the metatarsal head. Hammer toes often may be the result of excessive plantar flexion when forefoot splaying is excessive. Semirigid orthoses to control the rear foot can be very helpful in reducing the forefoot problem and reverse the attitude of the digits themselves. When shoe pressure causes irritation at the proximal interphalangeal joint with the formation of ulceration, soft cushioning materials with apertures to protect the ulcer can heal these lesions. Latex appliances made over a cast of the deformed toe can reduce pressure. Shoes made to a cast of the foot will provide pressure relief to all areas of bony prominence. These are especially useful if the patient is a poor surgical risk.

Soft-tissue changes are another very commonly seen pathology in forefoot lesions. These generally occur under the metatarsal heads and were mentioned briefly in the earlier paragraph. The usual changes include swelling under the involved bones and frequently present heavy callus formation (figure 35.4). Metatarsal bars and pads are very often used and can help a great many patients. Plastizote® or Spenco® reduces pressure and friction. When heavy callus produces an ulcer, cut-off paddings or felt or foam rubber relieves or reduces the force that causes the skin erosion. At times the only relief of pressure is an osteotomy performed at the metatarsal neck. Permitting the head to float erases the plantar stress and will allow the ulcer to heal. Naturally the medical status including the variability of the vascular bed must be considered. Adventitious bursae frequently accompany either hallux valgus or the condition found at the head of the fifth metatarsal referred to as "tailor's bunion," or bunionette. Bursae are the product of excessive pressure, either from shoes themselves or the splaying of the forefoot. In either case apertured pads of felt or layers of Reston® will reduce the

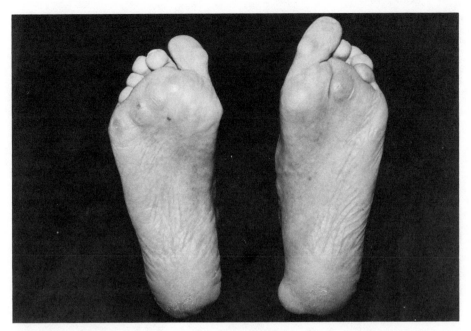

Figure 35.4.   Soft-tissue swelling under the metatarsal heads is very evident in this rheumatoid patient. Besides the submetatarsal lesions, note the nodules under the great toe and at the heel.

stress and bursa. Some arthritidies create swellings like bursae, and they must be treated by aspiration and possible excision. A rheumatoid nodule is a prime example.

NAIL CARE

The toenails, especially those of the great toe, can suggest the cause of the arthritis. The common arthritidies that manifest nail problems are Reiter's syndrome, psoriatic arthritis, and rheumatoid arthritis. Both Reiter's and psoriatic arthritis cause a lifting of the nail plate (onycholysis).[10] In the former a pustular nodule develops under the nail plate and lifts it, permitting subungual debris to form. The psoriatic patient forms small punctate depressions (pits) on the plate itself. The systemic component of the psoriasis affects the nail matrix, resulting in a thickened and irregular nail plate (figure 35.5). The nail bed also is involved, and the eventual pressure from both may lead to ulceration of the nail bed. The rheumatoid patient develops a nail plate that becomes detached at the proximal end (onychomadesis) and paronychia is the eventual result. Many patients present with the complaint of "ingrown toenails," especially of the great toes. Few actually have this entity.[11] The symptom of pain that is the major reason for

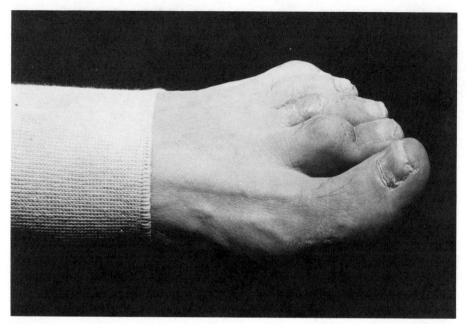

Figure 35.5.   Digital changes shown in 65-year-old man with psoriatic arthritis. Note the boutonniere deformity on the second toe of the left foot and the contracted digits on the right. Also the subungual debris characteristic of the disease is evident under the large toenail on the left, seen in the closeup view.

mentioning the nails has its genesis, in the majority of cases, in the thickened nail plate and the subungual debris. Sometimes the chief concern of the patient is the wearing of the toe box of the shoe. Initially the nails cause no distress; only when they become grossly deformed or incurvated with nail pressure in the sulci does the patient call this problem to the attention of the physician.

Nail plate problems in the arthritis patient should be treated conservatively. Referral to a podiatrist should be the first consideration. He may grind the thick nail plates and can painlessly trim the elongated and incurvated margins. This is accomplished by using a variety of steel burrs of varying coarseness. Pain is almost always relieved by thinning of the nail plate. Cosmetically the nail plate may be given a fairly normal appearance. The secondary infections that may be present can be controlled with local or systemic antibiotics. In the vast majority of patients nail problems can be managed without the necessity for traumatic surgery or special shoes.

SUMMARY

Foot problems that plague the person with arthritis call for the cooperation and treatment by many disciplines. The primary care physician has the responsibility to call upon each health professional. By early recognition and preventive treatment one ensures the best possible results and may avoid more drastic measures.

REFERENCES

1. Gerster TJ, et al. Talalgia: a review of 30 severe cases. J Rheum 1978:5(2):210–215.
2. Sbarbaro JL Jr., Katz WA. The feet and ankles in the diagnosis of rheumatic diseases. In: Katz WA, ed., Rheumatic diseases: diagnosis and management. Philadelphia: JB Lippincott, 1977, pp. 179–182.
3. Gainnestras NJ. Foot care: whither bound? Clin Orthoped Related Res 1972;85:5–6.
4. Inman VT. The joints of the ankle. Baltimore: Williams and Wilkins, 1976.
5. Freyberg RN. Physical and orthopedic management of rheumatoid arthritis. In: Hollander JI, McCarty DJ, eds., Arthritis and allied conditions. Philadelphia: Lea and Febiger, 1972, p. 567.
6. Root ML, Orien WP, Week JH. Normal and abnormal function of the foot. Los Angeles: Clinical Biomechanics, 1977, pp. 41–43.
7. Gamble FO, Yale I. Clinical foot roentgenology. Huntingdon, N.Y.: Robert E. Krieger, 1975, pp. 62–64.
8. Clayton ML. Surgery of the forefoot in rheumatoid arthritis. Clin Orthoped 1960; 16:136–138.
9. Kelikian H. Hallux valgus, allied deformities of the forefoot and metatarsalgia. Philadelphia: WB Saunders, 1965, pp. 294–296.
10. Bluefarb SM, Caro WA. Cutaneous manifestations of rheumatic diseases. In: Katz WA, ed., Rheumatic diseases: diagnosis and management. Philadelphia: JB Lippincott, 1977, pp. 235–236.
11. Snyder M, Hansen R. Ingrown toenails—fact or fancy. Ariz Med 1981;38 (Oct.):759–762.

ADDITIONAL READING

Bateman JE. Foot science: a selection of papers from the proceedings of the American Orthopedic Foot Society. Philadelphia: WB Saunders, 1976.
Fielding MD, ed., The surgical treatment of the hallux-abductor-valgus and allied deformities. Mt. Kisco, N.Y.: Futura, 1973.
Frankel VH, Nordin M. Basic biomechanics of the skeletal system. Philadelphia: Lea and Febiger, 1980.
Helal B. Metatarsal osteotomy for metatarsalgia. J Bone Joint Surg (B) 1975;57:187–192.

36

Rheumatoid Arthritis

Joseph Lee Hollander, M.D., M.A.C.P.

Rheumatoid arthritis is a common, painful, progressive disease, all too often producing disability. Because of the frequency of its development, it has been called "the great crippler." Unlike the rehabilitation problems presented by acute diseases such as poliomyelitis or even stroke, rheumatoid arthritis tends to be progressive and chronic with development over the months and years of more and more disabilities. The succession of relapses and partial remissions that occur spontaneously in the course of the disease makes it difficult to evaluate true progress in rehabilitation. Unreasonable optimism results from improvements in function for a time, only to be offset by a relapse that not only wipes out the gain but often brings the patient to a lower level of function than previously. This erratic and unpredictable course leads to discouragement not only to the physician and therapist, but, more important, to the long-suffering patient.

Physicians responsible for management of rheumatoid arthritis often feel frustration. Although considerable progress has been made in treatment of this disease, the cause of rheumatoid arthritis is still unknown and no cure is yet available.

This gloomy outlook on rheumatoid arthritis is presented only to give a realistic picture of the problem the disease presents to physician and therapist. I have been treating rheumatoid arthritis for 45 years and have been responsible for management of literally thousands of sufferers. I am as impatient with the cocksure young physicians who imply that proper treatment of the disease with aspirin in sufficient dose and bed rest almost always induces marked improvement or even remission of the disease, as with the pessimists who imply that nothing can be done for rheumatoid arthritis.

As evidence against both extremes, I have found that in more than half of the cases high-dose aspirin usage has either been inadequate to control the symptoms and signs of the disease, or that side effects such as tinnitus, gastric intolerance, or even bleeding that result from regular ingestion of more than twelve tablets of aspirin daily nullify most of its effectiveness.

Bed rest, although helpful for very acute polyarticular flares, has been often abused by overrestriction of activity in a moderately severe case, leading to weakness, muscle atrophy, and restricted motion of the involved joints. This necessitates very extensive and elaborate programs of rehabilitation for the newly invalided arthritis sufferer. Dr. Frank Krusen, one of the pioneers in physical medicine and rehabilitation, once said, "The day the arthritic goes to bed is the day he becomes a cripple."

Clearly the answer rests with *appropriate* therapy with an anti-inflammatory drug both tolerable and helpful for each patient and *adequate* rest balanced with exercise as tolerated to prevent muscle atrophy and restricted joint function.

OBJECTIVES OF TREATMENT

To those who take the pessimistic and nihilistic approach to treatment of rheumatoid arthritis, I can answer with the voice of experience that there is hardly a patient with the disease, however severe, who cannot be helped with some treatment measures. "Therapeutic resourcefulness" is the term applicable to management of this chronic disease. The physician and therapist should not expect the impossible but must seek ways to help the patient achieve the following objectives.

1. *Relieve suffering.* As much as possible, patients' pain should be relieved, whether by proper positioning, splints, application of heat or cold packs, or other physical therapy. Administration of analgesic drugs in minimum adequate dose is usually very helpful; narcotics and strong relaxants should be restricted to only the most acute and severe cases. Properly utilized acupuncture, transcutaneous electrical nerve stimulation (TENS), and other techniques for pain relief belong in the therapeutic armamentarium. Too much analgesia in active rheumatoid arthritis, however, may encourage the patient to abuse the inflamed joints. The proper degree of analgesia is the amount of pain relief that makes the disease *bearable* and permits a reasonable amount of activity without aggravation of the joint. Dependency and even addiction must be prevented, so overkill with too much analgesic is to be avoided. Pain is a *useful* symptom, telling where something is wrong. Blotting it out completely may remove the warning sign that can protect the diseased joint from further damage.

This admonition against abuse of analgesics does not mean the patients should suffer unremitting pain, particularly when it prevents sleep or wakens them from sleep. Even when pain persists, analgesics are needed, but when it simply hurts on starting to move, the pain is probably from the stiffness induced by long inactivity. A jingle used for instructing patients in this regard goes, "The oftener you move despite some pain, the less cause you will have to complain." This refers to frequent, mild, limbering activity, not to bouts of strenuous exertion. If it hurts to exercise and does not hurt to remain still, underexercise is the natural result.

2. *Suppress inflammation.* The sundry methods for analgesia can relieve or lessen pain but do *not* decrease the intensity of the inflammatory reaction. Anti-inflammatory drugs often act as analgesics, because they lessen the intensity of

swelling, heat, tenderness, and other signs of the inflammatory process, thus acting at a more fundamental level than merely decreasing pain perception. Chronic inflammation of joints and related structures is the cause of arthritic pain, with the process leading to tissue breakdown, destruction, and deformity. Complete suppression of inflammation is not feasible in rheumatoid arthritis, but even partial suppression of the destructive process slows the development of the granulation tissue (pannus), which erodes the cartilage and bone. Deterring joint destruction is a prime objective of rheumatoid arthritis therapy.

Anti-inflammatory measures are many. Rest of the inflamed part decreases inflammation. Splinting may facilitate local rest. Various forms of physical therapy, particularly cold packs or baths (cryotherapy) lessen the intensity of the inflammatory process. Liniments, surface heat, and gentle massage may decrease the deep hyperemia and congestion of inflamed joints by diversion of blood flow. Most of these measures are not feasible for continuous or long-term use in the active chronic inflammation of rheumatoid arthritis. They are discussed in detail elsewhere in this book.

Anti-inflammatory drugs chemically suppress inflammation by inhibiting leukocyte responses, by blocking formation of such mediators of inflammation as prostaglandins, and by slowing down the formation of antibodies. The most potent anti-inflammatory agents are the cortisone drugs. Their careful use is still advocated for severe and otherwise uncontrollable rheumatoid arthritis, but the side effects from continued use, particularly in older persons, often outweigh any benefits. Local use of cortisone drugs for severely inflamed joints is widely employed with benefit (see chapter 18).

The nonsteroidal anti-inflammatory drugs (NSAIDS) are many. The first of these, both in appearance on the drug scene and in priority for trial in rheumatoid arthritis therapy, is aspirin (and other forms of salicylate). No one can contest the fact that aspirin is the basic drug for treatment of rheumatoid arthritis. It is certainly the first anti-inflammatory agent, is universally available, is cheap, and usually is helpful in lessening inflammation if tolerated in sufficient dosage, usually 4 grams or more daily. Serum levels of salicylates may be readily measured in most laboratories; they should be in the range of 20–30 mg % for anti-inflammatory effect. The analgesic effect of aspirin, so commonly used for headaches, menstrual cramps, and relief of all sorts of minor pain, makes patients skeptical of its worth as an anti-inflammatory agent. The number of tablets required to achieve reduction of inflammation, the need for taking the drug every 4 hours, the frequent dyspepsia or ringing in the ears and even deafness induced by the large doses all detract from the practical value of aspirin and patients' acceptance and cooperation. To many patients, "It's just aspirin," without the mystery and hope for great improvement implicit in the use of other agents. Despite these drawbacks aspirin and its relatives should be tried first for treatment of rheumatoid arthritis.

For those in whom aspirin is inadequate or badly tolerated, the newer anti-inflammatory drugs have been a blessing. All of these so-called wonder drugs deserve that name not because they are wonderful, but because we *wonder* whether they are as good as aspirin, we *wonder* why they are so expensive, and we *wonder* what new side effects they will produce. New models appear at least yearly, the marketing claims for each exceeding all previous claims for others. Advantages may be definite, however, for those unable to benefit from adequate aspirin. All are more potent than aspirin; that is, less milligrams of drug are required for anti-inflammatory effect. Although indomethacin (Indocin) is more irritating to the stomach than aspirin, most of the others produce less gastric distress. Phenylbutazone (Butazolidin), the first superaspirin, has proved itself a potent anti-inflammatory agent but with both gastric irritating effects and sometimes bone marrow depressing action detracting from its widespread use. Chemical derivatives of propionic acid such as ibuprofen (Motrin), naproxen (Naprosyn), and fenoprofen (Nalfon) have been found effective and fairly well tolerated in some patients. Others have obtained greater benefit from indole acetic acid derivatives such as sulindac (Clinoril) or tolmetin (Tolectin). New models appear with bewildering frequency, and some do have advantage for patients who could not tolerate earlier drugs. Both sulindac and naproxen have an advantage in that only one tablet twice daily may give adequate anti-inflammatory effect for the 24-hour period. Newer drugs such as proxicam (Feldene) with a once-a-day dose regimen may even improve on this. Suffice it to say that the best of these for any given patient is the one most effective, most acceptable, best tolerated, and least expensive. Finding the best drug for each rheumatoid arthritis patient tests the therapeutic resourcefulness of the physician.

The so-called remittive drugs for rheumatoid arthritis will not be discussed in detail here. Gold salt therapy, hydroxychloroquine, penicillamine, immuno-suppressive drugs such as azathiaprine, cyclophosphamide, or methotrexate, and immune regulators such as levamisole have been widely employed in the treatment of rheumatoid arthritis, not as simple anti-inflammatory agents, but in more fundamental attempts to suppress the disease process and to induce an arrest or remission. Such agents can be effective but are best used by or supervised in consultation with experienced rheumatologists rather than by primary care physicians or allied health personnel alone because of insidious side effects and intricacy of monitoring patient effectiveness.

3. *Prevent contractures and other deformities.* In this important objective of rheumatoid arthritis treatment the physical and occupational therapists and the primary care physician must work as a team. Diligence in observing joint-function changes, decreasing range of motion, muscle tenderness and spasm, development of limp in walking, inability to rise from a chair, or other decreases in daily living functions is of prime importance. Repeated careful evaluation of each patient will quickly detect incipient spasm, weakness, tendon shortening, ligamentous laxity or tightening before they become established contractures. Decreasing muscle strength occurs rapidly in rheumatoid arthritis, often overnight with an acute flare. Frequent measurement of hand grip strength using the rolled blood pressure cuff inflated to 20-mm mercury on the manometer is a much neglected but important gauge of finger, hand, and wrist function including problems with the joints, muscles and tendons. Any marked drop in grip strength should be investigated promptly.

Hand deformities are far and away the most common ravages of rheumatoid arthritis and often begin and progress quite insidiously. Ulnar deviation of fingers from subluxations of the metacarpophalangeal (MCP) joints, a hallmark of rheumatoid arthritis, appears early and is easily noted. The slipping of the extensor tendons to the ulnar side of the MCP, together with stretching of the joint capsules and unequal pull of the intrinsic hand muscles set up this problem. If active swelling, tenderness, and stiffness of the joints are noted, increased application of anti-inflammatory measures is needed promptly—that is, increased amounts of drugs, physical therapy, or intra-articular steroid injections locally for severely inflamed joints. Splints, whether for resting or so-called working splints, may help prevent the development of deformities passively and decrease pain and inflammation when properly designed and fitted. Graduated active exercise for the weakened muscles must be instituted as soon as active inflammation subsides enough to permit it. Range-of-motion exercises as well as grip-strengthening exercises are taught so the patient repeats them frequently.

The same general principles apply to prevention of finger deformities, wrist deformities, elbow contractures, or shoulder capsular contractures. Promptness, patience, and perseverence are watchwords in prevention of rheumatoid deformities.

Neck and spinal contractures are also usually preventable if detected early. Physical therapy with heat, massage, and particularly with guided active range-of-motion exercises, frequently repeated as tolerated, may retain function.

Prevention of contractures and deformities of lower extremity joints must take into account that these are weight-bearing joints. In such joints stability as well as movability is important to retain. Rheumatoid arthritis causes erosions of joint margins and articular cartilages. Weakness of muscles controlling joint motion leads to stretching or attenuation of ligaments. Between erosion of bony margins, thinning of cartilage, and stretching of capsular ligaments, *instability of joints,* particularly knees, ankles and foot joints, is likely to develop, sometimes slowly and insidiously, often unexpectedly and rapidly. Again, regular monitoring of joint range and stability can detect such problems before they become well established.

More common in earlier stages than deformities or instability are *flexion contractures of hips or knees.* If the muscles are spastic and tender, hot compresses, traction, and even splints may be required. Whenever the joints themselves are swollen, tender, and stiff, prompt aspiration and corticosteroid injection can suppress the inflammation and permit painless motion often within 24 hours, with palliation persisting for weeks. This permits early resumption of painless graduated exercise for regaining range of motion and muscle strength. This method of management is far more rapid and dependable in preventing hip and knee contractures than older techniques.

Ankle and subtalar joint inflammation is likewise amenable to local steroid, and such joints seldom require splinting, only a suitable period of rest (abstinence from weight-bearing).

The joints of the feet often are inflamed and painful in active rheumatoid arthritis. When this occurs simultaneously in several of the tarsal joints, rest and local hot or cold applications may be helpful. Paraffin baths, warm compresses, and baking lamps may bring relief. Weight-bearing should be minimized or even avoided until this subsides. Deformities seldom are important in tarsal joints, but subtalar, talonavicular, and calcaneocuboid joints become unstable and very painful in many patients with long-standing rheumatoid arthritis of the feet.

Toe joint deformities are extremely frequent, painful, and disabling in rheumatoid arthritis. Hallux valgus (bunion deformity of the great toe) often develops early, soon followed by cock-up contractures of the second, third, and fourth toes, with dorsal subluxation of the proximal phalanges on the metatarsal heads. Shoe pressure pushes the metatarsal heads down, flattening the metatarsal arch, producing calluses underneath, with painful corns developing on the bent toe joints where they crowd up into the toe box of the shoe. To prevent this, acutely swollen joints should be injected with steroid as needed, shoes should fit loosely, and flexion exercises for toes should be started as soon as rest and physical therapy with hot soaks or paraffin permit. A properly fitting shoe is the best splint for an arthritic foot, with arch supports and foam rubber pads and other orthotics inserted by a competent podiatrist as needed. (See chapters 8 and 35.) For the severely deformed foot shoes made to a special cast or surgical intervention should be considered.

4. *Correct disabling deformities whenever possible.* No matter how carefully the program for prevention of deformities has been carried out, such deformities frequently occur. Many existed before the institution of the program, and others develop in spite of all reasonable measures to prevent them. Relatively minor deformities of fingers and toes are *not* very disabling. Modest restrictions of motion of wrists, elbows, shoulders, neck, back, hips, knees, and ankles may be hardly noticeable to the patient in daily activities so are *not* disabling deformities once the fire of the rheumatoid inflammation is under control. Such limitations are the charred timbers left by the fire. Unless motion of the affected joint has been restricted to the extent that it does perceptibly impair function, only gently limbering exercise should be continued as treatment.

If deformities of fingers, hands, or wrist are sufficient to impair grasp and dexterity, orthopedic help is needed. Reconstructive surgery for the rheumatoid hand is *not* done for cosmetic reasons, only to improve function.

If elbow or shoulder motion is so limited as to prevent motions of eating, dressing, or ordinary reaching, orthopedic correction may be needed. Joint surgery may salvage failures in arthritis treatment.

Although spinal deformities are rare in rheumatoid arthritis, neck problems, such as atlantoaxial subluxation, do occur in late and severe cases. Cervical collars may suffice in mild cases, but occipitocervical fusion may be needed if neurologic symptoms develop.

When arthritic destruction of *hip* joints has decreased function to the point that the patient has difficulty standing or sitting down, climbing or descending stairs, or walking any distance without pain in spite of canes or crutches to lessen the weight carried, then surgical replacement can salvage hip joints. Surgical replacement of damaged hip joints has become a standard procedure, with low failure rate. Thousands of arthritic hips have been replaced with plastic and metal prostheses with almost normal functional result and little pain. Maintaining maximum muscle strength and preventing flexion contractures preoperatively help to assure maximum success.

Knee joints that have been so eroded as to be grossly unstable should also be checked by a competent orthopedic surgeon, since knee surgery with replacement of such a knee is almost as dependable for salvage of function as hip surgery. Even knees that have been neglected and have flexion contractures of disabling degree can be repaired. Rehabilitation problems with patients after such repair surgery will be discussed later.

Ankle, subtalar, and tarsal joints that have become eroded and unstable and painful on standing and walking can also be greatly helped by reparative surgery, as can deformed toe joints.

The cardinal indications for joint surgery are persistent pain on use despite conservative treatment and loss of function sufficient to interfere with activities of daily living. Other conditions, such as severe cardiac or hypertensive disease, diabetes, or even marked obesity may mitigate against corrective surgery, but advanced age is rarely a contraindication. Corrective joint surgery has improved the outlook for even the most severely stricken victim of rheumatoid arthritis.

5. *Above all, preserve function.* The first four methods and objectives of treatment of rheumatoid arthritis can best be summed up in this fifth and overall objective. Because there is no cure for the disease, it is important that any treatment that can lessen the suffering and limitations imposed by the disease, decrease the damage it inflicts on the joints and other tissues, or repair its ravages should be considered in the management program. The comprehensive program is designed for each patient and varies with time and intensity of the disease. It would be inappropriate and wasteful to hospitalize a person with an early and fairly mild case of rheumatoid arthritis simply for rest and physical therapy and likewise inappropriate and wasteful to hospitalize the severe and late rheumatoid arthritis patient unless the person is in need of intensive rehabilitation, surgery, or some fairly complicated and potentially dangerous therapy. This does *not* mean that only the hospitalized rheumatoid patient should have intensive therapy but that most of the measures can be administered to out-patients or at home except when the patient becomes "arthritically decompensated." Patients who have been able to cope with the pain and disability, even though the rheumatoid inflammation is active, are compensating by living on in spite of it. When a flare occurs or the disability reaches a stage when he cannot manage even minimal functions of his activities of daily living, the patient becomes decompensated. This does *not* mean he or she has become a cripple, but this is the time when "all stops must be pulled," and treatment intensified to cope with the loss of function, hospitalizing if indicated, as noted before.

As mentioned earlier, there are very few rheumatoid arthritis patients who cannot be helped using one or more of the approaches to treatment discussed here. The patient in the late stages of rheumatoid arthritis, in whom the joint pain, stiffness, and decreased function are the charred timbers left by previously active fire of arthritic inflammation, obtains little benefit from anti-inflammatory drugs, but still needs analgesics, a well-designed program of physical and occupational therapy, and perhaps some corrective surgery, all designed to improve function. Even the bedfast arthritic derelict, so commonly seen in yesteryears but much rarer today, can be helped by surgery and intensive rehabilitation. Goals must be realistic, taking into account the status of the disease *and the motivation of the patient.*

THE PHYSICAL MANAGEMENT OF RHEUMATOID ARTHRITIS

At any stage of rheumatoid arthritis the correct amount of physical activity is the maximum amount tolerable without undue pain either during or following the exercise, balanced by the minimum amount of rest required before the activity can be repeated. This is the optimum ratio or balance of exercise and rest. Too little exercise leads to stiffness, weakness, and loss of function. Too much or too vigorous exercise produces more pain and even aggravation of the arthritis and muscle spasm. The ratio must be determined repeatedly. Patients must learn their individual exercise tolerance and need for rest. It is not the purpose of this discussion to enumerate all the corrective exercises used but to stress that exercise must be *limbering,* not strenuous. Rest must be adequate, not overlong. Both must alternate, so that exercise periods are not done once to exhaustion, necessitating a long rest period that allows stiffening. Many short limbering periods, interspersed with many short rest periods should be the order of the day for each rheumatoid arthritis patient. Exercise *as tolerated* is the rule of thumb for physician and therapist in prescribing activity. The exercise need not be calisthenics but regular daily activities or functional occupational therapy monitored to be sure range of motion is emphasized.

LIMITATIONS AND PRECAUTIONS IN TREATMENT

When mild to moderate activity is *painful,* use more rest, more medication, more physical therapy, or local corticosteroid injection as indicated before trying again. Exercise and resumption of normal function should not be a torture. Patience and persistence are needed.

In coping with *limited motion* in joints, refrain from forceful manipulation, except under anesthesia. Pain and spasm will increase if the stiffened joint is pushed too hard. Gentle, repeated movement is better tolerated and eventually more productive. Assisted active motion is better than manipulation (passive motion) unless the muscles are paralyzed, which is rare in rheumatoid arthritis.

Muscle weakness is almost invariably a part of active rheumatoid involvement. Overactivity will produce severe pain and discouragement, even muscle spasm and fasciculations. Again, gentle and repeated assisted active motion on the installment plan eventually produces improvement. Encouragement and sometimes even electrical stimulation are needed as well.

Coping with discouragement is one of the most difficult lessons to learn by physician, therapist, and patient. An optimistic attitude is needed by all, but it must be *reasonable* optimism. Setting initial goals too high leads to despair. Even when initial goals are attained, relapse may again send morale crashing down. Encouragement, continued interest, and *cautious* optimism must be repeatedly applied, day after day. Relapses must be put into perspective and not regarded as final. When the patient senses loss of interest, despair, or even discouragement in his physician or therapist, his or her own morale hits bottom. Motivation is always eroded by the long, rough road of rheumatoid arthritis. Reevaluations must be frequent enough to keep up interest and motivation but not so frequent as to become burdensome and dilute enthusiasm. Even when progress is only negative, some ray of hope can be found in the dismal picture or some new change made in the treatment program perhaps to bring some improvement. Here again therapeutic resourcefulness is needed. The overambitious patient must be gently restrained from overdoing, but the discouraged or poorly motivated patient must be frequently prodded, coaxed, and encouraged into doing more. Quick results should never be promised or expected, just hoped for.

Rehabilitation following joint surgery.   A few old-fashioned orthopedic surgeons place recently operated joints in casts for a matter of weeks. This often leads to fusion or decreased motion in the patient with rheumatoid arthritis. Early, graduated activity is to be encouraged, short of pain, danger to wound healing, or distortion of the corrected joint surfaces. Even casted extremities should be treated with a program of repeated muscle-setting exercises. Actual weight-bearing, however, must be at the discretion of the surgeon. Pain will always be the limiting factor for exercise of any rheumatoid arthritic joints.

SUMMARY

Although rheumatoid arthritis is a painful, usually chronic and often progressively worsening disease with no known cause or cure, there is *much* that can be done to help. The pain can be largely controlled by a variety of drugs, modalities of physical therapy, and other measures as outlined. The inflammation can often be suppressed to a substantial degree by a variety of anti-inflammatory drugs, and even some so-called remittive agents. These slow down the destruction from the disease, helping to prevent crippling. Contractures, muscle atrophy, and deformities can be largely prevented by adequate physical and occupational therapy and corrective exercises, aided by intra-articular steroids if needed. The most encouraging progress in treatment of rheumatoid arthritis has been the tremendous success in salvaging the function of destroyed joints by corrective surgery. Preservation of joint function in the rheumatoid arthritis patient can be accomplished during many years of treatment by patience, persistence, and by utilizing *as needed* the many modalities found to be effective. Cautious optimism should be maintained throughout.

REFERENCES

1. Lowman EW. Rehabilitation in arthritis. In: Hollander JL, ed., Arthritis and allied conditions, 8th ed. Philadelphia: Lea and Febiger, 1972, ch. 36, pp. 580–592.
2. Swezey RL. Physical management and rehabilitation of the arthritic patient. In: Hollander JL, ed., The arthritis handbook. West Point, Pa.: Merck, Sharp, and Dohme, 1974, pp. 85–104.
3. Policoff L. Physical medicine and rehabilitation in the management of the arthritic patient. In: Katz WA, Rheumatic diseases. Philadelphia: JB Lippincott, 1977, ch. 46, pp. 923–948.
4. Swezey RL. Rehabilitation aspects in arthritis. In McCarty DJ, ed., Arthritis and allied conditions, 9th ed. Philadelphia: Lea and Febiger, 1979, ch. 36, pp. 519–543.

37

Osteoarthritis

H. Ralph Schumacher, M.D.,
Karen Moutevelis, O.T.R., and
Nina Wolchasty, L.P.T.

Osteoarthritis is by far the most common type of arthritis. It is largely a mechanical problem with irregularity and then loss of the normally smooth articular cartilage. Pain thus occurs predominantly on use of the diseased joint(s) and is relieved by rest. Inflammation is a minor component. Physical measures to protect the diseased joint, maintain motion, and strengthen adjacent muscles are especially important since no systemic drug therapy has yet been proven to alter the disease process.

Osteoarthritis is most common in older patients but can occur at any age after joint abuse or trauma. It can also occur at an earlier age in patients with certain systemic (largely metabolic) diseases, like hemochromatosis, ochronosis, and acromegaly, that alter the normal cartilage structure.[1]

Not all musculoskeletal symptoms of arthritis in older patients are due to osteoarthritis. Rheumatoid and other inflammatory arthritis continue to occur at all ages. Severe proximal myalgias with an elevated sedimentation rate should suggest polymyalgia rheumatica that occurs typically after age 60. Periarticular problems such as bone diseases, calcific tendinitis, and bursitis can also produce mechanical pain on use. Significant osteoarthritis should be diagnosed by positive findings such as demonstration of joint crepitus, pain on joint motion, and bony overgrowth, not just by exclusion. Synovial effusions usually are noninflammatory, with leukocyte counts less than 2,000/mm³, Otherwise different diseases should be considered. Many older persons show osteoarthritic changes on x-ray but their symptoms may still be due to other coincidental diseases.

Before planning treatment, consider current symptoms and exactly what functional limitations or concerns these cause the patient. Much osteoarthritis needs no rehabilitative therapy. In examination, identify the patient's goals and, with the patient, determine whether they are realistic.

Remember that some physical measures may be good for one purpose but have potential risk for others. For example, walking is good for general conditioning and should be continued in most elderly osteoarthritis patients even if potentially accelerating hip or knee disease.

DRUG THERAPY

Nonnarcotic analgesics can be used for the occasional rest pain or pain that limits most activities. Severe pain, however, should be considered a warning that the symptomatic joint is not receiving optimal local and mechanical protection. Do not try to eradicate all pain with drugs. Some patients with osteoarthritis have some joint inflammation that may in part be due to calcium pyrophosphate or apatite crystals or to cartilage and bone fragments that develop in osteoarthritic joints.[2] These patients may especially benefit from use of aspirin or other nonsteroidal anti-inflammatory agents. It is usually safest to use drugs in 2-week trials to try to get some objective as well as subjective evidence of effect before continuing long-term use.

Intra-articular injections of depot corticosteroids, such as the longest acting, triamcinolone hexacetonide, do seem to decrease pain and effusions in osteoarthritic joints despite the absence of prominent inflammation.[3] The effect may last for weeks to months. Such injections may relieve pain while a good physical medicine and rehabilitation program is being started for certain joints but should not be relied on for frequent repeated use, because local steroid injections can accelerate cartilage destruction and increase instability.

APPROACH TO SPECIFIC SITES OF OSTEOARTHRITIS

Hands

Osteoarthritis in the hands typically affects the distal interphalangeal joints and the trapeziometacarpal joint of the thumb. The proximal interphalangeal joints may also be prominently involved, while the metacarpal phalangeal joints are rarely affected.

In osteoarthritis of the interphalangeal joints, the major difficulties arise from pain with activity and decreased hand function. Heat by immersion in warm water, paraffin wax treatments, or a recently introduced modality named Fluidotherapy, followed by range-of-motion exercises can be employed to relieve pain and increase joint mobility. Borrell et al. demonstrated that when compared with paraffin and hydrotherapy, Fluidotherapy generated higher intramuscular and intracapsular temperatures.[4] The effectiveness of such external heating of joints on pain relief has not been established, although patients often report some short-term relief of pain.[5]

"Pressure gradient" or cotton stretch gloves have also been recommended to alleviate stiffness in arthritic hands.[6,7] However, Swezey et al. report no subjective or objective benefits in patients with osteoarthritis in a controlled experimental study.[8]

An activities of daily living (ADL) evaluation should be administered to determine functional deficits. In the presence of ankylosis or flexion contractures that restrict finger flexion and decrease full-hand prehension, assistive devices such as built-up handles for utensils, razors, and writing devices may be necessary. Patients also may need to use both hands in grasping to allow ease and safety in lifting glasses or cups when eating and to hold objects too large or too heavy for just one hand to hold.

The trapeziometacarpal or fist metacarpal-carpal (MC-C) joint is a saddle joint that allows retroposition and opposition, adduction and abduction, and circumduction.[9] Tip pinch, lateral pinch, and especially, strong finger-to-thumb pinch are dependent upon good joint integrity. The trapeziometacarpal joint is important in both precision and power grip. As trapeziometacarpal disease develops, instability, crepitation, pain, and decreased movement result. An adaptation response may occur in which the individual avoids stressful pinch and painful movements.[10]

An on-site or simulated work evaluation may be necessary to determine the effect of the first MC-C osteoarthritis on the patient's job tasks. Adaptations in the work environment can often be made with the assistance of the employer to allow the patient to continue employment.

Thumb stability can be restored through the use of a thumb-stabilizing carpometacarpal splint.[5,11,12] (See figure 37.1.) This splint will restrict carpometacarpal and metacarpal phalangeal joint movement while allowing interphalangeal motion. The thumb must be splinted in abduction and should allow tip of finger to thumb prehension. The splint should be evaluated in use to detect inappro-

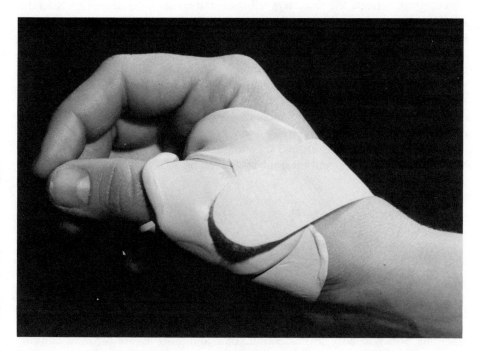

Figure 37.1.   Thumb-stabilizing carpometacarpal splint for use in painful arthritis.

priate fit or other problems. Mobility is compromised with this splint and it may initially feel awkward or confining. Nonetheless it can give considerable pain relief during activity. Patients can determine when splint use is most beneficial for symptomatic relief. Activities such as crocheting and knitting may become easier with the splint. Otherwise pain during prolonged unsupported positioning may interfere with these hobbies.

There are four surgical procedures to consider when conservative measures are insufficient to relieve first MC-C symptoms. They are:

Fusion of the trapeziometacarpal joint

Resection arthroplasty

Resection implant arthroplasty

Soft-tissue interposition arthroplasty

In general the implant is most successful, because it provides both motion and stability.

Shoulders

Osteoarthritis affects the shoulders, elbows, and wrists much less often than the hands. When it does occur in the shoulders, occupational therapy is directed toward maintaining and increasing range of motion and includes instruction in methods to reduce stress to the shoulders.[12] Patients should be instructed to wear loose-fitting clothes that are easy to don. Recommendations for adapting the work environment may also be necessary; in the home, reorganizing shelves so that frequently used items are within easy reach is helpful. Assistive devices that may be beneficial include long-handled bath sponges, reachers, extended combs, and dressing sticks. (See chapters 22 and 23.)

Spasm in the muscles around the shoulder joints is a common complication. Various heat modalities and local injections can be used.

The Spine

Osteoarthritis of the spine usually affects areas with the most mobility. These sites include the cervical and lumbar regions. In older patients the areas of involvement can be more diffuse and can be more disabling. Physical therapy is aimed at relieving symptoms of pain and stiffness secondary to adjacent soft-tissue involvement and at maintaining motion.

In the cervical spine, osteoarthritis typically produces spasm of the upper trapezius, which in turn, produces more pain and more loss of range of motion.

The goal of therapy is to break this cycle. Treatment usually consists of heat and a balanced program of rest and range-of-motion exercises. Often a soft cervical collar is worn to encourage the patient to hold the neck in slight flexion. Note that there is no support with the soft collar. One purpose of the collar is to encourage restriction of motion to decrease the strain on the cervical musculature. This is particularly important during activity. Patients should be cautioned, however, against continuous use of a cervical collar, because this could contribute to muscle atrophy and a further decrease in range of motion. A simple timetable such as 2 hours on and 1 hour off can prevent this potential problem. A cervical pillow may be used to support the neck and limit unusual positioning during sleep.[13] Lying prone as well as using more than one pillow should be avoided. Once pain subsides, patients should be instructed in isometric neck exercises to minimize disuse atrophy.

Often patients complain of radicular pain, which can result from nerve root irritation by osteophytes or prolapsed discs. Cervical traction in slight flexion is frequently helpful for pain relief. Jackson has stated that traction may prevent and eliminate adhesions between the dural sleeves of the nerve roots and adjacent structures by separation of the cervical vertebrae.[13] For some patients traction certainly helps to induce relaxation of tense muscles. The actual mechanisms of action are not known at this time. Traction should not be used in the presence of very painful spasm. Kraft et al. demonstrated that traction alone actually aggravated muscle spasm, whereas it was helpful if administered after other treatment with heat, massage, salicylates, and mobilization exercises.[14] Traction should be discontinued after eight to ten sessions if patients obtain no relief of their symptoms. Other modalities that can be considered for neck pain include cold applications, TENS, or biofeedback. (See chapter 19.)

Osteoarthritis in the lumbar region can cause severe pain in some patients. In the acute stage, bedrest in the semi-Fowler position (45° elevation of the upper half of the mattress) is the treatment of choice. Pelvic traction can be used, provided it does not increase patient discomfort. Since the amount of force generally applied is not enough to produce intervertebral distraction, pelvic traction mainly serves as a method for keeping patients in bed.[15,16] Heat is also used to relieve pain and muscle spasms. For those few patients in whom heat aggravates pain, icy massage may be tried. This should be considered only for patients who are receptive to the idea. Most arthritic patients prefer heat treatments. We have found no controlled studies on the use of these modalities.

As their symptoms subside, patients should be instructed in an active exercise program. Williams's back flexion exercises are most often prescribed. This regimen aims to strengthen both the abdominal and lumbar musculature. In a study conducted by Kendall and Jenkins, three different low-back exercise programs were compared. These included (1) exercises to increase range-of-motion and strength, (2) low-back flexion exercises along with standing exercises to work on pelvic tilting, and (3) back hyperextension exercises. Although some patients in each group improved, there was significantly greater improvement in the low-back flexion group. Symptoms were actually exacerbated in a number of patients in the hyperextension group.[17,18]

A lumbosacral corset or back brace can also be used in the treatment of the painful low back. Although such supports do not truly immobilize the spine, they do restrict motion and provide reminders to patients to avoid certain types of movements. They are particularly helpful in subacute conditions when patients are beginning to increase their daily activities. Weight reduction is indicated in obese patients to decrease an exaggerated lumbar lordosis. Patients who wear any type of back support must continue to exercise daily. They must also be instructed in proper body mechanics to enable them to modify their functional activities accordingly. Instruction in proper standing and sitting posture is essential. A firm mattress or use of a bed board is also recommended. Surgery is most often indicated when there is cord compression or root symptoms and signs that are not controlled with these conservative measures.

Hips

Osteoarthritis of the hip can be treated symptomatically with heat and range-of-motion exercises. Heat is applied in the form of hydrocollator packs, ultrasound, diathermy, or hydrotherapy. Patients can also be instructed to lie prone at least 1–2 hours each day to prevent the development of hip flexion contractures. Decreasing the weight-bearing forces through the use of crutches or canes is another major component of therapy. Such measures rarely give more than temporary relief; there are no controlled studies on these measures. An assessment of activities of daily living should be performed if hip (or knee) involvement limits function. Specific problems for the individual can be identified and goals of treatment established. Reducing joint stresses is essential, and this can be achieved through daily planning and organization as well as through the use of assistive devices. Patients should be instructed to limit standing and ambulation in the presence of severe, painful hip disease.

Assistive devices and equipment such as a bathtub bench, elevated toilet seats, elevated chairs, stocking aids, reachers, dressing stick, and long shoehorn might be considered in the presence of lower extremity disease, in order to increase independence and reduce joint stress.

Weight reduction is often advised in the patient with progressive disease partly in anticipation that surgery may be needed. When pain and limitation of ambulation significantly hamper activity, a total hip replacement is an effective alternative. Patients with osteoarthritis often have good bone mass that provides strong support for a joint prosthesis. When other joints are not involved, patients sometimes put their new joints through more abuse than do people with rheumatoid arthritis. Intertrochanteric osteotomies have been used for earlier hip osteoarthritis.[19] Heterotopic new bone formation has been a complication in some hip arthroplasties, limiting motion after an otherwise successful procedure.

Knees

Pain, loss of range of motion, atrophy of adjacent muscles, and instability are all common clinical manifestations of osteoarthritis of the knees. As the disease progresses, varus or valgus deformities may occur. The aims of rehabilitation include pain relief and maintenance of range of motion and strength. As in the case of osteoarthritis of the hips, heat is most often prescribed for relieving pain. A recent report by Taylor et al. suggests that TENS may be used as an appropriate alternative.[20] The results of this controlled study demonstrated that TENS provided effective short-term relief of pain. No long-term beneficial effects were achieved, but even short periods of pain relief may allow time for institution of good exercise or other programs. The effectiveness of ultrasound in relieving pain and stiffness in the osteoarthritic knee joint is currently being studied. Preliminary data indicate that there is no significant difference between patients receiving ultrasound and exercise and those receiving exercise therapy alone.[21] The stress of weight-bearing should be decreased through the use of a cane or crutches. In the presence of coincidental carpometacarpal disease, platform crutches should be considered to reduce thumb joint stress. Since normal walking produces a force three times that of the body weight at the tibial plateau, overweight patients should be encouraged to lose weight.[22] Stair-climbing should be decreased. The homemaker who must climb stairs repeatedly in the course of the day must learn to consolidate trips.

Knee cages with lateral supports can be used when there is painful lateral instability. A variety of orthopedic surgical procedures are available for osteoarthritis of the knee, but they are not yet as successful as most hip surgery. Osteotomies below the knees can be effective in early osteoarthritis with unicompartmental knee disease.

Feet

Deformities of the feet due to osteoarthritis are common with first metatarsophalangeal (MTP) involvement being of greatest concern. If hallux valgus results, orthopedic shoes with wide bunion lasts and a high toe box are the conservative treatment of choice. If pain persists, a bunionectomy can be performed. Spur formation and cartilage loss can prevent complete dorsiflexion of the great toe (hallux rigidus). Patients compensate for the lack of complete dorsiflexion by taking shorter steps and possibly putting more stress on other joints. Further treatment for this can consist of warms soaks, anti-inflammatory medication as for any osteoarthritis joint, and a hallux rigidus bar placed in the sole of the shoe to decrease the weight-bearing stress on the MTP joint. A rocker bottom shoe may also be used. Weight reduction and modification of activities are also recommended to decrease the stress of the painful metatarsal bones. Implant arthroplasty is considered when symptoms become severe and disabling.[23]

CONSIDER OTHER DISEASES

Especially in the elderly patient with osteoarthritis, possible adverse effects of interventions on other diseases have to be kept in mind. Even intra-articular steroids are absorbed to some degree systematically and can temporarily disturb the diabetic who is difficult to control. Nonsteroidal anti-inflammatory drugs can cause retention of sodium and worsen edema or hypertension. Severe cardiorespiratory disease may contradict orthopedic surgery under general anesthesia, but many patients in their 80s have still had successful major joint surgery. Exercise programs must be begun gradually in the older person with attention to any antecedent angina, respiratory difficulty, osteopenia, and so on. Heat must be used cautiously in feet of diabetics and persons with peripheral vascular disease who may have impaired circulation.

SUMMARY

The management of the patient with osteoarthritis requires a proper diagnostic work-up to establish the diagnosis and to establish a good therapeutic program. Medical therapy, exercise, physical modalities, careful planning of daily activities, and surgery all play important roles in the management of this disease. Various rehabilitation and physical medicine techniques (see table 37.1) can be used to good effect in the treatment of osteoarthritis. Because of the nonsystemic nature of the disease, the carefully planned treatment protocol is often successful and satisfying for both the patient and the health care team.

Table 37.1.   Summary

Rehabilitation and physical medicine techniques in the treatment of osteoarthritis

1. Carefully diagnose how much disability is due to joint pain, joint restriction, adjacent muscle spasm, or nerve root compression.
2. Evaluate functional ability and identify problems.
3. Use analgesics and anti-inflammatory agents sparingly in most patients.
4. Reduce adjacent muscle spasm with appropriate modalities.
5. Maintain range of motion and muscle strength.
6. Protect severely osteoarthritic joints with splints, use of assistive devices, and changes in activities.
7. Consider surgery to provide stability, decrease pain, and often maintain motion at severely involved joints.

REFERENCES

1. Schumacher HR. Secondary osteoarthritis. In: Moskowitz R, ed., Osteoarthritis. Philadelphia: WB Saunders, in press.
2. Schumacher HR, Gordon GV, Paul H, et al. Osteoarthritis, crystal deposition and inflammation. Semin Arth Rheum 1981;11:116-119.
3. Gordon GV, Schumacher HR. Electron microscopic study of depot corticosteroids crystals with clinical studies after intraarticular injection. J Rheum 1979;6:7-14.
4. Borrell RM, Parker R, Henley EJ, Masley D, Repinecz M. Comparison of in vivo temperatures produced by hydrotherapy, paraffin wax treatment and Fluidotherapy. Phys Ther 1980;60:1273-1276.
5. Swezey RL. Arthritis: rational therapy and rehabilitation. Philadelphia: WB Saunders, 1978.
6. Ehrlich GE, DiPiero AM. Stretch gloves: nocturnal use to ameliorate morning stiffness in arthritic hands. Arch Phys Med Rehab 1971;52:479-480.
7. Askari I, Moskowitz RW, Ryan C. Stretch gloves: a study of objective and subjective effectiveness in arthritis of the hands. Arth Rheum 1974;17:263-265.
8. Swezey RL, Spiegel TM, Cretin S, Clements P. Arthritic hand response to pressure gradient gloves. Arch Phys Med Rehab 1979;60:375-377.
9. Tubiana R, Valentin P. Opposition of the thumb. Surg Clin Am 1968;48:967-977.
10. Swanson A. Disabling arthritis at the base of the thumb. J Bone Joint Surg [A] 1972; 54:456-471.
11. Fess E. Hand splinting: principles and methods. St. Louis: CV Mosby, 1981.
12. Melvin J. Rheumatic disease: occupational therapy and rehabilitation. Philadelphia: FA Davis, 1978.
13. Jackson R. Syndrome of cervical nerve root compression. In: McCarty DJ, ed., Arthritis and allied conditions. Philadelphia: Lea and Febiger 1979, pp. 1023-1037.
14. Kraft GH, Johnson EW, LaBan MM. The fibrositis syndrome. Arch Phys Med Rehab 1968;49:155-162.
15. Lawson GA, Godfrey CM. A report on studies of spinal traction. Med Serv J Canada 1958;14:762-771.
16. Masturzo A. Vertebral traction for treatment of sciatica. Rheumatism 1955;11:62.
17. Kendall PH, Jenkins JM. Exercises for backache: a double-blind controlled trial. Physiother 1968;54:154-157.
18. Kendall PH, Jenkins JM. Lumbar isometric flexion exercises. Physiother 1968;54: 158-163.
19. Coventry MB. Osteotomy of the hip for degenerative arthritis. Mayo Clinic Proc 1969;44:505-514.
20. Taylor P, Hallett M, Flaherty L. Treatment of OA of the knee with TENS. Pain 1981; 11:233-240.
21. Wolchasty N. Unpublished work, Hospital of the University of Pennsylvania, Philadelphia.
22. Leach RE, Baumgard S, Brown J. Obesity: its relationship to osteoarthritis of the knee. Clin Ortho 1973;93:271-273.
23. Cracchiolo A, Swanson A, Swanson GD. The arthritic great toe metatarsophalangeal joint: review of flexible silicone implant arthroplasty from 2 medical centers. Clin Ortho 1981;157:64-69.

38

Spondyloarthropathies

Frank C. Arnett, Jr., M.D.

The spondyloarthropathies encompass a family of rheumatic diseases unified by a propensity to affect the axial skeleton, the absence of rheumatoid factor (seronegative), and a strong association with the genetic marker HLA-B27. Although once thought to be variants of rheumatoid arthritis, they are now appreciated as distinct disease entities with different pathogenesis, clinicoroentgenographic features, and courses.[1,2]

Ankylosing spondylitis is a predominantly spinal disease and, except for the hips and shoulders, infrequently affects peripheral joints. Spondylitis occurs in a primary form as ankylosing spondylitis and as a secondary complicating feature of psoriasis, inflammatory bowel diseases (ulcerative colitis and Crohn's disease), and Reiter's syndrome. (See table 38.1.) Sacroiliitis, proven by radiographs, is the hallmark of spondylitis, and a conclusive diagnosis is difficult without it.[3,4]

Reiter's syndrome is a peripheral arthropathy, classically associated with nongonococcal urethritis and conjunctivitis.[5] Some patients, however, perhaps a majority, have only the typical arthritis along with other discriminating clinical features that allow proper diagnosis (incomplete Reiter's syndrome).[6] Sacroiliitis or spondylitis occurs in 20–25 percent.[5-7]

Psoriatic arthritis is another primarily peripheral articular disease affecting 5–7 percent of persons with cutaneous psoriasis. Sacroiliitis or spondylitis, often clinically silent, occurs in approximately 20 percent.[8] Similarly, inflammatory bowel disease predisposes to both peripheral (20 percent) and axial (10 percent) forms of arthritis.[1,2,9,10]

HOST FACTORS

Ankylosing spondylitis and Reiter's syndrome most often affect young adults and children between the ages of 15 and 35 years. Males predominate, especially in Reiter's disease (the ratio of male victims to female is 9:1). Ankylosing spondylitis was once thought rare in women, but it has been underrecognized. Women and children are more likely to present with peripheral and cervical arthritis, which dominate the clinical picture and overshadow low-back complaints for long

Table 38.1. Clinical Features and HLA-B27 among the Spondyloarthropathies

	Commonly Affected Joints	Extra-articular Features	HLA-B27 Positive
Ankylosing spondylitis	Sacroiliacs Lumbar, thoracic, and cervical spines Hips, shoulders	Iritis 25 percent; cardiac conduction defects and/or aortic insufficiency (5 percent) Apical pulmonary fibrosis and cauda equina (rare)	90 percent
Reiter's syndrome (Reactive arthritis)	Knees, ankles, feet "Sausaged digits" Enthesopathies Heel pain Others	Nongonococcal urethritis Conjunctivitis Mucocutaneous lesions Scaling rash on soles and palms (keratodermia) Penile rash (balanitis) Painless oral ulcers Nail changes Fever, weight loss	75 percent
Psoriatic arthritis	Peripheral Distal interphalangeals, any others	Psoriasis	Normal frequency (8 percent)
	Sacroiliacs or spondylitis	Psoriasis	50 percent
Enteropathic arthritis	Peripheral Knees, ankles, wrists	Erythema nodosum Pyoderma gangrenosum Painful oral ulcers Fevers	Normal frequency (8 percent)
	Sacroiliacs or spondylitis	Same	30–50 percent

periods.[11,12] Similarly, psoriatic and enteropathic arthritis usually begin in young life but affect the sexes nearly equally.[8,9]

The hereditary tissue type, HLA-B27, is strongly associated with ankylosing spondylitis, Reiter's syndrome, and the spondylitis accompanying psoriasis and inflammatory bowel disease. (See table 38.1.) Peripheral psoriatic and enteropathic arthritis are not related to HLA-B27.[2,13] HLA-B27 occurs in 8 percent of the normal U.S. Caucasian and 2 percent of the black population and is inherited in a Mendelian dominant fashion.[13,14]

CHARACTER AND NATURAL HISTORY

Axial Arthritis (Spondylitis)

Regardless of clinical setting, spondylitis is characterized by a sterile inflammation of fibrocartilaginous and synovial joints as well as ligamentous structures of the spine. The disease usually begins in the sacroiliac joint, where it may remain or ascend into the lumbar, thoracic, and cervical segments. With time and persistent disease, articular structures develop bony fusion, and ligaments become calcified and ossified resulting in the syndesmophytes characteristically seen in x-rays, sometimes called the bamboo spine (illustrated in figure 38.1).[3,4,15] Secondary osteoporosis ensues and fracture may occur even with seemingly insignificant trauma.[16] In typical ankylosing spondylitis, hips or shoulders become involved in 30–50 percent of patients.[3] With progressive spinal involvement, the patient becomes stooped forward, with loss of lumbar lordosis and increasing thoracic and cervical kyphosis. Hip flexion contractures may develop, and shoulders may lose range of motion.

The natural history of spondylitis is highly variable. The majority of affected persons have mild disease that does not involve the entire spine. It is impossible to predict from the outset those who will progress into severe stages, however. Thus the preventive postural and exercise methods described later in this chapter should be presented to the majority.

Peripheral Arthritis (Reiter's Syndrome)

The peripheral articular features of the spondyloarthropathies are best typified by Reiter's syndrome. This oligoarthritis most commonly affects knees, ankles, and small joints of the feet in an asymmetrical fashion.[5,6] In addition to synovitis, inflammation of tendon and fascial insertions (enthesopathies) results in some of the most disabling features. Heel pain at the attachment of the plantar aponeurosis or Achilles tendon occurs in over 50 percent of patients, and discomfort in other nonarticular structures around the pelvis and rib cage is common.[5] In addition diffuse inflammation of digital structures results in painful "sausage" toes or fingers.[5] Unlike rheumatoid arthritis, where peripheral joints become

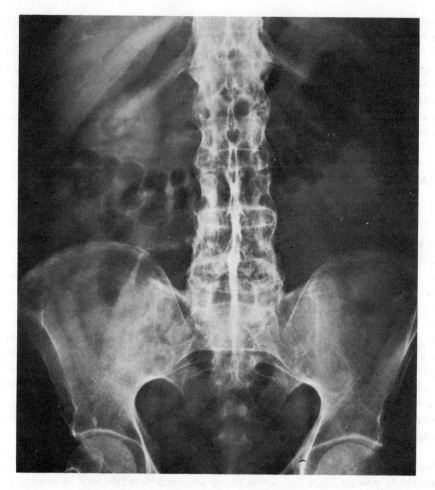

Figure 38.1. Anterior-posterior x-ray of pelvis and lumbar spine demonstrating bilateral fusion of sacroiliac joints and syndesmophyte formation between several vertebral bodies.

loosened and unstable, the lesions of the spondyloarthropathies promote bony fusion across joint structures. Thus progressive limitation of motion, fusion, and contracture characterize the peripheral as well as the spinal picture.

PHYSICAL EVALUATION

Axial Arthritis (Spondylitis)

Pain, stiffness, and progressive loss of spinal mobility typify ankylosing spondylitis. Unlike mechanical and degenerative processes, symptoms of inflam-

matory back disease are typically worse with rest and better with exercise. But-
tock pain, due to sacroiliitis, sometimes with sciatic-like radiation down the legs,
is frequently an early symptom, but neurologic deficits are absent.[3,4,17]

The physical examination is often normal early in the disease, or there may
only be tenderness with deep palpation or manipulation of the sacroiliac joints
(See table 38.2). As the disease ascends into upper spinal segments, loss of the
normal lumbar lordosis ensues, accompanied by decreased flexion, extension,
and lateral motion. There may be tenderness along vertebral structures as well as
significant paravertebral muscle spasm. A useful measure of lumbar flexion is the
Schober test. With the patient standing erect, a mark is made at the L-5, S-1 area
and another 10 cm above. When the patient bends forward in maximal flexion,
the distance between these two marks should normally increase to 15 cm. In
spondylitis, this is significantly impaired. The Schober test is most useful in
evaluating young people since it normally decreases with age. The distance from
finger to floor when the patient attempts to touch his toes is also a useful measure.

Thoracic and costovertebral involvement results in diminished ability to
expand the chest and a tendency to develop a kyphotic posture. Chest expansion
is measured by encircling the thoracic cage with a tape measure at the nipple line
and determining excursion from full expiration to inspiration. A value below
3 cm is definitely abnormal.

Cervical disease is characterized by progressive loss of all ranges of motion,
most prominently extension, and a fixed kyphosis resulting in significant functional impairment, especially visual. Sequential measurements of the distance
from occiput to wall, when the patient is positioned with heels against the wall
and fully extending his neck may detect progression of cervical kyphosis.

Table 38.2   Parameters in the Assessment and Follow-up of Ankylosing Spondylitis

General	Sacroiliac and vertebral tenderness
	Paravertebral muscle spasm
Lumbar	Loss of normal lordosis
	Decreased range of motion
	Abnormal Schober test (<5 cm)
	Decreased distance from finger to floor in toe-touching
Thoracic	Kyphosis
	Decreased chest expansion (<3 cm)
Cervical	Flexion deformity (occiput to wall)
	Decreased range of motion
Hips and shoulders	Pain and decreased range of motion

Peripheral Arthritis

The peripheral joint symptoms and signs in the spondyloarthropathies are similar to those in other inflammatory diseases. Special problems relate to a propensity for joints to rapidly loose range of motion and become fused or contracted. Inflammation and shortening of tendons and para-articular structures contribute to this tendency. Fusion of tarsal, metatarsal, and digital joints, along with severe heel pain and Achilles tendon shortening may produce foot deformity and dysfunction, the major cause of disability in Reiter's syndrome.[18,19] Psoriatic arthritis may cause similar problems, but small joints of the hands are more often affected.[8]

THERAPY AND MANAGEMENT

There are at this time no cures or means of preventing any of the spondyloarthropathies. Therapy and management therefore are aimed at (1) pharmacologic suppression of the pathologic inflammatory process, (2) the maintenance of as much articular function as possible, (3) the prevention of deformities and complications, and (4) the promotion of a relatively normal and productive life-style. Before any of these principles can be realized, the patient must understand the nature of the disease, its possible outcomes, and the reason for each modality of therapy. Frequent reinforcement is desirable since these diseases tend to be chronic, and disability or deformity often begins subtly and progresses slowly. Similarly the professional must assess each patient's life-style, goals, and motivations so as to help design a realistic management plan.[20]

Drug Therapy

Anti-inflammatory drugs of the nonsteroidal classes (salicylates, indomethacin, phenylbutazone, and others) are required in the majority of patients. These agents promote relief from pain, stiffness, and swelling, but it is not known whether they alter natural history of disease. It is likely, however, that they have a major impact on functional outcome since they allow more comfort in performing the exercises necessary for maintenance of function and prevention of deformity.

Intra-articular corticosteroids may be effective in reducing inflammation in refractory joints, but systemic steroids should be avoided except in special circumstances (severe uveitis). Attempts to relieve the heel pain of Reiter's syndrome with corticosteroid injections are rarely successful and are quite painful.

Rest and Posture

The institution of good sleeping habits early in the course of spondylitis is very important. A firm mattress and/or bed board is desirable. The prone position provides sustained extension to the spine but is only possible in those without significant fixed thoracic or cervical kyphosis. The supine position on a firm surface is next most desirable. Lying on the side in a curled attitude should be avoided. Pillows ought to be small or not used at all because they promote cervical kyphosis.

The patient should exert a conscious effort to maintain an erect posture when walking or standing. The use of firm, straight-backed chairs helps to prevent flexion spinal deformity. Splinting of certain severely affected peripheral joints (knees) at night may be necessary to prevent contracture in patients with Reiter's syndrome.

Exercises

Instruction, reinforcement, and interval reevaluation of a daily exercise program for patients with spondylitis, especially by a physical therapist, are key ingredients of management. The exercise should promote extension of all segments of the spine, as well as complete range of motion of the neck, shoulders, and hips. Swimming is an excellent method of accomplishing these ends. Cervical traction should not be used in patients with spondylitis. The osteoporosis and brittleness of the neck make fracture more likely, and spinal cord compression with quadriplegia may ensue. In fact it may be desirable for patients with cervical involvement to use protective soft collars in situations where unexpected injury may occur. Other assistive devices, including prism glasses and special footwear, may be needed.

PSYCHOSOCIAL

Several unique psychosocial issues arise in patients with spondyloarthritis. These relate primarily to the age and sex of the person most vulnerable, the young man; and to recent knowledge about the heritability of HLA-B27, the risk factor for these diseases.

Both ankylosing spondylitis and Reiter's disease usually begin in young adult life, a time when men are beginning careers and supporting families. A diagnosis of arthritis may threaten a young man's self-concept by bringing into question his youth, his virility, his productivity, and his future aspirations. Feelings of depression and hostility are common, and if they are severe, the patient may require professional counseling. The majority of patients, however, can be reassured by careful explanation of the disease process, the likelihood of mild or limited involvement, and the availability of therapeutic measures to relieve pain and preserve function. It should be emphasized that for the majority of patients with ankylosing spondylitis, no change in vocation is necessary, and productive lives are the rule. Those with Reiter's disease have an excellent chance of complete remission. Approximately 40–50 percent will have only a self-limited episode lasting 3 months to 1 year; another third may have a relapsing pattern of disease but be well in between. Only 15–20 percent of patients will have persistent arthritis and disability, usually from foot involvement.[19,20]

Genetic Counseling

Patients and their families frequently request information about the risk of arthritis in their children, and some wish to have HLA-B27 typing performed. Fifty percent of offspring can be expected to have B27 if one parent is positive (in the heterozygous state).[13] Twenty percent of B27 positive persons will develop disease.[21] Thus only 10 percent of children (0.50 ×0.20) would be expected to become affected.

One other situation is important to note. Reiter's syndrome may be triggered by diarrheal illnesses caused by Shigella, Salmonella, and Yersinia.[5,6] Patients or B27-positive relatives may desire advice regarding foreign travel in countries where these organisms are endemic. The likelihood of developing a significant reactive arthritis following exposure is 20 percent and a patient should be fully cognizant of this risk.[22]

Sexual Problems

Reiter's syndrome is considered by many to be a venereally acquired disease. The data supporting this concept are largely anecdotal and presumptive.[5] Nevertheless the stigma of presumed sexual misbehavior is frequently transmitted to the patient, often via health care professionals. Family members may become misinformed by lay articles and medical dictionaries. Thus the patient is subjected to added burdens of guilt and opprobrium that may stress a marriage or undermine family support. Every effort should be made to educate patients and family members about the facts and myths of this disease.

SUMMARY

The spondyloarthropathies include a group of inflammatory rheumatic diseases that may affect axial structures (spondylitis), peripheral joints, and tendon insertions (enthesopathy). Approach to therapy and management requires a knowledge of their natural histories and the realization that vigilant care over long periods may be necessary. Principles inherent to management include (1) patient understanding of the disease and the rationale for each of the steps to be taken, (2) anti-inflammatory drugs to relieve pain and stiffness, (3) attention to posture and sleeping habits, (4) daily exercises to maintain joint mobility and prevent deformity, (5) and psychosocial counseling as needed for some of the unique problems that occur in these diseases.

REFERENCES

1. Moll JMH, Haslock I, MacRae I, Wright V. Associations between ankylosing spondy-litis, psoriatic arthritis, Reiter's disease, the intestinal arthropathies and Behcet's syndrome. Med (Baltimore) 1974;53:343-364.
2. Wright V. Seronegative polyarthritis: a unified concept. Arth Rheum 1978;21: 619-633.
3. Rosen PS, Graham DC. Ankylosing (Strümpell-Marie) spondylitis: a clinical review of 128 cases. Arch Interam Rheum 1962;5:158-211.
4. Bluestone R. Ankylosing spondylitis. In: McCarty DJ Jr., ed., Arthritis and allied conditions. 9th ed. Philadelphia: Lea and Febiger, 1979, pp. 610-632.
5. Renlund DG, Kim WS, Arnett FC. Reiter's syndrome. Johns Hopkins Med J 1982; 150:39-44.
6. Arnett FC, McClusky OE, Schacter BZ, Lordon RE. Incomplete Reiter's syndrome: discriminating features and HLA-W27 in diagnosis. Ann Intern Med 1976;84:8-12.
7. Good AE. Involvement of the back in Reiter's syndrome. Ann Intern Med 1962; 57:44-59.
8. Moll JMH, Wright V. Psoriatic arthritis. Semin Arth Rheum 1973;3:51-78.
9. Haslock I, Wright V. The musculoskeletal complications of Crohn's disease. Med (Baltimore) 1973;52:217-225.
10. Enlow RW, Bias WB, Arnett FC. The spondylitis of inflammatory bowel disease: evidence for a non-HLA linked axial arthropathy. Arth Rheum 1980;23:1359-1365.
11. Resnick D, Dwosh IL, Goergen TG, Shapiro RF, Utsinger PD, Wlesner KB, Bryan BL. Clinical and radiographic abnormalities in ankylosing spondylitis: a comparison of men and women. Radiol 1976;119:293-297.
12. Arnett FC, Bias WB, Stevens MB. Juvenile-onset chronic arthritis: clinical and roent-genographic features of a unique HLA-B27 subset. Am J Med 1980;69:369-376.
13. Woodrow JC. Histocompatibility antigens and rheumatic diseases. Semin Arth Rheum 1977;6:257-276.
14. Khan MA. Clinical application of the HLA-B27 test in rheumatic diseases. Arch Intern Med 1980;140:177-180.
15. Cruickshank B. Pathology of ankylosing spondylitis. Bull Rheum Dis 1960;10: 211-214.
16. Hunter T, Dubo H. Spinal fractures complicating ankylosing spondylitis. Ann Intern Med 1978;88:546-549.
17. Calin A, Porta J, Fries JF, Schurman DJ. Clinical history as a screening test for anky-losing spondylitis. JAMA 1977;237:2613-2614.
18. Fox R, Calin A, Gerber RC, Gibson D. The chronicity of symptoms in Reiter's syn-drome. Ann Intern Med 1979;91:190-193.
19. Csonka GW. Long-term follow-up and prognosis of Reiter's syndrome. Ann Rheum Dis 1979;38:(Suppl 1):24-28.
20. Calin A, Marks S. Management of ankylosing spondylitis. Bull Rheum Dis 1981; 31:35-38.
21. Calin A, Fries JF. Striking prevalence of ankylosing spondylitis in "healthy" W27 positive males and females. New Engl J Med 1975;293:835-839.
22. Woodrow JC. Genetics of B27-associated diseases. Ann Rheum Dis 1979;38:(Suppl 1):135-141.

Rash

Sweats

how many joints
were effected

age

39

Juvenile Rheumatoid Arthritis

F. Paul Alepa, M.D.

The general development of a rehabilitation program for a patient with juvenile rheumatoid arthritis requires an understanding of the nature and characteristics of the disease and the disabilities it may cause. Of equal importance is that the illness has its onset between the ages of 2 and 15 years. This is a time of rapid physiologic and psychosocial growth and development. Prolonged illness and physical and functional disabilities can have a profound effect on each area of development.

Juvenile rheumatoid arthritis is a disease with great variability, suggesting that it represents more than one entity.[1,2] It is a general term used for idiopathic chronic inflammatory arthritis with onset under the age of 16 years. At present there are five subgroups of the disease that differ as to the number of joints involved, presence of systemic manifestations, complications, course, and outcome. The number of joints involved within the first 6 months of disease establishes the major categories. (See table 39.1.) The polyarticular type with a total involvement of five or more joints occurs more commonly (60–80 percent) than the pauciarticular type, which by definition has four or fewer joints affected.

The polyarticular group can be further subdivided into three groups. Daily high fever spikes and rash are prominent symptoms of the systemic onset subgroup (Still's disease).[3,4] It can occur at any age and is only slightly more common in boys than girls. The prognosis is good. Remission occurs in 90 percent of the children, usually without significant articular disabilities, within 2 years of onset. The remaining 10 percent, however, have major articular disabilities, are frequently short in stature, and may continue to have active arthritis into early adulthood. In addition to the articular problems, the daily spiking afternoon fevers, if not adequately controlled by appropriate medication, can be quite disabling. This is particularly true in younger children, who often become extremely irritable, fatigued, and fretful as their temperature rises. Loss of appetite and significant weight loss may add to the problem.

In the remaining two subgroups of the polyarticular type, systemic manifestations are mild or completely absent. The major manifestation is inflammatory polyarthritis. The two subgroups are readily distinguished by the presence of

439

Table 39.1. Clinical Classification of Juvenile Rheumatoid Arthritis

Group and Subgroups	Age at Onset	Sexual Predominance	Systemic Manifestations			Chronic Iridocyclitis (%)	Laboratory (%)		Significant Physical Disabilities (%)
			Fever (°F)	Rash (%)	Joints		ANA	RF	
Polyarticular									
Systemic	2–15	Equal	101–105	90	Large Small	> 5	> 5	0	20
Articular Seronegative	2–15	Girls	98.6–101	Rare	Large Small	> 5	25	0	10
Articular Seropositive	10–15	Girls	98.6–101	0	Large Small	> 5	75	100	70
Pauciarticular									
Early onset	2–6	Girls	98.6	0	Large	50	60	0	Rare
Late onset	10–15	Boys	98.6	0	Large, SI	0	0	0	20

a positive serum test for rheumatoid factor. The rheumatoid-factor-positive, polyarticular subgroup carries the worst prognosis. Seventy percent of those youngsters will enter adult life with major articular disabilities. The onset of arthritis is usually between the ages of 10 and 15 years, and girls are more prone to be victims, by a 2:1 or 3:1 ratio. Fortunately less than 10 percent of all children with juvenile rheumatoid arthritis belong to this subgroup.

In the nonsystemic, rheumatoid-factor-negative subgoup the onset of disease may occur at any age; it occurs more commonly in girls than boys. The prognosis is far better than in the rheumatoid-factor-positive subgroup but slightly worse than those with systemic onset. About 20 percent of these children enter adult life with significant articular disabilities.

The pauciarticular group, the other major division, has at present two subgroups differing in the age of onset and the sexual predominance. The early-onset subgroup occurs most often in girls ages 2 to 6 years. The articular involvement is usually insidious, affecting large joints of the lower extremity. Progression to severe disabling arthritis is extremely rare. However, flexion contractures are a frequent residual consequence. Linear overgrowth of the bones of the involved joints is common and may contribute to the maintenance of flexion contractures, particularly of the knee. The major complication occurring in the early-onset subgroup is that of asymptomatic persistent or recurrent chronic iridocyclitis; which occurs in over 50 percent of these patients. As many as 20 percent of the children with eye involvement develop ocular damage that may lead to blindness. Slit-lamp examination by an ophthalmologist is the only means of diagnosing and following chronic iridocyclitis. A serum test for antinuclear antibody (ANA) can be used to identify the children of this subgroup who have the greatest risk of developing chronic iridocyclitis. Almost 90 percent of juvenile rheumatoid arthritis patients with iritis have a positive test for ANA.[5] Chronic iridocyclitis, although occurring most frequently in the early-onset pauciarticular subgroup (50 percent) also occurs in the polyarticular group, with an incidence of less than 10 percent. This eye disorder is frequently asymptomatic until irreversible damage has been done, thus the frequent need for ophthalmologic study.

In the late-onset pauciarticular subgroup, the majority of patients are boys, with the most common onset being between the ages of 10 and 15 years. The arthritis is often mild and episodic. Large joints such as the hips, knees, ankles, and shoulders are commonly involved. Systemic complaints are rare. The majority of these boys have a positive HLA B-27 cell surface antigen. They often develop ankylosing spondylitis or Reiter's syndrome in their postpuberty years. Sacroiliac and back symptoms do not usually occur under the age of 16.

REHABILITATION IN CHILDREN

The objective of rehabilitation of the child with juvenile rheumatoid arthritis is to minimize disabilities and to maintain or restore the patient to as normal a functional state as possible. This does not differ from the objective of rehabilitation in the adult with arthritis, except that in childhood the normal functional state itself is rapidly changing. Physical, psychosocial, and educational abilities are all rapidly expanding as the dependent child moves toward becoming a self-sufficient, productive adult.

Prolonged illness and physical disabilities can have a profound effect on psychosocial and educational development. The effect will vary in individual patients. It depends on such factors as the age of the child when the illness begins, the severity, chronicity, and outcome of the disease, the patient's response to the situation, and the environment surrounding the patient. The physician responsible for the patient's care must continually assess the patient's physical, psychosocial, educational, and environmental needs in order to devise a practical rehabilitation program with specific goals directed at the identified problems in each of the four areas. The skills of a variety of professions such as ophthalmologists, physiatrists, physical and occupational therapists, social workers, psychologists, psychiatrists, counselors, marriage counselors for the parents, orthopedic surgeons, podiatrists, dentists, and educators may be required. The physician caring for the patient must maintain good communication with all the participants. Progress must be monitored and the program or the methods altered as needed. Thoughtful consideration must be given to the cost of the program and to the amount of time required of both the patient and the parents. A good working relationship with the parents in addition to the patient is necessary in order to encourage active and constructive participation in the program.

Playing and interacting with peers is extremely important in the psychosocial and educational development of children. Time for such activities must be maintained, because they are part of a sound rehabilitation program. This may also help ensure the patient's cooperation with the more formalized part of the program.

Physical Assessment

In assessing the needs in the four areas—physical, psychosocial, educational, and home environment—the easiest to identify are the physical problems. The frequent occurrence of the asymptomatic chronic iridocyclitis, which requires slit-lamp examination for early detection, makes periodic ophthalmologic examination necessary in all juvenile rheumatoid arthritis patients except the pauciarticular late-onset HLA-B27-positive boys. The early-onset pauciarticular girls have the greatest risk (50 percent) and should be given a slit-lamp examination every 3 to 4 months. The polyarticular subgroups with a much lower incidence can be safely examined every 6 to 9 months. The pauciarticular late-onset HLA-B27-positive boys do not develop chronic iridocyclitis and therefore do not require the periodic eye examination. They may however develop an acute iridocyclitis. Unlike the chronic form, this is symptomatic at onset, at which time ophthalmologic examination and treatment can be instituted.

Abnormalities of the musculoskeletal system are the most common of the physical problems requiring rehabilitative efforts. During the phase of active arthritis with varying degrees of inflammation, the objective should be to maintain the range of motion, muscular strength, and normal joint position while at the same time sparing the joints from excessive use and trauma. The more inflamed and painful the joint (particularly if weight-bearing), the less active use should be allowed. Complete bed rest and restriction of all physical activities is rarely, if ever, warranted. However, regular short rest periods can be helpful in allowing the patient to be more physically active during the remainder of the day. Resting splints for use at night may decrease joint discomfort and at the same time help maintain correct joint position. Prolonged immobilization by casting should not be routinely used as it leads to muscle atrophy and flexion contractures. The use of lightweight rigid wrist splints will enable the patient to use fingers and hands more actively while resting the wrists. The splint that holds the wrist in the functional 10° "cocked-up" position ends just before the metacarpophalangeal joint and does not markedly interfere with finger and thumb motion. Custommade splints work best, but if custom fitting is not possible, readymade wrist splints can be altered for use in older children.

Range-of-motion and specific muscle-strengthening exercises should be done twice a day with special emphasis on involved joints and their muscles. Even when the joints are acutely involved, gentle passive range-of-motion and isometric exercise can usually be tolerated and should be done. The parents and school-aged patients can be instructed in the performance of these exercises by a physiotherapist. While complete parental responsibility for the exercises will be necessary in preschool patients, the older child who has received instruction should ideally require only minimal parental supervision. Visits with the therapist every 4 to 6 weeks will allow for reassessment of the progress and of changing needs. More active muscle-strengthening exercises and postural exercises are added as the amount of joint inflammation and pain decreases. Often therapists experienced in working with children can make a game out of the exercise program, thus making the exercises fun. Attainable goals should be set for each interval of time and between visits with the therapist.

Swimming and range-of-motion exercises done in a heated pool are effective and pleasant. The buoyancy of the water allows for easier and greater mobility. The warmth of the heated pool encourages muscle relaxation and also leads to a decrease in stiffness. The patient feels freer, the activity is enjoyable, and the exercises get done. Heated pools are now more readily available. In many locations the YMCA and public schools have special pool times for disabled individuals. Special arrangements can often be made with commercial health spas or private clubs.

Significant loss of motion and contractures are common and often early complications in juvenile rheumatoid arthritis. The joints most affected are the neck, the proximal and distal interphalangeal joints, the wrist, elbows, knees, and subtalar joints. Range-of-motion exercises are extremely important in preventing loss. The use of splints, primarily at night, to hold the joint in a functional position, minimizes the occurrence of functionally abnormal position and contracture. Once the range of motion is lost or a functionally abnormal position has occurred, it is difficult and often impossible to correct. A greater effort will be required, and the end result is more often to stop progression rather than to achieve significant reversal. The patient and the parents must be aware of this in order to avoid disappointment and total abandonment of the exercises. Once severe contractures of the distal interphalangeal joints and of the elbows are well established, there is no point in continuing various stretching exercises or splinting techniques except to prevent progression. In contrast, adequate correction of severe flexion contractures of the knees can often be attained by serial casting. The cast is applied with the knee extended as fully as possible with gentle pressure. Once the plaster is dry, the cast is bisected so that it can be removed and reapplied with ease.

Depending on the severity of the contracture, the cast is worn all day or just at night. Muscle strengthening, stretching, and range-of-motion exercises are done several times each day with the cast removed. A new cast is applied every 7 to 10 days, with each cast extended slightly further to maintain improvement and lessen the contracture. Keeping and dating the used casts produces an excellent record of the progress.

As mentioned earlier, cock-up splints for the wrist are very helpful in preventing flexion contractures of this joint. If ankylosis cannot be prevented with the range-of-motion exercises, the cock-up splint will ensure that the hand fuses in the most functional position.

Total joint replacement, particularly of the hips, is best delayed until closure of the epiphyseal plates has occurred and bone growth has ceased.[6] Regaining motion in a postsurgical joint is more difficult in a juvenile than in the adult and requires a highly motivated and cooperative patient.[7]

Involvement of the cervical spine with arthritis often leads to marked limitation of motion, particularly of extension. Range-of-motion exercises frequently cause muscle spasm and pain and cannot be used in painful situations. X-rays of the cervical spine should always be obtained prior to instituting any exercise if clinical evidence of involvement is present. If the range of motion is decreasing, efforts to maintain the best possible static functional position are necessary. The head should be maintained in a neutral position and not allowed to become permanently flexed. This can be achieved by avoiding prolonged periods of neck flexion. A small pillow such as a so-called cosmetic pillow gives support to the cervical spine in the supine position while not causing flexion and should replace the usual pillow. The use of an inclined table for reading and writing eliminates the need for head flexion. The television must be placed so it can be comfortably viewed with the head in neutral or slightly extended position. A totally unacceptable but quite common practice is lying in bed or on a sofa with the head held in flexion by a pillow while watching the TV at coffee table height. A soft collar may be useful not only to relieve discomfort, but also to remind the patient to avoid neck flexion when up and about.

Growth disturbances are a unique feature of juvenile rheumatoid arthritis. Both local and generalized growth defects are seen. Generalized growth retardation occurs in children with prolonged active polyarticular disease. No specific treatment is available other than attempting to control the disease activity and maintaining good nutrition. The prolonged use of systemic corticosteroids, which have a very limited place in the therapy of juvenile rheumatoid arthritis, appears to make this problem worse.

Selective growth retardation also occurs. Perhaps the most apparent of these is undergrowth of the jaw, which leads to varying degrees of micrognathia (receding chin). Children with prolonged, active polyarticular disease beginning between the ages of 4 and 10 are at greatest risk. Dental and cosmetic problems are the result. Abnormal bite, crowding of teeth, and abnormal location of tooth eruption require appropriate dental care. The micrognathia, if severe enough to alter bite and appearance, can be corrected by intraoral surgery, which is usually done after the age of 16, when all growth in the area is completed.

Localized overgrowth and undergrowth are frequent in children with limited joint disease, most commonly in the pauciarticular group. Mild arthritis can lead to accelerated epiphyseal growth, while more severe inflammation may retard the growth. Unequal leg lengths can result from this growth disturbance. Leg-length inequality of greater than ½ inch can cause abnormal gait, abnormal muscle usage, pelvic tilt, scoliosis, and abnormal weight-bearing on the joints of the lower extremities. In addition the knee of the long leg may be held in flexion, leading to permanent contracture. Such deformity is difficult to correct if the leg-length difference is not also remedied. This can usually be accomplished with a simple shoe lift.

The child's gait should be monitored periodically. Clothing should be limited to underwear or shorts and a halter when observing so that spine and limb movement can be seen. Abnormalities should be noted, their cause defined, and appropriate therapy implemented if practical. Watching the child walk is extremely helpful in recognizing foot problems.[8] Ankle, subtalar tarsal, and metatarsal involvement is common and frequently leads to ankylosis and abnormal foot positions. Podiatric care with corrective shoes and appliances can promote proper alignment.

Psychosocial Assessment

Monitoring the psychosocial development of the patient is somewhat more difficult. The child should be encouraged to participate as fully as is physically possible in the normal activities of his or her peer group. Every effort must be made to enable the child to go to school. Home schooling should be avoided, and at no time should parental convenience be the deciding factor. Home schooling should be reserved only for the most severely disabled patients and then only when absolutely necessary. The child should be treated as normally as possible within the family and at school. Household responsibilities commensurate with the patient's age and physical abilities should be assigned.

The use of various appliances and training by occupational therapists will enable the child to be more independent. The disabled child will at times use the disability to get what he wants. This in itself is not abnormal. The family must recognize such manipulative behavior and cooperate with the patient only when they believe the demands are reasonable and justified.

Feelings of insecurity, dependence, lack of self-esteem, and poor self-body image are all common emotional problems facing the child or adolescent. The majority appear to handle these difficulties fairly well, at least in terms of being able to function in society. On a more intimate level, males with significant physical disabilities commonly remain single with few, if any, sexual experiences. In contrast, females with similar degrees of disabilities have a near normal sexual life and commonly marry.[9]

Education Assessment

Formal schooling is one of the most important aspects of childhood and dominates children's life-style for many years. The school-age child with juvenile rheumatoid arthritis may have special needs and requirements in order to attend, learn, and function in a school setting. In most cases necessary adjustments can be achieved with thoughtfulness, imagination, and good communication. The amount of physical activity the child can undertake must be clearly defined by the physician and communicated to all those who need to know. The accessibility of classrooms, lunchroom, and restrooms should be assessed by the parents and school officials. The height and suitability of the desk and chair and the height of water fountains and the lavatory fixtures must be considered. Special arrangements may be needed for aiding the child in using the restroom. The occupational therapist may be of great help in devising solutions for specific problems. A simple tape recorder can be used in place of writing for tests and homework, if hand use is a major limitation. Special exercise programs devised by the physical therapist can be done by the patient in place of the usual physical education activities.

Learning and social problems recognized by the teachers should be brought to the attention of the parents and the physician so that solutions can be sought. The child's teachers must attempt to treat the child as normally as possible. Problem behavior cannot be dismissed because the patient "has an illness."

Home Environment

The family unit is of prime importance in childhood. The development in a child of a chronic illness that may lead to severe disability places great emotional stress on the family. Yet the responsible family members will be expected to provide the proper leadership and supervision to meet the patient's special physical, emotional, financial, and time needs. All of this must be done while at the same time maintaining the necessary home ambiance for normal child-rearing. The parents will require sufficient information as to the nature of the child's illness, the therapy, and the likely duration and outcome. Selected written material specifically prepared by the physician or obtained from the American Juvenile Arthritis Organization of the Arthritis Foundation is useful in augmenting the oral discussions. Information can be obtained from your local Arthritis Foundation chapter. (See the appendix to chapter 10 for addresses.) The information given should be to acquaint, reassure, and alleviate the anxiety of the unknown rather than being pedantic, detailed, and scientific. The physician caring for a number of children with juvenile rheumatoid arthritis may find it helpful to establish a parent group that families may contact as a support group. Parent-patient groups organized by the Arthritis Foundation currently exist in many areas of the country and can be a valuable resource.

The parents must have a clear idea of the objectives and specific goals of the rehabilitation program and the amount of leadership, supervision, and observation they must provide. They must be aware of the importance to childhood development of self-image, self-esteem, increasing autonomy, and the necessity of normal play, school attendance, and peer activities. The educational process should be a continuing one, as specific needs or problems arise that may require special attention.

Emotional disturbances of varying severity and marital discord are frequent among the parents.[10] Mothers often have deep-seated guilt feelings, believing themselves somehow responsible for their child's arthritis. They become overprotective and preoccupied with caring for the patient. Fathers rarely verbally object if their wives behave in this manner but, rather, become more emotionally isolated from the problem and less supportive of their wives. Recognition of these problems and instituting the appropriate measures may be critical for maintaining a healthy home environment.

SUMMARY

Rehabilitation of the patient with juvenile rheumatoid arthritis requires an understanding of the nature and characteristics of this heterogeneous disease and the disabilities it may cause. In developing the program, the physical, psychosocial, educational, and home environmental needs of the patient should be assessed. Specific goals should be targeted and progress carefully monitored. A high level of cooperation and communication must be maintained between the patient, the parents, the school, and those providing health care. Management must be optimistic, for the prognosis for the majority is excellent and much can be accomplished for those with more severe disabilities. The program must facilitate active participation in normal childhood activities in the usual environment. It is important that the parents and the child understand that the illness must be looked after but not focused on to the exclusion of normal, everyday activities.

REFERENCES

1. Calabro JJ, Holgerson WB, Sonpal GM, Khoury MI. Juvenile rheumatoid arthritis: a general review and report of 100 patients observed for 15 years. Semin Arth 1976; 5:257-298.
2. Ansell B. Chronic arthritis in childhood. Ann Rheum Dis 1978;37:107-120.
3. Calabro JJ, Marchesano JM. Fever associated with juvenile rheumatoid arthritis. New Engl J Med 1967;276:11-18.
4. Calabro JJ, Marchesano JM. Rash associated with juvenile rheumatoid arthritis. J Pediat 1968;72:611-615.
5. Schaller JG, Johnson GD, Holborow EJ, Ansell BM, Smiley WK. The association of antinuclear antibodies with chronic iridocyclitis of juvenile rheumatoid arthritis (Still's disease). Arth Rheum 1974;17:409-416.
6. Bisla RS, Inglis AE, Ranawat CS. Joint replacement surgery in patients under thirty. J Bone Joint Surg (A) 1976;58:1098-1104.
7. Singsen BH, Isaacson AS, Bernstein BH, Patzakis MJ, Kornreich HK, King KK, Hanson V. Total hip replacement in children with arthritis. Arth Rheum 1978;21:401-406.
8. Dhanedraw M, Hutton WC, Klenerman L, Witemeyer S, Ansell BM. Foot function in juvenile chronic arthritis. Rheum Rehab 1980;19:20-24.
9. Hill RH, Herstein A, Walters K. Juvenile rheumatoid arthritis: follow-up into adulthood—medical, sexual, and social status. Can Med 1976;114:790-796.
10. Henoch MJ, Batson JW, Baum J. Psychosocial factors in juvenile rheumatoid arthritis. Arth Rheum 1978;21:229-233.

40

Connective Tissue Diseases

Evelyn V. Hess, M.D., F.A.C.P

The diseases usually included under the heading connective tissue diseases, or collagen diseases, are systematic sclerosis (SS), polymyositis (PM) dermatomyositis (DM), systemic lupus erythematosus (SLE), and a syndrome called mixed connective tissue disease (MCTD). A very heterogeneous group of disorders and syndromes called the vasculitidies are also usually included but because they infrequently have joint involvement, they will not be discussed here. It should be noted, however, that many of the principles and practices of therapy applicable to the major connective tissue diseases are also appropriate for the vasculitidies and the many other subgroups of collagen disorders.

Review of English-language textbooks and monographs for both generalists and specialists and for medical students and physicians reveals a dearth of information and recommendations for rehabilitative aspects of treatment for patients with systemic sclerosis (scleroderma), polymyositis, and SLE. The information provided ranges from a few specific references to physical and occupational therapy in one or two of the disorders, to general references to the need for supportive care, to no mention of these important therapy components. Review of English-language textbooks for physical and occupational therapists, nurses, and social workers reveals little or no reference to these specific collagen diseases. Even in textbooks on rheumatic disease for members of the arthritis health professions, there is a surprising dearth of information on rehabilitative aspects in the often very short chapters on these specific diseases. A review of the syllabuses of a number of allied health professional undergraduate and graduate schools reveals limited attention to these aspects, if indeed the disorders are even mentioned. There is an obvious concentration on rheumatoid arthritis and more obvious joint diseases, to the detriment of the other collagen disorders.

Many of these patients have joint involvement that is often similar to that seen in rheumatoid arthritis and deserve appropriate therapy. Each disease has its own special characteristics requiring a specific approach to rehabilitation. This chapter reviews and synthesizes what is known and recommended from a wide range of the literature and includes personal recommendations from experience at a number of centers where these diseases are treated.

Each disease is reviewed under the following headings, and reference is made to the appropriate referral if indicated: general review, primary care physician, physical and occupational therapy, nursing, nutritionist/dental care, social worker/counseling, podiatrist/prosthetist, community resources.

SYSTEMIC SCLEROSIS

Systemic sclerosis (SS), also called progressive systemic sclerosis (PSS), or scleroderma, is a generalized disorder of connective tissue and small blood vessels that nearly always involves the skin. Other organs such as the lung, heart, kidneys, intestinal tract, and esophagus are frequently involved, and muscle and joints are symptomatic to a variable degree. The reported incidence is roughly twelve cases per million people annually.[1] Women are affected three times more frequently than men, and the first symptoms usually appear between 30 and 50 years of age. The disease is very uncommon in children. No specific etiology is yet known and treatments are not definitive. Since the disease tends to run a chronic course, treatment of the specific organ involvement and general supportive measures are the main objectives of therapy. A small number of patients succumb to renal, cardiac, pulmonary, or gastrointestinal involvement. A subset of the disease is called by the acronym CREST, because the patients have calcium deposits, Raynaud's phenomenon, esophageal problems, scleroderma, and telangiectasia. This subset of patients tends to have less severe disease.

The primary care physician. The physician needs to keep in mind the World Health Organization definition of rehabilitation: "the combined and coordinated use of medical, social, educational and vocational measures for training and retraining the individual to the highest possible level of functional ability."[2] Continuous sympathy and support are essential. Attention to Raynaud's phenomenon if it is present is important, with constant reminders to avoid cold and keep the body warm, wear gloves or mittens, avoid cuts and injuries, use special soaps or bath oils to help excessive dryness of the skin. Smoking should be discouraged. Renal or other severe organ involvement may necessitate consultation with a rheumatologist or other specialist.

Physical therapy. The peripheral joints may be stiff and painful. These symptoms may be helped by exercise, massage, moist heat, and paraffin baths. Care should be taken if the circulation is severely compromised. It is best if the patient actively exercises the involved areas. Frequent repetition of the exercises also improves the circulation. Rest splints may be of some value if there is arthritis. Muscle inflammation and occasionally muscle atrophy occur. The severity can be determined by electromyography and the appropriate physical or occupational therapy program determined.

Nutritionist and dental care. Particular care is needed in patients who manifest severe bowel involvement or evidence of malabsorption. They may require skilled nutritional counseling. It is important to remember that oral disease can occur because of restriction in mouth opening, dry mouth, and dental decay. Regular dental care is essential.

Counseling. Patients with SS, especially if they have severe skin and joint involvement may need a complete functional assessment and counseling for suitability to continue or to change occupations. Whenever possible, life-style should be as normal as possible. Advantage should be taken of the U.S. Department of Health and Human Services Social Security Administration Revised Medical Criteria for Determination of Disability, which were published in the Federal Register in 1982. The specific criteria for musculoskeletal disability is reviewed in volume 47. Section 10.05 defines SS as "a) Advanced limitation of use of hands due to sclerodactyly or limitation in other joints or, b) significant visceral manifestations of digestive, cardiac or pulmonary impairment."

Podiatrist. Because of the poor circulation and occasionally Raynaud's phenomenon in the feet, careful podiatric care is an excellent preventive measure for infection and chronic ulcers in the feet.

Community resources. Information on the disease and patient club meetings can be obtained from local chapters of the Arthritis Foundation (see the appendix to chapter 10) or the United Scleroderma Foundation (P.O. Box 350, Watsonville, Calif. 95077).

MIXED CONNECTIVE TISSUE DISEASE

In recent years a syndrome termed *mixed connective tissue disease* has been described and accepted by rheumatologists.[3] Patients with this syndrome have characteristics of SS, polymyositis, SLE, and occasionally rheumatoid arthritis. They require from their primary care physician and allied health professionals evaluation and therapy as determined by the predominant disease components they manifest. The syndrome is often more benign than the specific collagen diseases dealt with in this section. However, in an increasing number of these patients, the syndrome is evolving into one of the better defined diseases, most often systemic sclerosis.

POLYMYOSITIS

This is an inflammatory disease of skeletal muscle, which when the inflammation involves the skin, is called dermatomyositis. The disease occurs most frequently between the ages of 30 to 50, with a 2:1 ratio of females to males. The incidence is similar to SS. The specific cause is not known and specific cure is not yet available. In a few patients the disease is related to an underlying cancer. Immunologic mechanisms are involved in the pathogenesis. The overall mortality rate is presently about 15 to 30 percent and death (excluding those secondary to cancer) is usually due to severe muscle weakness resulting in lung or esophageal problems.[4] As well as muscle and skin involvement, there may be Raynaud's phenomenon, arthralgias, subcutaneous calcification, and pulmonary and cardiac involvement. A special type of dermatomyositis occurs in children.

The primary care physician. The physician's concerns are similar to those for patients with SS. Fatigue is an important symptom, and suitable rest periods are important. The muscle weakness occurring well into treatment can be steroid related or due to failure of therapy. Medical therapy includes the use of cortico-steroids and cytotoxic agents. Special attention to swallowing difficulties and the prevention of aspiration by appropriate bed posturing is important. Patients with this disorder should be seen in consultation at rheumatic disease centers to help determine the extent of disease involvement and to plan therapy.

Physical and occupational therapy. When the patient is hospitalized, chest physiotherapy with appropriate suctioning may be necessary. General strengthening exercises for all muscle groups when disease activity is controlled are essential. The exact role of muscle exercise is controversial.[5] Some studies have shown that exercise can increase inflammation.[5] Gentle, graded exercises under strict supervision are best. Muscle strength must be built up to avoid future disability and all concerned should realize that this may be a slow process. Recently S.A. Hyde has described resistive exercises using techniques of proprioceptive neuromuscular facilitation.[5] This approach has not yet been fully accepted. If the joints are involved, range-of-motion exercises and gait training are indicated. This occupational and physical therapy approach is an important part of the management of the subacute and chronic stages of the disease.

Counseling. Assessment of the patient's work potential or change of work with appropriate counseling is an important part of management. Advantage should be taken of Social Security Disability benefits when indicated.

Nursing. Patients with polymyositis are frequently hospitalized, and skilled nursing care is essential. The nurse and other members of the health care team have an excellent opportunity to provide information to the patients and to play a sympathetic and supportive role.

Community resources. The local chapters of the Arthritis Foundation can supply information on the disease and on patient education meetings.

SYSTEMIC LUPUS ERYTHEMATOSUS

Systemic lupus erythematosus (SLE) is a disorder in which inflammation of the small and sometimes medium-size blood vessels of the body causes a large number of clinical signs and symptoms. Many immunologic abnormalities are present, so it is considered the prototype of autoimmune disease. The incidence is about 3 per 100,000 and in the United States about 500,000 have the disease at any time. It occurs most frequently between ages 15 and 40 years and the female/male ratio is probably 8/1.[6] The specific cause or causes are not yet known and it therefore lacks specific therapies. Most therapy is aimed at controlling the inflammatory and immunologic reactions. It occurs in children and in the elderly as well. A subset of the disease is related to certain drugs, for example hydralazine. Many organ systems can be involved, especially renal, cardiac, pulmonary, hematologic, and central nervous system. The joint and muscle involvement is similar to rheumatoid arthritis. Today SLE has a good prognosis.

The primary care physician. Close supervision is necessary except in the very mild forms of the disease. Most patients need a consultation at some time with a rheumatologist or a nephrologist. Many have frequent hospitalizations. It is important to pay attention to stress, fatigue, incriminating drugs, excessive sun exposure—all of which may cause or worsen the disease. It is vital to be optimistic about prognosis, for at the present time up to 94 percent of the patients are alive at five years.[6] Since multiple systems and organs may be involved, the patients may need the help of a wide range of health professionals. It is important for all concerned to provide information and to be optimistic with the patient. Many of the recommendations for SS and polymyositis apply also to SLE. Since SLE patients are often young women, they will need advice about sex and pregnancy. If they become pregnant, the obstetrician should be consulted as early as possible. Medical treatment includes the use of anti-inflammatory, antimalarial, corticosteroid, and cytotoxic drugs, depending on what organ system is involved and how severe the involvement is. Some patients require no medication. The rheumatologist can help guide this decision.

Physical/occupational therapy. Joint and muscle disease is common, but fortunately deforming arthritis occurs infrequently. In some patients the joint involvement is due to a capsulitis, which may cause severe damage, including ulnar drift in the hands. Splints and other procedures as used for rheumatoid arthritis may be indicated. Serious disability is unusual, however. Myositis if present needs muscle-strengthening exercises and a regime to prevent muscle contractures as in polymyositis.

Counseling. Patients with SLE are very often quite ill, with profound fatigue but without necessarily appearing ill. They need constant reassurance, and counseling may be necessary to treat and prevent depression. Since most of these patients lack the physical deformities often seen in SS and polymyositis, they should be encouraged to work and to remain at their occupations. They frequently are very productive members of the community. When indicated, referral for Social Security Disability should be made. SLE is defined in the 1982 USDHHS Social Security Administration Revised Medical Criteria for Determination of Disability, volume 47, section 10.04 as follows: "With frequent exacerbations demonstrating involvement of renal, cardiac or pulmonary or gastrointestinal or central nervous systems."

Community Resources. Chapters of the Arthritis Foundation have literature and patient education classes for SLE. Two other organizations, the Lupus Foundation of America (11673 Holly Springs Drive, St. Louis, Mo. 63141) and the American Lupus Society (23751 Madison Street, Torrance, Calif. 90505) also have local chapters and educational material.

SUMMARY

The major collagen diseases—systemic sclerosis, polymyositis, and systemic lupus erythematosus—are all multisystem diseases. Therapy and management of

454   REHABILITATION TECHNIQUES

these disorders need many members of the health care team. The employment of proper treatment and management results in a decrease in morbidity and mortality, with an improvement of function with appropriate rehabilitation. Educating patients and their families about the diseases is very important.

REFERENCES

1. Kurland LT, Hauser WA, Ferguson RH, Holley KE. Epidemiological features of diffuse connective tissue disorders in Rochester, Minnesota, 1951–1967, with special reference to systemic lupus erythematosus. Mayo Clin Proc 1969;44:649–663.
2. World Health Organization (WHO). The international classification of impairment, disabilities and handicaps: a manual of classification relating to the consequences of disease. Geneva: WHO, 1980.
3. Sharp GC. Mixed connective tissue disease: current concepts. Arth Rheum 1977;20: 5181–5185.
4. Pearson CM. Polymyositis and dermatomyositis. In: McCarthy DJ, ed. Arthritis and allied conditions. 9th ed. Philadelphia: Lea and Febiger, 1979, p. 755.
5. Hyde SA. Physiotherapy in rheumatology. Oxford: Blackwell Scientific Publications, 1980.
6. Rothfield NF. Systemic lupus erythematosus: clinical and laboratory aspects. In: McCarty DJ, ed. Arthritis and allied conditions. 9th ed. Philadelphia: Lea and Febiger, 1979.

ADDITIONAL READINGS

Bluestone R, ed. Rheumatology. Boston: Houghton Mifflin, 1980.
Currey H, ed. An introduction to clinical rheumatology, 3rd ed. Philadelphia: JB Lippincott, 1980.
Woolf D, ed. Rehabilitation in the rheumatic diseases. Clin Rheum Dis (London) 1981;7(2).

41

Septic Arthritis

Eric P. Gall, M.D.

Septic arthritis is a common disease both in pediatric and adult ages. Concepts regarding management of this disorder have shifted over the past decade. Medical management is preferred to surgery and consists of nonsurgical drainage of the affected joint, proper antibiotic therapy, and physical measures in the vast majority of patients.

Although only the treatment of acute suppurative bacterial arthritis is discussed in this chapter, there are a number of other important syndromes with differing clinical features. Table 41.1 summarizes the common infectious causes of joint disease. They include acute bacterial arthritis, including gonococcal arthritis, the chronic slow-growing organisms, osteomyelitis, viral arthritis, and infections having special considerations.

Table 41.1. Common Varieties of Infectious Arthritis

Acute bacterial arthritis
Gonococcal arthritis
Chronic septic arthritis
Tuberculous arthritis
Fungal arthritis
Osteomyelitis
  Acute
  Chronic
Viral arthritis
  Hepatitis
  Rubella
  Arbovirus
  Other
Infections in special circumstances
  Postoperative infections
    Infected joint prostheses
  Immunocompromised host
  Diabetic arthropathy (neurogenic with infection)
  Spinal infections

CLINICAL PRESENTATION

Recognition of septic arthritis is crucial to the proper management of the disorder. Table 41.2 outlines the key features that should lead the clinician to consider this diagnosis with a high degree of clinical suspicion at all times. An agressive approach to diagnosing infections is the key to success. While none of the listed signs and symptoms are pathognomonic in and of themselves (with the exception of a positive culture), all of them should lead to a careful consideration of joint infection.

Patients with gout, pseudogout, rheumatoid arthritis, and other diseases may have fever and chills due to the inflammatory nature of their disease. Nonetheless such a finding should heighten the clinician's sensitivity to the possibility of infection. Many patients are predisposed to infection, particularly joint infection, because of an underlying condition. Such underlying causes are also noted in table 41.2.

The diagnosis of septic arthritis in a patient with rheumatoid arthritis is particularly difficult. The "out-of-phase joint" or failure to respond to therapy in a single joint, when others respond, suggests superimposed infection. Loosening and pain of total joint prosthesis also should cause concern in such a patient. The delay in diagnosis along with the abnormal leukocyte function in such patients leads to poor prognosis even with therapy. Therapy in these cases is usually more aggressive than in uncomplicated septic arthritis.

Table 41.2.   Suspect Septic Arthritis

Arthritis associated with fever or chills
Patients with arthritis and known infections outside the joint
Patients with arthritis and typical associated skin rash
  Gonococcal rash
Patients who are immunocompromised
  Drug-related (steroids, cytotoxic drugs)
  Disease-related (disseminated tumor, hypogammaglobulinemia)
Persistent joint inflammation not responding to standard treatment
Monoarticular arthritis
A prior joint infection (known by patient's history)
Recent injection into joint (especially through cellulitis)
Prior surgical procedure in joint (especially prosthesis)
A history of
  Drug abuse
  Diabetes
  Sickle cell disease
  Rheumatoid arthritis
Typical radiographic findings (*diffuse* loss of bone cortex)
Low sugar in joint fluid
Synovial fluid white count greater than 50,000/mm^3
Positive culture results

Physicians caring for patients with a so-called "well-diagnosed disease" that is not responding to therapy should suspect arthritis. Symptoms of many patients with joint infections mimic other disorders, including gout and rheumatoid arthritis. Monoarticular involvement is a particular signal to suspect infection. All such joints should be aspirated and cultured if possible.

DIAGNOSIS

Definitive diagnosis of septic arthritis requires demonstration of the offending organism by microscopy and particularly by culture. This is usually accomplished by joint aspiration, the techniques of which are beyond the scope of this chapter but are covered in other sources.[3,4] Gram stains and special stains as indicated (AFB, fungal) are done, and cultures for all appropriate organisms are carried out. Careful and prompt handling of specimens as well as communication with the microbiology laboratory regarding specimen handling is requisite. In some situations synovial fluid culture has a poor yield in growing organisms.[5] This is particularly true with gonococcus (multiple other sites are also cultured), acid-fast bacilli, and fungal organisms. In the latter situations synovial and/or affected bone biopsies are done for better recovery of the offending organism. Cultures of blood, obvious sources of hematogenic spread and metastatic infections, can all help to identify the infection.

Synovial fluid cell-count, differentials, and sugars (compared to serum values) help to generate suspicion of infection. Occasionally no organism is isolated and antimicrobial therapy is instituted on clinical grounds alone. This should be the rare exception, and quick, extensive, multiple cultures should be performed before beginning a therapy.

Radiologic studies may or may not be helpful in diagnosing septic arthritis. The finding of diffuse cortical bone loss in a joint, in contrast to focal erosions, is often strongly suggestive of infection.[6] This finding may not be radiographically apparent early in the septic joint except in the most virulent infections. Loosening of prosthetic joints may also alert the clinician to the possibility of infection in a painful joint months or years after total joint replacement.[7] Such infections are often associated with normally nonpathogenic bacteria such as staph epidermidis and alpha strep. Biopsy may be required for definitive culture. Other radiographic findings are less definitive in nature.

TREATMENT

The treatment of septic arthritis requires a comprehensive approach. Clinical suspicion, early diagnosis, and correct identification of the offending organisms are requisite. The treatment program for septic arthritis is compared to the structure of a pyramid (figure 41.1). A strong foundation of proper diagnosis is supplemented with definitive therapy in a logical progression. Only after the lower

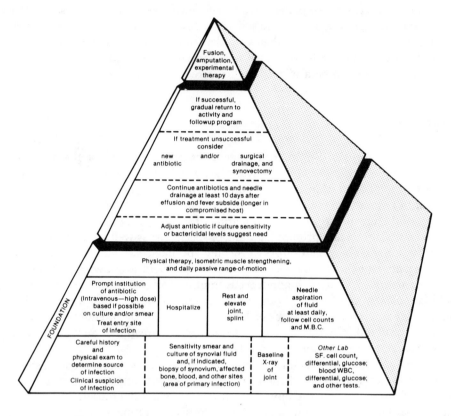

Figure 41.1. Treatment pyramid for septic arthritis.

portions of the structure are firmly in place should the upper reaches of the pyramid be added, and then only if they are needed. The top of the pyramid is more costly, experimental, and is associated with higher morbidity and more side effects.

One can guess as to the most likely organisms based on patient presentation, but this never substitutes for definitive identification. Nonetheless one is often forced to begin treatment before culture and sensitivities are available. Almost all joint infections require hospitalization because of the seriousness of both local and systemic consequences. In almost all situations intravenous antibiotics are required to achieve adequate blood and joint concentrations. Some authors advocate oral antibiotics for uncomplicated gonococcal arthritis.[8] However, many of these patients are unreliable, and since serious consequences may arise from partially treated infections, it is safer to hospitalize these patients for intravenous therapy. Intra-articular antibiotics are almost never used for two reasons. First, adequate synovial fluid levels are achieved by intravenous antibiotics in virtually all cases.[9] Also local intrasynovial installation of antibiotics frequently causes a chemical synovitis.[10] Response to therapy is measured by decreased synovial fluid white counts, increased patient well-being, and antibiotic minimal bactericidal concentrations in the fluid. Once culture and sensitivities have been obtained, adjustments may be made in either the type or dose of antibiotics.

The merits of surgical drainage versus medical needle drainage of infected joints have been argued in the literature extensively. Most recent literature favors a medical approach.[9,11] This approach requires initially tapping the involved joint on a daily basis following the following parameters:

Minimal bacteriocidal concentration

Cell count

Amount of fluid

Culture of fluid

Patient well-being

When recovery is underway and the effusion is sterile, cell counts and fluid volume alone can be followed. Arthrocentesis is done on a daily basis (or more often if reaccumulation is rapid enough). Theoretically much of the joint damage comes from the accumulation of white blood cells and lysosomal enzymes in the septic joint; thus fluid removal is essential in preventing joint damage.

Occasionally medical therapy is not successful or not indicated and surgical debridement is resorted to. Surgical drainage usually includes synovectomy and joint debridement. The indications for surgical drainage of the septic arthritic joint are as follows:

Joint is inaccessible to needle drainage (like the hip).

Fever is persistent.

Synovial fluid white cell count remains elevated.

Pus cannot be removed or is local.

Osteomyelitis is present.

Antibiotic does not penetrate fluid.

Certain infections that do not respond to nonsurgical therapy (such as coccidioidomycosis).

Antibiotic therapy and drainage of the joint are successful only in relation to the promptness of the diagnosis and institution of therapy.[13] Special attention must be paid to the source of infection. Frequently sinus, pulmonary, genitourinary, abraded skin, and other sources of infection cause hematogenous or local spread of infection into a joint. These sources obviously must be located and eradicated. While eradication of infection may be accomplished by the principles outlined here, lack of attention to physical factors may lead to prolonged morbidity or a poor functional result.

Prescription of rest as a time-honored therapy for the inflamed or infected joint dates back to the work of John Hunter in the eighteenth century.[14] Most clinicians put the joint at rest during the acute inflammatory portion of the septic arthritis. Indeed our unit routinely splints and elevates the involved joint until inflammation subsides, putting the joint through daily passive range of motion, then placing the joint back in a splint. The physical therapist and sometimes the occupational therapist as well as the nursing staff are intimately involved with patient care from the onset of therapy. While range-of-motion exercise is done only once daily, isometric muscle exercises are repeatedly performed to maintain muscle strength until the patient is fully mobilized. This activity is supervised by the therapist or nurse.

There has long been some belief in the advantage of active exercise early in the treatment of septic arthritis. Williams in 1919 suggested early exercise after arthrotomy for septic arthritis.[15] In the same year Everidge used a hinged, Thomas splint to eliminate gravity in the septic knee and immediate active motion.[16] Good results were reported in 201 patients with this method in an uncontrolled study.[17] In modern times Ballard et al. found that early active motion after surgery resulted in better range of motion. Salter, Bell, and Keeley showed healing of cartilage defects in rabbits with septic arthritis undergoing active motion.[19] Nonetheless in nonsurgically treated patients, the use of active exercise early in the treatment regimen is untested and not advisable until further studies are done. The need for intermittent passive motion is suggested, especially in those with underlying rheumatoid arthritis, which is subject to fusion. Unfortunately there are very few controlled studies in the physical modalities for treatment of these disorders.

The entity of postinfectious synovitis is well described in patients who exercise early in the course of the disease. The medically treated patient who moves the affected joint throughout the day and particularly who bears weight on an involved joint will experience initial improvement and decrease in symptoms. This improvement may be slower than in an unexercised joint, although there are no data to support this contention. After initial improvement, however, persistent low-grade synovitis is present for several days and sometimes weeks after the infection has subsided. This prolongs morbidity and confuses the issue as to whether the infection is under control. For this reason, until studies suggest otherwise, a conservative approach to active exercise is suggested. Once the infection has subsided, gradual return to normal activity is in order.

SUMMARY

The patient with septic arthritis has a life-threatening disease that requires a high degree of clinical suspicion, prompt and accurate diagnosis, and a comprehensive treatment program. A team approach to care is essential as in all types of arthritis. Particular attention to details of medical and physical treatment will lead to full recovery in the great majority of patients who are properly diagnosed early in the illness. Patient and family education will lead to better compliance with the treatment protocol and, it is hoped, to a greater degree of long-term success. Nonsurgical treatment approaches are preferred in the majority of patients at this time.

REFERENCES

1. Myers AR, Miller LM, Pinals RS. Pyarthrosis complicating rheumatoid arthritis. Lancet 1969;2:714–717.
2. Starkebaum G, Jeminez RAHA. Effect of immune complexes on human neutrophil phagocyte function. J Immunol 1982;128:141–147.
3. McCarty DJ. Arthritis and allied conditions, 9th ed. Philadelphia: Lea and Febiger, 1979.
4. Steinbrocker O, Neustedt DH. Aspiration and injection therapy in arthritis and musculoskeletal disorders. Hagerstown, Md.: Harper & Row, 1972.
5. Schumacher HR, Kulka JP. Needle biopsy of the synovial membrane—experience with the Parker-Pearson technique. New Eng J Med 1972;286:416–419.
6. Resnick D, Niwayama G. Diagnosis of bone and joint disorders. Philadelphia: AB Saunders, 1981, p. 3.
7. Ibid, vol. 1.
8. Hunter-Handsfield H, Wesner PJ, Holmes KK. Treatment of the gonococcal arthritis-dermatitis syndrome. Ann Int Med 1976;84:661–669.
9. Schmidt FR, Parker RH. Ongoing assessment of therapy in septic arthritis. Arth Rheum 1969;12:529–534.
10. Argen RJ, Welson CH, Wood P. Suppurative arthritis clinical features of 42 cases. Arch Int Med 1966;117:661.
11. Goldenberg DL, Brandt KD, Cohen AS, Cathcart ES. Treatment of septic arthritis. Arth Rheum 1975;18:83–90.
12. Boyer AS, Cherow AW, Louie JS, Gage LB. Sternoarticular pyarthrosis due to gram negative bacilli. Arch Int Med 1977;137:108–140.
13. Newman JH. Review of septic arthritis throughout the cantibiotic era. Ann Rheum Dis 1976;35:198–205.
14. Keiter A. Menders of the maimed. London: Oxford University Press, 1919.
15. Williams C. Treatment of purulent arthritis by wide arthrotomy followed by immediate active mobilization. Surg Gyneocol Obst 1919;28:5461.
16. Everidge J. A new method of treatment of suppurative arthritis of the knee-joint. Brit J Surg 1918–1919;6:566–578.
17. Heberling JA. A review of 201 cases of suppurative arthritis. J Bone Joint Surg 1941; 23:917.
18. Ballard A, Burkholter WE, Mayfield AW, Dehne E, Brown P. The functional treatment of pyogenic arthritis of the adult knee. J Bone Joint Surg (Am) 1975;57:1119.
19. Salter RB, Bell RS, Keeley FW. The protective effect of continuous passive motion in articular cartilage in acute septic arthritis. Clin Orthop Related Res 1982;159:223–247.

42

Nonarticular Rheumatism

John T. Boyer, M.D.

The term *nonarticular rheumatism* (NAR) enjoys wide use in rheumatology and implies the aches, pains, stiffness, and tenderness, both local and generalized, that haunts mankind but strictly speaking is not arthritis. Confusion arises from the fact that a clinician seldom tells his patient, "you have nonarticular rheumatism" and is more likely to diagnose "tendinitis," "bursitis," or "ordinary arthritis." Worse, physicians often attribute NAR symptoms to osteoarthritis because of a patient's advanced age or thoracic spine osteophytes, thus distracting themselves and other members of the health care team from treatment that is more effective. The situation is further confounded by the practice of some rheumatologists of using "NAR" only as a generalization for regional syndromes (rotator cuff tears, bicipital tendinitis, tennis elbow), while others confine its use to syndromes of diffuse symptoms (fibrositis, polymyalgia rheumatica, psychogenic rheumatism). While I favor a definition that includes all musculoskeletal symptoms other than arthritis, this chapter will be confined to general remarks on tendinitis, bursitis, myofasciitis, and that controversial entity known generally as fibrositis, leaving specific examples to be considered in the chapters on regional disorders.

ACUTE NAR

Sudden and transient examples of NAR include strains, bruises, and minor muscle tears, usually, but by no means always having an obvious, external cause and generally responding to rest, time, and simple analgesics or nonsteroidal anti-inflammatory drugs. In the examples that follow, only chronic NAR is addressed and the notion "chronic" is arbitrarily limited to conditions persisting longer than 3 weeks.

CHRONIC NAR

Clinical Features

Chronic NAR frequently has its beginning in an acute traumatic pain that simply does not go away. NAR may also arise without apparent cause, sometimes gradually over days to weeks and sometimes abruptly, perhaps overnight. Patients usually describe an ache that grows in both distribution and intensity. An appreciation of swelling, usually apparent only to the patient, is probably a misinterpretation of the tenderness and stiffness that occur. There is a tendency for pains that begin proximally to spread distally (the shoulder-hand syndrome; the hip-foot syndrome). Patients will frequently note that persistent motion of the painful area often produces relief temporarily. By the time the patient seeks professional help, however, he or she usually tries to move the painful area as little as possible. Objective signs of inflammation, such as redness, warmth, and swelling, are rare, although pain and tenderness may be severe. Systemic manifestations such as fever, anorexia, and nausea sometimes occur at the beginning of symptoms, probably because certain acute viral illnesses may trigger NAR, but they are absent during the chronic stages. Fatigue, loss of sleep, and decreased energy are often present, as is the case in most pain syndromes.

Table 42.1 contains a list of body areas and the regional syndromes of NAR commonly associated with them. Fibrositis, a generalized NAR, is considered separately.

Table 42.1.   Body Areas and "Regional Syndromes of NAR"

	Tendinitis	Bursitis	Myofasciitis
Occiput	Muscle insertion Headaches		
Jaw			Masseter "tense jaw"
Neck			Wry Neck or torticollus
Shoulder	Biceps tendinitis	Subdeltoid bursitis	Trapezius pain
Elbow	Tennis elbow Lateral epicondylitis Golfer's elbow Medial epicondylitis	Olecranon bursitis	
Wrist	Extensor tendinitis		
Thumb	de Quervain's tendinitis		
Back			Most back pain
Hip area	Quadriceps tendinitis	Trochanteric bursitis	Sacral attachments
Knee	Hamstring tendinitis	Anserine bursitis	
Ankle	Achilles tendinitis Peroneus tendinitis	Pre-Achilles bursitis	Plantar fasciitis

Pathology

Rarely, tendinitis, bursitis, and myofasciitis occur as truly inflammatory conditions with local redness, warmth, and obvious swelling on physical examination and with manifestations of edema formation, blood vessel dilatation, and inflammatory blood cell infiltration on microscopic study. Bacteria, viral, and fungal infestations may be the cause of such obvious inflammation and mandate antimicrobial therapy. Occasionally a rheumatic condition affects extra-articular tissues, as in rheumatoid disease, Reiter's disease, and perhaps gout. Many examples of NAR with true inflammation are of unknown cause and are unassociated with any generalized syndrome (calcific biceps tendinitis; de Quervain's syndrome).

By far the most common finding in NAR, however, is normal tissue: no swelling; no redness; no warmth; and no microscopic changes; only pain and tenderness. *Most chronic NAR is a pain syndrome*, and the cause and mechanism of this pain are unknown. It occurs so frequently in the wake of an injury or strain or temporary illness that it *seems as if* the pain is a memory of pain one cannot lose: a habit or conditioned reflex. Consider "phantom pain": if one can experience chronic pain in the "foot" that was amputated long ago, one can appreciate how one might experience pain in a normal structure, still present, but injured long ago.

Physical Findings

Table 42.2 contrasts the features of NAR or extra-articular pain with true arthritis or intra-articular pain. Tenderness occurs only over the tendon, bursa, or muscle involved and is therefore "trigger point" in nature in NAR. (See figure 42.1.) In arthritis, except when the inflammation is intense, as in septic arthritis or gout, tenderness comes from inside the joint, is less available to the probing hand, and is more vague or general.

The most valuable test of NAR versus arthritis is the study of motion in the afflicted area. Inside a raw, inflamed arthritic joint, pain is induced whenever motion rubs the two surfaces together, either in active motion (the patient uses his muscle) or passive motion (the patient *relaxes* while the examiner moves the joint). In NAR joint interiors are normal, and no pain is induced by rubbing mo-

Table 42.2.   Features of NAR and Arthritis

	NAR	*Arthritis*
Inflammation	Rarely	Usually
Tenderness	Trigger point	General/vague
Pain on motion	Active only	Active and passive

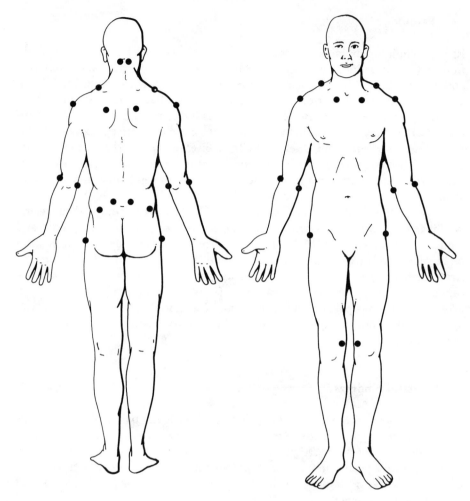

Figure 42.1.   Trigger points.

tion of the joint surfaces unless external structures are disturbed by contraction of one's own muscles to create the motion. Thus the main distinction on physical examination between NAR and arthritis is that *only active motion hurts in NAR whereas in arthritis both active and passive motion hurt.* The art of examination depends upon the physician's ability to get the patient to relax sufficiently for passive motion assessment.

Treatment

For NAR without obvious inflammation the two goals of therapy are to *distract the patient from his pain* and to *return the symptomatic part to active motion.* Pain relief distractors popular among various therapists include the following:

Heat

Cold

Heat and cold

Massage

Ultrasound

Diathermy

Acupuncture

Trigger-point injections with
   Local anesthetics
   Steroids
   Both

Stretching/manipulation

Linaments

Mustard plaster

Transcutaneous stimulation

DMSO

Such disparate modes of therapy seem to be held together conceptually only by the common ability of each to distract. All except steroid injections lack the ability to inhibit inflammation. Some are believed to "increase blood flow" (whatever that is good for). But they all alter pain perception in some way that allows the patient to "de-focus" for a valuable period of time. The value of distraction therapy is not confined to NAR, of course, and it is useful in any situation featuring pain.

Active exercise and power building are the most important aspects of NAR treatment. Though sometimes a period of assistive or passive motion exercises is necessary to relieve contracted tissues (in frozen shoulder or stiff finger, for example), eventually the conservative program or resistive exercise, escalated gradually over several weeks is successful. The rationale for this therapy is that it generally works. Since most NAR is a pain syndrome in normal structures, perhaps power building is the ultimate distractor. Total rest of the painful part is usually successful in relieving pain also, but all too frequently total rest programs eventuate in atrophy, pain, or restriction of motion, local edema formation, spreading of pain to adjacent areas, and reflex sympathetic dystrophy such as the shoulder-hand syndrome.

The art of therapy is to persuade the patient to use resistive exercises even if pain occurs. The use of distractors for this is very important. Oral analgesics or local anesthetics to facilitate comfortable exercise are of inestimable value. It is also helpful to the therapist, as well as the patient, to follow the aphorism: "If it's arthritis, baby it; if it's NAR, bully it." For the former, use splints, passive range-of-motion exercise, and isometric exercise. For the latter, use hard massage and power building. For the naive patient it is very helpful to be told that some pain (arthritis) is to be heeded and given in to, but that other pains (NAR) are harmless or even trivial and are to be ignored or overcome.

FIBROSITIS

Fibrositis is a term used to describe a syndrome of general body aching pain and tenderness, usually in the proximal pectoral or pelvic girdle muscles but sometimes including the distal extremities. Generalized trigger-point tenderness, fatigue, sleep aberrations, depression, and disability are characteristic though no abnormalities of x-ray, blood test or objective abnormalities on physical examination are present. Secondary gain is often a prominent feature. Chronicity and resistance to treatment are the rule, although deterioration and deformity never occur. Synonyms include fibromyositis, myofasciitis, and psychogenic rheumatism. Fibrositis is separated from other syndromes of pain previously considered by the fact that it is generalized rather than regional, constant rather than episodic, and almost totally resistant to treatment rather than eminently responsive. Fibrositis is one of the major causes of permanent disability today.

Clinical Features

Fibrositis afflicts men and women in about equal proportions, usually starting between the ages of 30 and 60 and persisting through old age. Health service practitioners tend to treat patients only in the earlier years, however, when diagnostic studies and medical sources of relief are sought diligently. The need for professional support of legal disability status is also an important factor. In the declining years patients become disillusioned with the medical system and generally bear their pain more stoically without medical help.

As with regional syndromes of NAR, the onset of fibrositis usually occurs with a major accident or illness with local signs of pain. Apparent recovery or partial recovery is then followed by an unaccountable relapse, with spreading of pain over neck, shoulders, arms, back, hips, and thighs. Tenderness, especially in trigger-point areas is invariable, and pressure on these produces a "jump sign" (an exaggerated withdrawal or grimace). Any body motion may induce similar exaggerated pain and patients markedly reduce physical activity, many retiring to bed and chair. Significantly, muscle atrophy does not occur, although weakness is common. Brief displays of strength can usually be prompted by the examiner, but the muscle set rapidly gives way and exhaustion follows. Indeed fatigue is a cardinal feature of fibrositis and any physical effort is usually followed by required rest for hours to days.

Sleep is almost always disturbed, staying asleep being more difficult than falling asleep, the same pattern seen in depressive syndromes. In fact overlap with depression is common in fibrositis, with the prognosis improving in proportion to the degree of depression present.

Two psychologic features are almost always striking. First, the patient's focus on pain is inordinate, usually greater than among patients with more obvious sources of pain such as arthritis, burns, and cancer. Patients cannot be distracted from pain for more than a short time and often find that they tire friends and family, thus greatly constricting social contact. Usually a spouse or other "nurturing" individual—alone—remains as a source of comfort and support. Often the visit to the clinic or physical therapy unit involves both the patient and this nurturing individual.

The second feature is a "locus of control" almost completely outside of self. Patients with fibrositis usually see themselves as completely at the mercy of their pain and believe they cannot overcome or become the masters of their fate. Only secondarily, allowing the pain also to control others (spouse, employer), does one see this locus return to the patient, which accounts for the categorization of fibrositis as an affliction of secondary gain. It is *not*, however, an example of malingering, a deliberate medical deception. Patients with fibrositis suffer not only before the physician, but in the privacy of their homes. The secondary gain is obtained at high cost to physical comfort.

Treatment

Therapy in this disorder is discouraging, both to patient and to therapist. First, there is no known organic lesion to correct. Second, with secondary gain so prominent in the determination of symptoms, motivation is missing. What good is a disorder of secondary gain if one might recover? Patient education, overcoming antagonisms, and simple "support" are the major areas of treatment available.

Patient Education

As the patient enters the therapist's office he usually expects, even anticipates, a diagnosis of rheumatoid arthritis or similar serious organic illness. He accepts drug therapy or other, passive program with full cooperation. He may have had considerable experience and disappointment previously. He may have been told his illness is psychological in origin. He may be skeptical or even bitter. I believe it is helpful to set up one's dialogue with the patient with a review of what is known about fibrositis.

First, it is not a crippling or progressive disease. The patient can be secure in this knowledge.

Second, it probably is not a disease at all, but merely a pain syndrome. As with headache, in fibrositis one can look wonderful and feel terrible. The x-rays, laboratory results, and physical examination are normal. Yet there is pain. People accept this view of headache. The patient should accept this view of fibrositis.

Third, the pain is learned. It is imprinted in memory like the ABCs. One can not stop the feeling of the first any more than forget the second. The analogy to phantom pain mentioned earlier for regional NAR is equally applicable here. This point is key in preparing the patient for the intellectually confusing (and threatening) discussion of the psychologic factors involved in the pain. One emphasizes that fibrositis is not a problem in character. Rather, the pain took root in an initial trauma or organic disease, now long gone, that imprinted with pain.

Fourth, one points out how pain has now taken over the control of the patient's life and that this is not healthy. The therapist can often point to the subtle influence of legal disability and Workman's Compensation in facing the continuation of symptoms. Similarly the organization of home life is often dominated by deference to pain. The desirability of regaining control over one's own life can be mentioned. The futility of treatment when there are environmental factors conspiring to keep one ill is appreciated in this view even by the least insightful patient.

Fifth, the disappointment patients feel after seeing doctors or other therapists is dealt with frankly. Since fibrositis, like headaches, is a pain syndrome without organic lesion, inflammation, or break in tissue continuity, treatment in the usual sense is without benefit. Physicians deal best with sickness, whereas fibrositis can be said to be a lack of wellness. The emphasis now is to put the problem back into the patient's control.

Antagonisms

In no other condition are therapist-patient antagonisms more likely to occur. Though the following words are never spoken, the thoughts represent an unspoken progression to conflict:

Patient	Therapist
I feel terrible.	You look great.
Can't you see I'm suffering?	Stop grimacing!
I can't work!	You're lazy!
You don't help me.	You don't need help.
You're a quack!	You're a crock!

This silent dialogue obviously leads nowhere. The patient continues to search for a more concerned therapist, while the therapist may actually become enraged at the prospect of having to see such a patient again, perhaps because therapists are understandably frustrated by patients who do not respond to therapy.

Support

Because insight therapy is so unsuccessful and the somatic symptoms so persistent, the wise therapist will do well to isolate the fibrositis patient's problems intellectually and to expect and accept the fact of very little response over the long periods of time patients seek help. A lighthearted attitude of support and a gentle attempt to focus the patient's attention away from pain while encouraging continued involvement with life do more than any medication. Agreeing with the patient that he needs extra rest, but with a continuing trade-off for light exercise, is also of great help. Finally, major life decisions should be resolved and depression minimized through pharmacologic and psychologic treatment for maximum benefit. Few patients with fibrositis are "cured," but many live a reasonably normal existence.

SUMMARY

I have always admired some aphorisms used in dermatology in the pre-World War II era, which went like this: If it's dry, wet it. If it's wet, dry it. And if zinc oxide and sulfur don't cure it, it doesn't exist!

In that spirit, I'll offer these summary aphorisms to NAR:

1. If it hurts on both active and passive motion, it's arthritis.
2. If it hurts on active, but not on passive motion, it's NAR.
3. Once chronic (over 3 weeks), if it's arthritis, baby it; if it's NAR, bully it.
4. If you feel antagonistic toward the patient, consider a diagnosis of fibrositis.

REFERENCES

1. Primer on the rheumatic diseases. JAMA (Suppl.) 1973;224:746–751.
2. Smith HA. Fibrositis and other diffuse musculoskeletal syndromes. In: Kelley WN, Harris ED, Ruddy S, Sledge CB, ed., Textbook of rheumatology. Philadelphia: WB Saunders, 1981, pp. 485–493.
3. Pinals RS. Traumatic arthritis and allied conditions. In: McCarty DJ, ed., Arthritis and allied conditions, 9th ed. Philadelphia: Lea and Febiger, 1979, pp. 985–1000.

INDEX